Extracellular Vesicles and Exosomes as Therapeutic Agents

Extracellular Vesicles and Exosomes as Therapeutic Agents

Guest Editor

David J. Rademacher

MDPI

Basel • Beijing • Wuhan • Barcelona • Belgrade • Novi Sad • Cluj • Manchester

Guest Editor
David J. Rademacher
Department of Microbiology
and Immunology
Loyola University Chicago
Chicago, IL
USA

Editorial Office
MDPI AG
Grosspeteranlage 5
4052 Basel, Switzerland

This is a reprint of the Special Issue, published open access by the journal *Biomedicines* (ISSN 2227-9059), freely accessible at: https://www.mdpi.com/journal/biomedicines/special_issues/G80M0Y7964.

For citation purposes, cite each article independently as indicated on the article page online and as indicated below:

Lastname, A.A.; Lastname, B.B. Article Title. *Journal Name* **Year**, *Volume Number*, Page Range.

ISBN 978-3-7258-5561-2 (Hbk)
ISBN 978-3-7258-5562-9 (PDF)
https://doi.org/10.3390/books978-3-7258-5562-9

Cover image courtesy of David J. Rademacher

Contents

About the Editor

David J. Rademacher

David J. Rademacher graduated with a Bachelor's degree in Psychology from Hamline University in 1994, a M.S. degree in Behavioral/Systems Neuroscience in 1999 from the University of Wisconsin-Milwaukee, and a Ph.D. in Behavioral/Systems Neuroscience in 2001 from the University of Wisconsin-Milwaukee. He is a member of the Department of Microbiology and Immunology at Loyola University Chicago and manages the Core Microscopy Facility. David has extensive experience with synaptic quantification and light and electron microscopy. He has spent decades studying the neurobiological underpinnings of stress, major depressive disorder, addiction, and neurodegenerative diseases. David has made several important contributions to our understanding of the endocannabinoid signaling system, discovered the first ever synaptic map due to the retrieval of a context-drug memory, characterized synaptic changes in striatal circuitry in Parkinsonism, dyskinesia, and as a result of striatal graft implants. Currently, David uses his expertise in confocal, super-resolution, and transmission electron microscopy to image a wide range of specimens in support of the innovative research of dozens of investigators.

biomedicines

Editorial

Editorial of the Special Issue: Extracellular Vesicles and Exosomes as Therapeutic Agents

David J. Rademacher

Department of Microbiology and Immunology and Core Microscopy Facility, Stritch School of Medicine, Loyola University Chicago, Maywood, IL 60153, USA; drademacher@luc.edu; Tel.: +1-414-628-9063

1. Introduction

Membrane-enclosed particles, known as extracellular vesicles (EVs), are ubiquitously present in organisms, including animals, plants, and microorganisms [1,2]. EVs are classified according to their size and origin as apoptotic bodies, microvesicles, or exosomes (EXs) [1–3]. EXs, the most extensively studied EVs, are enclosed in a single phospholipid bilayer and are secreted by all cell types [1,3–5]. EXs are usually 30 to 150 nm in diameter and are formed by fusion of the multivesicular body and the inward invagination of the endosomal membrane [1,3–5]. EXs are present in body fluids such as saliva, amniotic fluid, breast milk, urine, and plasma [6]. They are essential for intercellular communication because they change the functions of recipient cells by delivering a variety of biologically active cargo, including proteins, lipids, and nucleic acids [7,8].

The use of EXs as a delivery strategy for therapeutic cargo has become increasingly popular, in part, because they overcome many of the challenges encountered by other approaches. EXs exhibit a high degree of stability and biocompatibility with minimal immunogenicity [9]. The delivery-to-target efficiency is higher for EXs than conventional approaches because they can traverse biological barriers, such as the blood-brain barrier (BBB) [10,11]. EXs can selectively target tissues or cells and reduce off-target effects because of their inherent tropism based on their cells of origin [12]. EXs provide a protective environment for the encapsulated cargo, safeguarding it from degradation [13]. Furthermore, because EXs are the primary way that stem cells exert their biological effects, the use of stem cell-derived EXs preserves the therapeutic potential of stem cells while avoiding any potential harm from the cells [14,15]. Importantly, systemic administration of EXs derived from a variety of cell types often results in their primary accumulation in the liver and spleen, with less than 1% of that administered reaching the desired target [12,16]. Consequently, several engineering approaches have been developed to improve targeting and increase the accumulation of EXs in the target tissue and/or cells.

2. Recent Developments in the Use of Extracellular Vesicles and Exosomes as Therapeutic Delivery Systems

2.1. Genetic Engineering of EXs

Genetic engineering has been used to modify exosomal surface proteins to better target EXs to tissues and cell types of interest, since even slight variations in exosomal tetraspanin complexes have a significant impact on target cell selection. Transfecting genes expressing a targeting moiety with exosomal membrane components is one method of genetically altering EX-producing cells. Through the natural EX biogenesis process, the cells transfected with these vectors produce surface-modified EXs that express the targeting moieties. EXs produced from genetically engineered cells stably display the introduced targeting moiety on their surface [17]. For example, Wang and colleagues [18] genetically engineered stem cell-derived EXs loaded with a ferroptosis inhibitor to target M2 microglia. The genetically engineered EXs exhibited M2 microglia targeting specificity in vitro and in vivo, inhibited ferroptosis in M2 microglia, and improved neurological function in ischemic stroke-affected mice [18]. A fusion protein, consisting of rabies virus glycoprotein (RVG), a protein that binds nicotinic acetylcholine receptors, and lysosomal membrane-associated protein 2B, an exosomal membrane protein, was transfected into 293T cells. The cells produced EXs with RVG embedded in the exosomal membrane [19]. As neurons and glia express receptors that bind to RVG on their cell surface, systemic administration of RVG-expressing EXs resulted in a two-fold increase in brain EX accumulation compared to systemic administration of non-engineered EXs [19].

2.2. Chemical Modifications of EXs

To make therapeutic EXs more targetable, their surface can be directly engineered through chemical modifications. One such approach is click chemistry. Click chemistry utilizes covalent interactions between an alkyne and an azide residue to form a stable triazole linkage, which can be applied to attach targeting moieties on the surface of EXs [20,21]. For example, Jia and colleagues [22] used click chemistry to conjugate the RGERPPR peptide (RGE) to the exosomal membrane. The engineered EXs delivered therapeutic cargo to intracranial tumors because RGE binds specifically to neuropilin-1 (NRP-1), which is overexpressed in glioma cells and is either not expressed at all or expressed at a low level in normal neurons and other tissues [22]. Chen and coworkers [23] used click chemistry to attach a targeting peptide to the surface of macrophage-derived EXs. These engineered EXs targeted bone tissue and released anti-microbial peptides, thereby relieving osteomyelitis without adverse effects in a rat model [23].

2.3. Combinatorial Approaches

Hybrid Nanoparticles

As an alternative to genetic engineering of parent cells or EXs and chemical modification of EXs, targeting ligands conjugated to polyethylene glycol (PEG) have been used to produce EXs in which the targeting ligand is expressed in the exosomal membrane. For example, nanobodies specific for epidermal growth factor receptor (EGFR), upregulated in a variety of solid tumors, were conjugated to phospholipid-PEG derivatives to produce nanobody-PEG-micelles [24]. Nanobody-PEG-micelles were expressed in the exosomal membrane when they were incubated with EXs; this had no effect on the size distribution, protein composition, or morphology of EXs. The PEGylated and targeted EXs increased the binding to tumor cells overexpressing EGFR and were retained in the circulation for six times longer than unmodified EXs [24].

Diacyl-chain phospholipids self-assemble in aqueous solutions to form spherical vesicles called liposomes [25]. Liposomes expressing tLyp-1 (CGNKRTR), which has a high affinity to NRP-1 to target glioma cells, were created and fused with EXs, which have an enhanced ability to cross the BBB, in part because of the expression of transferrin receptors on the EX's surface, to create hybrid liposome-EX nanovesicles with an enhanced ability to cross the BBB and target brain tumors [26,27]. Compared with liposomes and EXs, the hybrid nanovesicles demonstrated an increased ability to cross the BBB and accumulate in glioma in mice [26].

In a fascinating study, adipose-derived mesenchymal stem cell (ADSC) EXs and gelatine nanoparticle (GNP) hydrogel combined to form a stable meshwork because of the opposing charges of the two substances. In a rat skull defect model, the skull bone formation produced by the GNP hydrogel-ADSC EX mixture was substantially greater than that of the GNP- and sham-treated groups [28].

Liu and colleagues [29] created a nanocomplex, referred to as REXO-C/ANP/S, which was comprised of a core and a shell. The core, referred to as C/ANP/S, was comprised of: (a) curcumin, a small molecule that disrupts α-synuclein aggregates; (b) small interfering RNA targeting *SNCA* to downregulate α-synuclein synthesis; and (c) a reactive oxygen species (ROS)-responsive polymer, poly(2-(dimethylamino)ethyl acrylate, which encapsulates curcumin and enables ROS-responsive drug release. The shell, termed REXO, was comprised of: (a) immature dendritic cell-derived EXs; and (b) RVG peptide, a targeting peptide embedded in the exosomal membrane to enhance delivery across the BBB and target neurons. In a mouse model of Parkinson's disease, the REXO-C/ANP/S nanoparticles decreased α-synuclein aggregates in diseased neurons [29].

2.4. Large-Scale EX Production Approaches

The quality and quantity of secreted EXs are reduced in conventional two-dimensional, static cultures, as these cultures cannot replicate the in vivo environment, including fluidic stimuli [30]. To overcome these limitations, Huang and coworkers [31] developed a method of culturing genetically engineered mesenchymal stromal cells to increase the production of EXs rich in hepatocyte growth factor (HGF) for improved wound healing. Two structured polydimethylsiloxane layers were used to construct a microfluidic chip, which was a crucial part of their culturing technique. The top layer had herringbone grooves, and the bottom layer had a micropillar array. By disrupting the laminar flow, these structures produced a turbulent vortex that improved waste removal and nutrient delivery. In addition, the bottom micropillar layer provided a large number of cell adhesion sites. The EX yield obtained from cells cultured on the microfluidic chip was ~14 times that obtained from cells cultured in a conventional, two-dimensional static cell culture flask. Furthermore, the EXs derived from microfluidic chip-cultured cells were abundant in HGF and aided in wound healing [31].

Contrary to conventional, static cell culture conditions, a flat-plate bioreactor was used to increase EX production. The chamber in the flat-plate bioreactor was seeded with cells. The culture medium was delivered to the chamber via a peristaltic pump, which produced laminar flow conditions. The flow introduced shear stress to the cells, which opened calcium channels, leading to increased calcium influx [32]. Prior studies have shown that increasing intracellular calcium concentration increases EX yield [33]. A closed-loop system was used to collect and recirculate the culture medium, which ensured a continuous exchange of oxygen and nutrients while eliminating waste. The bioreactor produced ~7 times more EXs than static culture conditions, while preserving the quality and therapeutic efficacy of the EXs [32].

2.5. Milk and Plant EXs

Milk- and plant-derived EXs have gained popularity recently despite advancements in the mass production of EXs derived from cultured cells. Milk is a particularly dense source of EXs, with concentrations in milk exceeding 10^{12} EXs per milliliter [34]. Due to their stability, scalability, ability to cross biological barriers, and between-species biocompatibility, recent research has focused on the development of milk EXs as a drug delivery platform. Milk EXs are non-immunologic oral delivery vehicles for gene editing agents, peptides, small molecules, and bioactive RNA cargo [35–37]. However, the isolation and characterization of milk EXs is complicated by the fact that milk contains a variety of nanoparticles besides EXs [38]. Continued research is crucial to harness the full potential of milk EXs in clinical and therapeutic contexts.

Similar to milk-derived EXs, plant-derived EXs represent a potentially rich source of useful EXs. Plant-derived EXs are thought to be used as a means of intercellular communication and immune regulation to protect plants from pathogenic attacks [39]. Notably, the size distribution, density, morphology, and surface electric charge of EXs derived from plants are comparable to those derived from mammals [40]. Like mammalian cell-derived EXs, they contain lipids, proteins, and RNAs, which reflect their plant sources, such as grapes, ginger, and apples [41–43]. The techniques used to isolate EXs from plants are not very different from those used to isolate EXs produced by cultured mammalian cells [44]. Plant EXs are safe [42] and their production is more scalable and cost-effective than EXs derived from mammalian cells [45]. Ongoing research is needed to establish standardized plant EX extraction protocols and evaluate long-term safety for clinical applications.

3. Contributions to This Special Issue

In this Special Issue, Mecocci and colleagues [46] described the anti-microbial and anti-inflammatory effects of cow colostrum-derived EXs in an in vitro model of neonatal calf diarrhea caused by *Escherichia coli* infection. Their results present the fascinating prospect that colostrum-derived EXs may provide an alternative to antibiotics in combating drug-resistant bacterial infections. Schepici and coworkers [47] provided a comprehensive review of the regenerative effects of mesenchymal stromal/stem cell-derived EXs in spinal cord injury and a summary of the preclinical studies on their therapeutic potential. Mohammad and colleagues [48] examined the effects of exercise-induced EXs on trophoblasts in vitro, highlighting their potential role in maternal–fetal communication during pregnancy. Rademacher [49] described the dual role of EXs in Parkinson's disease, as both a contributor to disease progression and a potential therapeutic tool. In Parkinson's disease, EXs act as mediators of disease progression by spreading toxic proteins and promoting neuroinflammation. However, their natural role in intercellular communication and ability to deliver therapeutic agents make them a promising tool for developing next-generation therapies [49]. Wang and coworkers [50] investigated the role of EXs derived from osteogenic-differentiated human bone marrow-derived mesenchymal cells (hBMSCs) in the rescue of the osteogenic ability of hBMSCs impaired by hypoxia. They discovered that EXs derived from hBMSCs cultured in normoxia restored the osteogenic capacity of hBMSCs that had been compromised by hypoxia, offering a possible treatment approach for bone regeneration in hypoxic conditions [50]. The literature on the effects of physical cues on stem cell-derived EXs to treat peripheral neuropathy was reviewed by Berry and colleagues [51]. They concluded that physical cues such as electrical stimulation, mechanical agitation, and conductive materials greatly improved the production, quality, and therapeutic potential of stem cell-derived EXs. These improvements make EXs more effective in treating peripheral neuropathy [51]. The efficiency and quality of artificial EXs produced by T cells using two different induction techniques—cytochalasin B, a chemical inducer, and ultrasonication, a physical inducer—were compared by Zmievskaya and colleagues [52]. Garaeva and colleagues [53] discovered that EXs loaded with exogenous, recombinant heat shock protein 70 derived from grapefruit triggered an anti-tumor immune response in both in vitro and in vivo models of colorectal cancer, highlighting the potential of plant-derived EXs as effective therapeutic cargo delivery vehicles. Jones and coworkers [54] determined the efficacy of lyophilized EXs derived from human adipose stem cells in promoting healing from traumatic brain injury, underlining their potential for storage at room temperature and clinical application. Finally, Salih and colleagues [55] investigated the expression of the microRNAs let-7a-5p and miR-21-3p in EXs derived from the serum of non-small-cell lung cancer patients, highlighting their potential as diagnostic biomarkers.

4. Future Research

High production costs, a high level of technical expertise, and challenges differentiating genetically engineered EXs from naturally occurring EXs in biological fluids are some of the drawbacks of genetically engineered EXs, despite their many benefits such as improved targeting precision, effective therapeutic delivery, and decreased off-target effects. Further research and optimization are needed to make them more feasible for clinical applications. Chemically modified EXs offer several advantages, including enhanced targeting, versatility, retention of the natural properties of the EXs, and the ability to cross biological barriers. The technical difficulties of both covalent and non-covalent EX modifications, the possible loss of native protein function in the EX membrane, and the difficulty in scaling up chemical modification techniques to large-scale production are the drawbacks of chemical modification of EXs. Future studies should focus on addressing these issues. Potential disruption of the exosomal membrane during production, the possibility of an immunological reaction, and regulatory ambiguity surrounding their classification—which makes approval more difficult—are some of the difficulties with hybrid nanoparticles. Clear regulatory frameworks, scalable production methods, and improved engineering techniques are essential to tackle these challenges. Future developments in isolation technologies, engineering methods, and standardization protocols are required to enable scalable EX production for clinical applications, even though recent advancements in the large-scale production of EXs, such as the use of microfluidic chips and bioreactors, are encouraging. Despite the fact that milk EXs are non-immunologic oral delivery vehicles for a range of therapeutic substances, a major obstacle is the transfer of isolation techniques from the laboratory to the industrial production process. In addition, there are no detailed pharmacokinetic studies, and the complex composition of milk makes it difficult to isolate high-purity milk EXs. To address these issues, improvements in isolation techniques, scalable production methods, and thorough safety and efficacy studies are needed. Despite the fact that plant EXs are safe [42] and can be produced more cheaply and efficiently than EXs produced by mammalian cells [45], preclinical and clinical research are required to confirm their therapeutic efficacy, optimize dosages, and assess long-term effects before they can be used successfully in clinical settings.

Funding: This research received no external funding.

Institutional Review Board Statement: Not applicable.

Informed Consent Statement: Not applicable.

Data Availability Statement: Not applicable.

Conflicts of Interest: The author declares no conflicts of interest.

References

1. Zaborowski, M.P.; Balaj, L.; Breakefield, X.O.; Lai, C.P. Extracellular Vesicles: Composition, Biological Relevance, and Methods of Study. *Bioscience* **2015**, *65*, 783–797. [CrossRef] [PubMed]
2. Yáñez-Mó, M.; Siljander, P.R.; Andreu, Z.; Zavec, A.B.; Borràs, F.E.; Buzas, E.I.; Buzas, K.; Casal, E.; Cappello, F.; Carvalho, J.; et al. Biological properties of extracellular vesicles and their physiological functions. *J. Extracell. Vesicles* **2015**, *4*, 27066. [CrossRef] [PubMed]

3. Borges, F.T.; Reis, L.A.; Schor, N. Extracellular vesicles: Structure, function, and potential clinical uses in renal diseases. *Braz. J. Med. Biol. Res.* **2013**, *46*, 824–830. [CrossRef]
4. Bebelman, M.P.; Smit, M.J.; Pegtel, D.M.; Baglio, S.R. Biogenesis and function of extracellular vesicles in cancer. *Pharmacol. Ther.* **2018**, *188*, 1–11. [CrossRef]
5. Raposo, G.; Stoorvogel, W. Extracellular vesicles: Exosomes, microvesicles, and friends. *J. Cell Biol.* **2013**, *200*, 373–383. [CrossRef]
6. Tabatabai, T.S.; Alizadeh, M.; Rezakhani, L.; Tabatabai, T.S.; Ehterami, A.; Kloucheh, S.G.; Kebria, M.M.; Vaez, A.; Salehi, M. Unlocking the potential of EXOs in regenerative medicine: A comprehensive review. *Tissue Cell* **2025**, *97*, 103068. [CrossRef]
7. Cocucci, E.; Meldolesi, J. Ectosomes and exosomes: Shedding the confusion between extracellular vesicles. *Trends Cell Biol.* **2015**, *25*, 364–372. [CrossRef]
8. Meldolesi, J. Exosomes and Ectosomes in Intercellular Communication. *Curr. Biol.* **2018**, *28*, R435–R444. [CrossRef]
9. Kim, H.; Jang, H.; Cho, H.; Choi, J.; Hwang, K.Y.; Choi, Y.; Kim, S.H.; Yang, Y. Recent Advances in Exosome-Based Drug Delivery for Cancer Therapy. *Cancers* **2021**, *13*, 4435. [CrossRef]
10. Samanta, S.; Rajasingh, S.; Drosos, N.; Zhou, Z.; Dawn, B.; Rajasingh, J. Exosomes: New molecular targets of diseases. *Acta Pharmacol. Sin.* **2018**, *39*, 501–513. [CrossRef]
11. Gomez-Molina, C.; Sandoval, M.; Henzi, R.; Ramirez, J.P.; Varas-Godoy, M.; Luarte, A.; Lafourcade, C.A.; Lopez-Verrilli, A.; Smalla, K.H.; Kaehne, T.; et al. Small Extracellular Vesicles in Rat Serum Contain Astrocyte-Derived Protein Biomarkers of Repetitive Stress. *Int. J. Neuropsychopharmacol.* **2019**, *22*, 232–246. [CrossRef]
12. Wiklander, O.P.; Nordin, J.Z.; O'Loughlin, A.; Gustafsson, Y.; Corso, G.; Mager, I.; Vader, P.; Lee, Y.; Sork, H.; Seow, Y.; et al. Extracellular vesicle in vivo biodistribution is determined by cell source, route of administration and targeting. *J. Extracell. Vesicles* **2015**, *4*, 26316. [CrossRef]
13. Akuma, P.; Okagu, O.D.; Udenigwe, C.C. Naturally Occurring Exosome Vesicles as Potential Delivery Vehicle for Bioactive Compounds. *Front. Sustain. Food Syst.* **2019**, *3*, 23. [CrossRef]
14. Yousefi Dehbidi, M.; Goodarzi, N.; Azhdari, M.H.; Doroudian, M. Mesenchymal stem cells and their derived exosomes to combat Covid-19. *Rev. Med. Virol.* **2022**, *32*, e2281. [CrossRef]
15. Phinney, D.G.; Pittenger, M.F. Concise Review: MSC-Derived Exosomes for Cell-Free Therapy. *Stem Cells* **2017**, *35*, 851–858. [CrossRef]
16. Mirzaaghasi, A.; Han, Y.; Ahn, S.H.; Choi, C.; Park, J.H. Biodistribution and Pharmacokinectics of Liposomes and Exosomes in a Mouse Model of Sepsis. *Pharmaceutics* **2021**, *13*, 427. [CrossRef] [PubMed]
17. Zhang, M.; Zang, X.; Wang, M.; Li, Z.; Qiao, M.; Hu, H.; Chen, D. Exosome-based nanocarriers as bio-inspired and versatile vehicles for drug delivery: Recent advances and challenges. *J. Mater. Chem. B* **2019**, *7*, 2421–2433. [CrossRef] [PubMed]
18. Wang, Y.; Liu, Z.; Li, L.; Zhang, Z.; Zhang, K.; Chu, M.; Liu, Y.; Mao, X.; Wu, D.; Xu, D.; et al. Anti-ferroptosis exosomes engineered for targeting M2 microglia to improve neurological function in ischemic stroke. *J. Nanobiotechnol.* **2024**, *22*, 291. [CrossRef] [PubMed]
19. Kim, M.; Kim, G.; Hwang, D.W.; Lee, M. Delivery of High Mobility Group Box-1 siRNA Using Brain-Targeting Exosomes for Ischemic Stroke Therapy. *J. Biomed. Nanotechnol.* **2019**, *15*, 2401–2412. [CrossRef]
20. Smyth, T.; Petrova, K.; Payton, N.M.; Persaud, I.; Redzic, J.S.; Graner, M.W.; Smith-Jones, P.; Anchordoquy, T.J. Surface functionalization of exosomes using click chemistry. *Bioconjug. Chem.* **2014**, *25*, 1777–1784. [CrossRef]
21. Nwe, K.; Brechbiel, M.W. Growing applications of "click chemistry" for bioconjugation in contemporary biomedical research. *Cancer Biother. Radiopharm.* **2009**, *24*, 289–302. [CrossRef]
22. Jia, G.; Han, Y.; An, Y.; Ding, Y.; He, C.; Wang, X.; Tang, Q. NRP-1 targeted and cargo-loaded exosomes facilitate simultaneous imaging and therapy of glioma in vitro and in vivo. *Biomaterials* **2018**, *178*, 302–316. [CrossRef] [PubMed]
23. Chen, Y.; Dong, J.; Li, J.; Li, J.; Lu, Y.; Dong, W.; Zhang, D.; Dang, X. Engineered macrophage-derived exosomes via click chemistry for the treatment of osteomyelitis. *J. Mater. Chem. B* **2024**, *12*, 10593–10604. [CrossRef] [PubMed]
24. Kooijmans, S.A.A.; Fliervoet, L.A.L.; van der Meel, R.; Fens, M.; Heijnen, H.F.G.; van Bergen en Henegouwen, P.M.P.; Vader, P.; Schiffelers, R.M. PEGylated and targeted extracellular vesicles display enhanced cell specificity and circulation time. *J. Control. Release* **2016**, *224*, 77–85. [CrossRef]
25. Wu, X.; Dai, X.; Liao, Y.; Sheng, M.; Shi, X. Investigation on drug entrapment location in liposomes and transfersomes based on molecular dynamics simulation. *J. Mol. Model.* **2021**, *27*, 111. [CrossRef]
26. Wang, R.; Wang, X.; Zhao, H.; Li, N.; Li, J.; Zhang, H.; Di, L. Targeted delivery of hybrid nanovesicles for enhanced brain penetration to achieve synergistic therapy of glioma. *J. Control. Release* **2024**, *365*, 331–347. [CrossRef]
27. Ma, Y.; Zhang, J.; Rui, Y.; Rolle, J.; Xu, T.; Qian, Z.; Gu, Y.; Li, S. Depletion of glioma stem cells by synergistic inhibition of mTOR and c-Myc with a biological camouflaged cascade brain-targeting nanosystem. *Biomaterials* **2021**, *268*, 120564. [CrossRef]

28. Li, R.; Li, D.; Wang, H.; Chen, K.; Wang, S.; Xu, J.; Ji, P. Exosomes from adipose-derived stem cells regulate M1/M2 macrophage phenotypic polarization to promote bone healing via miR-451a/MIF. *Stem Cell Res. Ther.* **2022**, *13*, 149. [CrossRef] [PubMed]
29. Liu, L.; Li, Y.; Peng, H.; Liu, R.; Ji, W.; Shi, Z.; Shen, J.; Ma, G.; Zhang, X. Targeted exosome coating gene-chem nanocomplex as "nanoscavenger" for clearing alpha-synuclein and immune activation of Parkinson's disease. *Sci. Adv.* **2020**, *6*, eaba3967. [CrossRef]
30. Cao, J.; Wang, B.; Tang, T.; Lv, L.; Ding, Z.; Li, Z.; Hu, R.; Wei, Q.; Shen, A.; Fu, Y.; et al. Three-dimensional culture of MSCs produces exosomes with improved yield and enhanced therapeutic efficacy for cisplatin-induced acute kidney injury. *Stem Cell Res. Ther.* **2020**, *11*, 206. [CrossRef]
31. Huang, J.; Chen, H.; Luo, Z.; Nie, M.; Wang, J.; Lu, L.; Zhao, Y. Genetically Engineered Stromal Cell Exosomes from High-Throughput Herringbone Microfluidics. *ACS Nano* **2025**, *19*, 10568–10577. [CrossRef] [PubMed]
32. Kang, H.; Bae, Y.H.; Kwon, Y.; Kim, S.; Park, J. Extracellular Vesicles Generated Using Bioreactors and their Therapeutic Effect on the Acute Kidney Injury Model. *Adv. Healthc. Mater.* **2022**, *11*, e2101606. [CrossRef]
33. Taylor, J.; Azimi, I.; Monteith, G.; Bebawy, M. Ca^{2+} mediates extracellular vesicle biogenesis through alternate pathways in malignancy. *J. Extracell. Vesicles* **2020**, *9*, 1734326. [CrossRef]
34. Marsh, S.R.; Pridham, K.J.; Jourdan, J.; Gourdie, R.G. Novel Protocols for Scalable Production of High Quality Purified Small Extracellular Vesicles from Bovine Milk. *Nanotheranostics* **2021**, *5*, 488–498. [CrossRef]
35. Munagala, R.; Aqil, F.; Jeyabalan, J.; Gupta, R.C. Bovine milk-derived exosomes for drug delivery. *Cancer Lett.* **2016**, *371*, 48–61. [CrossRef]
36. Aqil, F.; Munagala, R.; Jeyabalan, J.; Agrawal, A.K.; Kyakulaga, A.H.; Wilcher, S.A.; Gupta, R.C. Milk exosomes—Natural nanoparticles for siRNA delivery. *Cancer Lett.* **2019**, *449*, 186–195. [CrossRef] [PubMed]
37. Yan, C.; Chen, J.; Wang, C.; Yuan, M.; Kang, Y.; Wu, Z.; Li, W.; Zhang, G.; Machens, H.G.; Rinkevich, Y.; et al. Milk exosomes-mediated miR-31-5p delivery accelerates diabetic wound healing through promoting angiogenesis. *Drug Deliv.* **2022**, *29*, 214–228. [CrossRef] [PubMed]
38. Holt, C.; Carver, J.A.; Ecroyd, H.; Thorn, D.C. Invited review: Caseins and the casein micelle: Their biological functions, structures, and behavior in foods. *J. Dairy Sci.* **2013**, *96*, 6127–6146. [CrossRef]
39. Malhotra, H.; Sheokand, N.; Kumar, S.; Chauhan, A.S.; Kumar, M.; Jakhar, P.; Boradia, V.M.; Raje, C.I.; Raje, M. Exosomes: Tunable Nano Vehicles for Macromolecular Delivery of Transferrin and Lactoferrin to Specific Intracellular Compartment. *J. Biomed. Nanotechnol.* **2016**, *12*, 1101–1114. [CrossRef]
40. Iriawati, I.; Vitasasti, S.; Rahmadian, F.N.A.; Barlian, A. Isolation and characterization of plant-derived exosome-like nanoparticles from Carica papaya L. fruit and their potential as anti-inflammatory agent. *PLoS ONE* **2024**, *19*, e0304335. [CrossRef]
41. Cai, Q.; Qiao, L.; Wang, M.; He, B.; Lin, F.M.; Palmquist, J.; Huang, S.D.; Jin, H. Plants send small RNAs in extracellular vesicles to fungal pathogen to silence virulence genes. *Science* **2018**, *360*, 1126–1129. [CrossRef]
42. Rutter, B.D.; Innes, R.W. Extracellular Vesicles Isolated from the Leaf Apoplast Carry Stress-Response Proteins. *Plant Physiol.* **2017**, *173*, 728–741. [CrossRef]
43. Alzahrani, F.A.; Khan, M.I.; Kameli, N.; Alsahafi, E.; Riza, Y.M. Plant-Derived Extracellular Vesicles and Their Exciting Potential as the Future of Next-Generation Drug Delivery. *Biomolecules* **2023**, *13*, 839. [CrossRef]
44. Mun, J.G.; Song, D.H.; Kee, J.Y.; Han, Y. Recent Advances in the Isolation Strategies of Plant-Derived Exosomes and Their Therapeutic Applications. *Curr. Issues Mol. Biol.* **2025**, *47*, 144. [CrossRef] [PubMed]
45. Wang, Q.; Zhuang, X.; Mu, J.; Deng, Z.B.; Jiang, H.; Zhang, L.; Xiang, X.; Wang, B.; Yan, J.; Miller, D.; et al. Delivery of therapeutic agents by nanoparticles made of grapefruit-derived lipids. *Nat. Commun.* **2013**, *4*, 1867. [CrossRef] [PubMed]
46. Mecocci, S.; De Paolis, L.; Zoccola, R.; Fruscione, F.; De Ciucis, C.G.; Chiaradia, E.; Moccia, V.; Tognoloni, A.; Pascucci, L.; Zoppi, S.; et al. Antimicrobial and Immunomodulatory Potential of Cow Colostrum Extracellular Vesicles (ColosEVs) in an Intestinal In Vitro Model. *Biomedicines* **2022**, *10*, 3264. [CrossRef]
47. Schepici, G.; Silvestro, S.; Mazzon, E. Regenerative Effects of Exosomes-Derived MSCs: An Overview on Spinal Cord Injury Experimental Studies. *Biomedicines* **2023**, *11*, 201. [CrossRef]
48. Mohammad, S.; Bhattacharjee, J.; Tzaneva, V.; Hutchinson, K.A.; Shaikh, M.; Fernandes da Silva, D.; Burger, D.; Adamo, K.B. The Influence of Exercise-Associated Small Extracellular Vesicles on Trophoblasts In Vitro. *Biomedicines* **2023**, *11*, 857. [CrossRef]
49. Rademacher, D.J. Potential for Therapeutic-Loaded Exosomes to Ameliorate the Pathogenic Effects of alpha-Synuclein in Parkinson's Disease. *Biomedicines* **2023**, *11*, 1187. [CrossRef]
50. Wang, C.; Stockl, S.; Pattappa, G.; Schulz, D.; Hofmann, K.; Ilic, J.; Reinders, Y.; Bauer, R.J.; Sickmann, A.; Grassel, S. Extracellular Vesicles Derived from Osteogenic-Differentiated Human Bone Marrow-Derived Mesenchymal Cells Rescue Osteogenic Ability of Bone Marrow-Derived Mesenchymal Cells Impaired by Hypoxia. *Biomedicines* **2023**, *11*, 2804. [CrossRef]

51. Berry, D.; Ene, J.; Nathani, A.; Singh, M.; Li, Y.; Zeng, C. Effects of Physical Cues on Stem Cell-Derived Extracellular Vesicles toward Neuropathy Applications. *Biomedicines* **2024**, *12*, 489. [CrossRef] [PubMed]
52. Zmievskaya, E.A.; Mukhametshin, S.A.; Ganeeva, I.A.; Gilyazova, E.M.; Siraeva, E.T.; Kutyreva, M.P.; Khannanov, A.A.; Yuan, Y.; Bulatov, E.R. Artificial Extracellular Vesicles Generated from T Cells Using Different Induction Techniques. *Biomedicines* **2024**, *12*, 919. [CrossRef] [PubMed]
53. Garaeva, L.; Komarova, E.; Emelianova, S.; Putevich, E.; Konevega, A.L.; Margulis, B.; Guzhova, I.; Shtam, T. Grapefruit-Derived Vesicles Loaded with Recombinant HSP70 Activate Antitumor Immunity in Colon Cancer In Vitro and In Vivo. *Biomedicines* **2024**, *12*, 2759. [CrossRef]
54. Jones, B.; Patel, R.; Wang, B.; Evans-Nguyen, T.; Patel, N.A. Lyophilized Small Extracellular Vesicles (sEVs) Derived from Human Adipose Stem Cells Maintain Efficacy to Promote Healing in Neuronal Injuries. *Biomedicines* **2025**, *13*, 275. [CrossRef]
55. Salih, D.J.; Reiners, K.S.; Loizzi, D.; Ardò, N.P.; Santantonio, T.A.; Sollitto, F.; Hartmann, G. Expression Analysis of let-7a-5p and miR-21-3p in Extracellular Vesicles Derived from Serum of NSCLC Patients. *Biomedicines* **2025**, *13*, 2060. [CrossRef]

biomedicines

MDPI

Article

Expression Analysis of let-7a-5p and miR-21-3p in Extracellular Vesicles Derived from Serum of NSCLC Patients

Dian Jamel Salih [1,2,*], Katrin S. Reiners [3], Domenico Loizzi [4], Nicoletta Pia Ardò [4], Teresa Antonia Santantonio [5], Francesco Sollitto [4] and Gunther Hartmann [3]

1 Department of Medical and Surgical Sciences, University of Foggia, Via Napoli, 121, 71122 Foggia, Italy
2 Department of Anatomy, Biology and Histology, College of Medicine, University of Duhok, Zakho Way, Duhok 42001, Iraq
3 Institute of Clinical Chemistry and Clinical Pharmacology, University Hospital Bonn, 53127 Bonn, Germany; kreiners@uni-bonn.de (K.S.R.); gunther.hartmann@uni-bonn.de (G.H.)
4 Institute of Thoracic Surgery, Department of Medical and Surgical Sciences, University of Foggia, 71122 Foggia, Italy; domenico.loizzi@unifg.it (D.L.); nicoletta.ardo@gmail.com (N.P.A.); francesco.sollitto@unifg.it (F.S.)
5 Infectious Diseases Unit, Department of Clinical and Surgical Sciences, University of Foggia, 71122 Foggia, Italy; teresa.santantonio@unifg.it
* Correspondence: dian.salih@unifg.it; Tel.: +39-3463610192

Abstract: Background/Objectives: Despite the significant advancements made in the diagnosis of lung cancer, the traditional diagnostic methods remain limited because they are often invasive, expensive, and not suitable for regular screening, creating a need for more accessible and non-invasive alternatives. In this context, the analysis of miRNAs in EVs and free circulating microRNA may be used as liquid biopsies in lung cancer to identify individuals at risk. This study aimed to compare miRNA profiles in the serum and EVs derived from lung cancer patients by focusing on Let-7a-5p and miR-21-3p. **Materials and Methods:** Serum and EVs were isolated from lung cancer patients and healthy controls. EVs were characterized using nanoparticle tracking analysis, electron microscopy, and Western blotting for surface markers (CD63, CD81, TSG101). Total miRNA levels were quantified in the serum and EVs, and specific miRNAs (hsa-let-7a-5p and hsa-miR-21-3p) were analyzed using RT-qPCR. Statistical analysis evaluated miRNA expression across clinicopathological features, including age, gender, smoking status, tumor stage, cancer type, and EGFR mutation status. **Results:** Total miRNA levels were significantly enriched in EVs compared to the serum. Let-7a-5p was downregulated in EVs from patients with advanced-stage lung cancer (Stage III–IV) compared to those with early-stage cancer and controls ($p < 0.05$), while no differences were observed in the serum. Conversely, miR-21-3p was significantly upregulated in EVs and serum from advanced-stage patients ($p < 0.01$) and in adenocarcinoma compared to squamous cell carcinoma ($p < 0.05$). No significant differences were observed for age, gender, or smoking status. **Conclusions:** Our findings highlight the differential expression of miRNAs in EVs and the serum, emphasizing the diagnostic potential of EV-associated Let-7a-5p and miR-21-3p in lung cancer. These results suggest that EVs are a more robust source for miRNA biomarkers compared to the serum.

Keywords: lung cancer; extracellular vesicles; miRNA; let-7a; miR-21

1. Introduction

Lung cancer is still the leading cause of cancer deaths worldwide due to its late diagnosis. Early detection significantly improves prognosis by reducing mortality and enhancing survival rate, adding to successful treatment by focusing on detecting asymptomatic patients. However, the diagnostic techniques currently available have major limitations, especially in the early detection of cancer [1].

CT has a high false-positive rate, indicating the presence of cancer when the reality is otherwise, and sputum cytology is only of limited sensitivity in locating minute lung tumors that are in the peripheral regions of the lungs. Therefore, these methods are not particularly effective in the early detection of lung cancer [2]. Considering these limitations, there is an urgent need for non-invasive and reliable biomarkers for the early-stage detection of lung cancer.

Recent extensive studies have identified microRNAs (miRNAs) as potential biomarkers for the diagnosis, prognosis, and targeted therapy of lung cancer. miRNAs are a class of highly conserved small non-coding RNAs, varying between 18 and 25 nucleotides in length [3], that modulate gene expression at the post-transcriptional level by binding to the complementary 3′ untranslated region (3′UTR) of target mRNAs, thereby facilitating mRNA degradation or inhibiting protein synthesis [4].

Bioinformatics algorithms predict that miRNAs regulate more than 60% of the protein-coding genes in the human genome. One miRNA can regulate numerous target mRNAs, just as one mRNA is regulated by several miRNAs. Thus, miRNAs are important in many biological processes, including gene regulation, apoptosis, hematopoietic development, and the maintenance of cell differentiation [5,6].

Multiple studies indicate the dysregulation of miRNAs involved in the pathogenesis of different cancers, including lung cancer, through the regulation of various biological processes such as cell proliferation [7], differentiation [8], angiogenesis [9], and apoptosis [10]. Specific miRNAs have oncogenic or tumor-suppressing potential, and their altered expression profiles in cancer patients serve as diagnostic biomarkers [11].

Previous investigations have reported that a variety of differentially expressed miRNAs in lung cancer may have potential as diagnostic biomarkers. For example, studies have pointed out that several miRNAs such as miR-21, miR-106a, miR-10b, miR-328, miR-155, let-7, and miR-103 are usually dysregulated in lung cancer patients [12–14].

These miRNAs have been found in several body fluids, such as the plasma and serum, and thus are accessible for non-invasive diagnostic tests. Bai et al. [13] found that miR-21 was significantly overexpressed in the serum of NSCLC patients compared with healthy controls, indicating a possible role as a diagnostic biomarker. Similarly, Xue et al. [15] reported elevated levels of miR-21 and miR-155 in the plasma of lung cancer patients, correlating with a poor prognosis.

MicroRNAs are unstable in body fluid and susceptible to degradation by ribonucleases (RNases) present in the bloodstream, which can affect their reliability as diagnostic biomarkers. Due to their instability, researchers are investigating alternative sources of miRNA that are more stable and less susceptible to degradation [16]. Recently, extracellular vesicles (EVs) have gained increasing attention in biomedical research as a promising solution to this problem due to the cargo composition of miRNAs in EVs and their stability in body fluids [6].

EVs are small, heterogeneous, membrane-bounded vesicles released by different cell types into the extracellular environment, contributing to intercellular communication. EVs are enriched with proteins, lipids, and nucleic acids, including DNA, mRNA, and miRNA. Based on their size and biogenesis, they have been categorized into exosomes, microvesicles, and apoptotic bodies [17]. The miRNA cargo of EVs reflects the molecular signature of their parental cell, hence becoming attractive candidates for the non-invasive diagnosis of cancer. Also, the miRNA packaged within EVs is more stable and reliable than free miRNA in plasma or serum because the phospholipid bilayer encapsulated in EVs protects them from the RNases degradation in body fluids [18].

Several studies have investigated the miRNA profiles of EVs derived from lung cancer patients and proved their potential in diagnostics. Rabinowits et al. [19] found that the miRNA profiles of EVs derived from plasma and tumor tissues of NSCLC were distinct from those of healthy individuals, with upregulated levels of 12 specific miRNAs, including miR-21, miR-210, and miR-223, meaning that the profile of plasma exosomal miRNAs parallels that of tumor-derived miRNAs. Similarly, Wu et al. demonstrated that serum EV miRNA-96 expression was higher in lung cancer patients than in controls and displayed a correlation with the stage of the cancer [20]. Although EV miRNA has tremendous potential, further studies are required to confirm the above findings and to develop reliable diagnostic assays.

However, there are still technical challenges in the isolation and characterization of EVs, necessitating the need for standardized protocols to ensure reproducibility and accuracy in miRNA detection. The aim of this study was to investigate the microRNA profile in EVs isolated from lung cancer by quantifying and comparing the total miRNA levels in the serum and EVs to assess their diagnostic potential. Subsequently, we focused on two specific miRNAs previously reported to be dysregulated in serum and lung cancer tissues, namely miR-let-7a, functioning as a tumor suppressor, and miR-21, identified as oncogenic, which were isolated and analyzed separately in both serum and EVs.

2. Materials and Methods

2.1. Patients' Samples

Whole blood samples from 37 patients with lung cancer and 37 healthy controls who showed no evidence of cancer or other diseases were collected before treatment at Foggia Hospital in the south of Italy. Venous blood samples (3 mL) were collected in coagulation-promoting tubes. The samples were allowed to coagulate in an upright position for 30 min without being disturbed and then centrifuged at 2500× g for 10 min at 20 °C. The top layer containing serum was carefully transferred to a 15 mL reaction tube and centrifuged at 3200× g for 20 min at 20 °C. Finally, the serum was transferred into a fresh 1.5 mL reaction tube or cryotube without disturbing the pellet and filtered with a 0.45 μM filter, and the serum samples were stored at −80 °C until needed.

2.2. Isolation of EVs by Size Exclusion Chromatography

EVs were isolated from serum samples by means of size exclusion chromatography (SEC) using sepharose-based qEV columns (iZON Science, Christchurch, New Zealand) according to the manufacturer's recommendations and previously published methods [18].

Briefly, the columns were removed from a 4 °C environment and slowly adapted to room temperature, the 20% ethanol storage solution was removed, and the column was flushed one to two times with 10 mL of PBS. The serum samples were thawed on ice and centrifuged for 10 min at 1500× g at 10 °C, and the supernatant was transferred to new Eppendorf tubes and subjected to another centrifugation for 10 min at 10,000× g at 10 °C. Each serum sample was transferred to a new Eppendorf tube and stored at −80 °C or processed directly. For frozen samples, an additional centrifugation at 10,000× g for 10 min at 10 °C was performed after thawing and immediately prior to SEC to remove aggregates potentially formed during storage. A 0.5 mL aliquot of serum was applied to the qEV column, and the flow-through was discarded. Then, 3900 μL of Hank's balanced salt solution (HBSS) was applied, and the flow-through was discarded. Another 3 × 500 μL of HBSS was applied and the flow-through was collected and protease inhibitor was added. Finally, the 1.5 mL samples of the collected EVs were subjected to ultracentrifugation at 130,000× g for 2.5 h at 4 °C. The supernatant was carefully removed, leaving 115 μL. This was used to carefully resuspend the pellet by pipetting for 5 min. EV suspensions were kept at −80 °C until further application.

2.3. Nanoparticle Tracking Analysis

The particle size distribution and concentration of EVs were assessed using nanoparticle tracking analysis (NTA), following established protocols [3]. Briefly, EV suspensions were diluted in HBSS buffer to obtain a final measurement volume of 1 mL, with dilution ratios ranging between 1:50 and 1:2000. The working concentration was optimized by ensuring a particle count of approximately 140–200 per frame. Each analysis consisted of two measurement runs, scanning 11 distinct positions, and capturing 30 frames at each position. Data acquisition was carried out under standardized conditions, including automatic focus adjustment, a fixed camera sensitivity of 79, a shutter speed of 70, auto-detected scattering intensity, and a chamber temperature of 24 °C. Recorded videos were processed using ZetaView Software (version 8.05.11 SP1, Particle Metrix, Meerbusch, Germany) on the ZetaView PMX-120 instrument, applying the following analytical thresholds: a minimum area of 5, a minimum brightness of 30, and a maximum area of 1000. The system hardware consisted of a CMOS camera and an integrated 40 mW, 488 nm laser source.

2.4. Transmission Electron Microscopy (TEM)

Transmission electron microscopy (TEM) was employed to confirm and analyze the morphology and size of EVs. For sample preparation, 3 μL of the EV suspension was placed onto glow-discharged copper grids coated with pioloform carbon and left to adsorb for 5 min. The grids were subsequently rinsed twice with drops of deionized distilled water. Negative staining was carried out by applying two successive 4 μL drops of 0.5% aqueous uranyl acetate. After excess stain was carefully removed with filter paper, the grids were air-dried prior to imaging. The vesicles were visualized using a JEOL JEM-1400 transmission electron microscope operated at 80 kV. Digital images were acquired with a Megaview III camera system and processed using iTEM software 5.2.

2.5. Western Blotting

Proteins from the extracellular vesicles were extracted using 1 × RIPA lysis buffer composed of 50 mM Tris-HCl (pH 7.6), 150 mM NaCl, 1% Triton X-100, 0.5% sodium deoxycholate, 0.1% SDS, and supplemented with a protease and phosphatase inhibitor cocktail. The protein was estimated using the BCA protein assay kit (ThermoFisher, Waltham, MA, USA, Cat#: 23227), and 5X Laemmli buffer was added to the lysate solution. Then, equal volumes of protein (50 μg) for each sample were prepared by separating them via 10% SDS-PAGE and then transferring them onto 0.45 μM nitrocellulose membranes (Sigma-Aldrich, ST. Louis, MO, USA, GE10600003). The membranes were blocked in 5% BSA in TBS-T for an hour at room temperature after being rinsed four times for five minutes each time with TBS buffer, followed by immunoblotting with primary antibodies of interest. The following antibodies were used: CD9 (1:1000. rabbit monoclonal, Abcam, Cambridge, UK, Cat#: ab92726), CD81 (1:1000. mouse monoclonal, Cat#: sc-166029), flotillin-1 (1:5000. mouse monoclonal, BD Biosciences, San Jose, CA, USA, Cat#: 610821), and TSG101 (1:5000. mouse monoclonal, Santa Cruz, CA, USA, Cat#: sc-7964). Membranes were again washed another four times for five minutes with TBS-T, and HRP-conjugated secondary anti-mouse antibody (1:10,000. mouse monoclonal, Cell signaling, Danvers, MA, USA, Cat#: 7076) was added for 1 h at room temperature. The detection of protein bands was carried out with an enhanced chemiluminescence (ECL) reagent (GE Healthcare Life Sciences, Chicago, IL, USA), and the resulting signals were captured and analyzed using the Odyssey Fc imaging system (LI-COR Biosciences, Lincoln, NE, USA).

2.6. Isolation of miRNAs

The EVs, after purification, were transferred to RNase-free tubes. Total RNA, including miRNA, from 100 μL of EVs and 200 μL of serum was extracted utilizing the QIAGEN miRNeasy Micro Kit (Qiagen, Hilden, Germany) in accordance with the manufacturer's instructions. RNA was eluted in 30 μL of RNase-free water provided with the kit. The NanoDrop One spectrophotometer (Thermo Fisher Scientific, Waltham, MA, USA) was employed to assess the concentration and purity of the eluted RNA. RNA purity was evaluated with the absorbance ratio OD260/OD280.

2.7. miRNAs Reverse Transcription and Expression by qRT-PCR

Following miRNA extraction, miRNA quantification was performed by using RNA samples with equal volumes for cDNA synthesis using miRCURY LNA RT kit according to the manufacturer's protocol (Qiagen, Hilden, Germany). Quantitative RT-PCR (qRT-PCR) was performed by using a QuantStudio 5 (ThermoFisher Scientific, Waltham, MA, USA) with miRCURY LNA SYBR Green PCR Kit (Qiagen, Hilden, Germany). Among the various target miRNAs, we focused on two microRNAs that have previously been reported as being altered in serum or lung cancer tissue samples: miR-let-7a-5p, identified as a tumor suppressor miRNA, and miR-21-3p, classified as an oncogenic miRNA. miR-103a-3p was selected as the internal control because it is consistently expressed in healthy populations and has not been reported to show alterations in lung cancer (Table 1). The PCR reactions were carried out in duplicate with 60 cycles of denaturation (10 s at 95 °C), annealing (60 s at 56 °C), and elongation (30 s at 54 °C) after an initial enzyme activation (2 min at 95 °C). The expression levels of EV miRNA in the serum and free circulating miRNA of patients with lung cancer were compared with those of healthy controls. The expression levels of the target miRNAs were normalized to the miR-103a, and the calculation was performed using the comparative $2^{-\Delta\Delta Ct}$ method.

Table 1. Primers used in this study.

Product Name	Sequence	GeneGlobe Id
hsa-let-7a-5p	5′UGAGGUAGUAGGUUGUAUAGUU	YP00205727
hsa-miR-21-3p	5′CAACACCAGUCGAUGGGCUGU	YP00204302
hsa-miR-103a-3p	5′AGCAGCAUUGUACAGGGCUAUGA	YP00204063
UniSp6		YP00203954

Normalization was performed using miR-103a, which has been reported to show stable expression across diverse tissue types and pathological conditions, including cancer. In a previous work from our group, systematic screening identified miR-103a and miR-484 as reliable endogenous reference miRNAs in serum and extracellular vesicle studies [3,17]. In our present dataset, miR-103a expression did not differ significantly between NSCLC patients and controls, supporting its use as an internal normalizer.

2.8. Statistical Analysis

All statistical analyses were performed using SPSS version 22.0 (IBM, Armonk, NY, USA), while figures and graphs were generated with GraphPad Prism version 10.1.2 (GraphPad Software, San Diego, CA, USA). To assess the adequacy of this sample size, we conducted a post hoc power analysis using the two-sample t-test model. Assuming a medium-to-large effect size (Cohen's d = 0.7) and a significance level of 0.05, the analysis indicated a statistical power of approximately 0.84, which exceeds the commonly accepted threshold of 0.80. The results are expressed as average ± SD. One-way ANOVA and Student's t-test were used to analyze the statistical significance of the differences between the groups. A threshold of $p < 0.05$ was considered statistically significant.

3. Results

3.1. Participant Characteristics

In the present study, from January 2023 to December 2023, serum samples from a total of 37 lung cancer patients who visited the Thoracic Surgery Department at the A.O.U. Polyclinic in Foggia, Italy, and 37 healthy controls (HC) were investigated. Among them were 31 patients with adenocarcinoma and 6 with squamous cell carcinoma. In lung cancer patients, samples were prospectively collected at a time prior to any treatment. The clinicopathological characteristics of the participants are shown in Table 2.

Table 2. The characteristics of the participants.

Groups		Patients		Healthy Control	
		No. 37	%	No. 37	%
Age	<60	10	27.03	16	43.24
	>60	27	72.97	21	56.76
Gender	Male	22	59.46	24	64.86
	Female	15	40.54	13	35.14
Smoking	Non-Smokers	17	45.95	15	40.54
	Former smokers	15	40.54	9	24.32
	Current smokers	5	13.51	13	35.14
TNM stages	Stage I	8	21.62		
	Stage II	14	37.84		
	Stage III	9	24.32		
	Stage IV	6	16.22		
Type of Cancer	AD *	31	83.78		
	SCC *	6	16.22		
EGFR statue	EGFR wild type	32	86.49		
	EGFR mutant	5	13.51		

* AD: adenocarcinoma, SCC: squamous cell carcinoma.

3.2. EVs Are Significantly Enriched in NSCLC Patient Serum

Circulating EVs were isolated from the serum of patients with lung cancer and healthy controls by means of size exclusion chromatography (SEC). The EV-enriched fractions were characterized by their size, morphology, concentration, and protein markers.

The NTA results showed that the diameter of EVs isolated from the serum of patients and healthy individuals primarily ranged between 50 and 200 nm in diameter

(Figure 1a–c). The median size of EVs in lung cancer patients was significantly smaller (116 ± 9.91 nm) compared to healthy controls (128 ± 7.63 nm) (Figure 1c). Quantification of EVs by NTA revealed that the concentration of EVs in lung cancer patients ($7.99 \pm 0.85 \times 10^{10}$ particles/mL) was significantly higher compared to healthy controls ($3.58 \pm 0.42 \times 10^{10}$ particles/mL) ($p \leq 0.01$), representing an approximately 2.2-fold increase (Figure 1d). TEM analyses revealed a majority of vesicles in the expected size range of 70–150 nm, which is characteristic of small EVs, from both NSCLC patient serum and that of healthy controls (Figure 1e). In addition, the protein concentration of the EV samples was evaluated. No significant differences were observed regarding the protein concentration of EVs from patient (349 ±25.7 µg/mL) or HC serum (307 ± 28.43 µg/mL) (Figure 1f). However, the higher protein concentrations of the patient EV samples reflect the higher number of EVs isolated from 0.5 mL of patient serum.

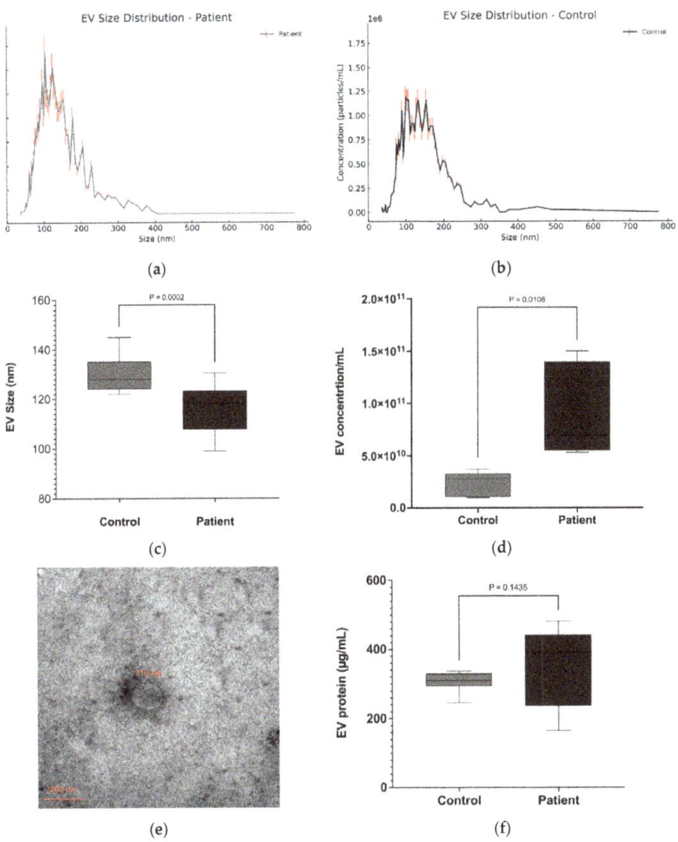

Figure 1. Characterization of EVs derived from lung cancer patients. NTA was used to analyze the size and concentration of EVs. (**a–c**) EV size: Representative measurements of lung cancer patient (**a**) and healthy control (**b**) EVs showing the size range of the isolated EVs. (**c**) Median sizes of EVs from lung cancer patients (116 ± 9.91 nm) and healthy individuals (128 ± 7.63 nm). (**d**) EV concentrations in lung cancer patients ($7.99 \pm 0.85 \times 10^{10}$ particles/mL) and in healthy controls ($3.58 \pm 0.42 \times 10^{10}$ particles/mL) particles/mL. (**e**) TEM image of EVs derived from patient serum. EVs, negatively stained with 2% uracyl acetate after removal of moisture, showed the expected size and shape of small EVs (30–150 nm in diameter). (**f**) EV protein quantification. n = 37.

3.3. Western Blot Analysis Confirms Purity of EVs Isolates

To ensure the successful enrichment and purity of EVs after SEC isolation, EVs were analyzed by means of Western blot to confirm the presence of EV markers and absence of proteins indicating contamination. In accordance with the Minimal Information for Studies of EVs 2024 (MISEV) [21], several known EV markers, including CD9, CD81, Flotillin-1, and TSG101, were observed in the purified serum EVs of patients with lung cancer and healthy individuals. Meanwhile, the endoplasmic reticulum marker calnexin was absent in our isolated EV samples, indicating their purity (Figure 2).

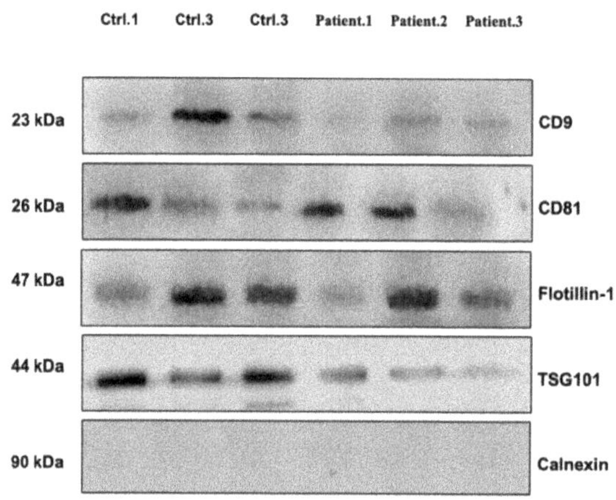

Figure 2. Immunoblotting assay for EV markers detected CD9, CD81, Flotillin-1 and TSG101 in EVs derived from lung cancer patients and healthy controls. Calnexin was used as a negative control.

3.4. miRNAs Are Targeted into EVs

In the present study, we isolated miRNAs from EVs and free-circulating serum in both lung cancer patients and healthy controls. EVs were isolated from 500 µL of serum, while free-circulating miRNA was extracted from 200 µL of serum, and in both cases, RNA was eluted in 30 µL of buffer. The average concentration of EV-derived miRNA in lung cancer patients was 78.53 ± 55.74 ng/µL, compared to 16.78 ± 8.82 ng/µL in free-circulating serum. Among the healthy controls, EV miRNA concentration averaged 69.61 ± 48.46 ng/µL, while free-circulating miRNA measured 12.36 ± 5.61 ng/µL. When normalized to serum input volume, these correspond to 4.71 ng/µL serum for patient-derived EV miRNA and 2.39 ng/µL serum for free serum miRNA (Figure 3a). Similarly, in healthy controls, EV miRNA yielded 4.18 ng/µL serum, while the free-circulating fraction yielded 1.85 ng/µL serum (Figure 3b). These findings confirm a consistent and significant enrichment of miRNAs in the EV compartment compared to the free-circulating serum fraction in both patients and healthy individuals.

Interestingly, the amount of miRNA in the patient EV samples was considerably higher compared to the miRNA content of EVs from healthy controls. However, the data indicates that there was no significant difference between the miRNA concentrations in the EVs of patients with lung cancer and those of healthy individuals ($p = 0.76$), nor between the miRNA concentrations in the serum of patients and those of healthy individuals ($p = 0.39$).

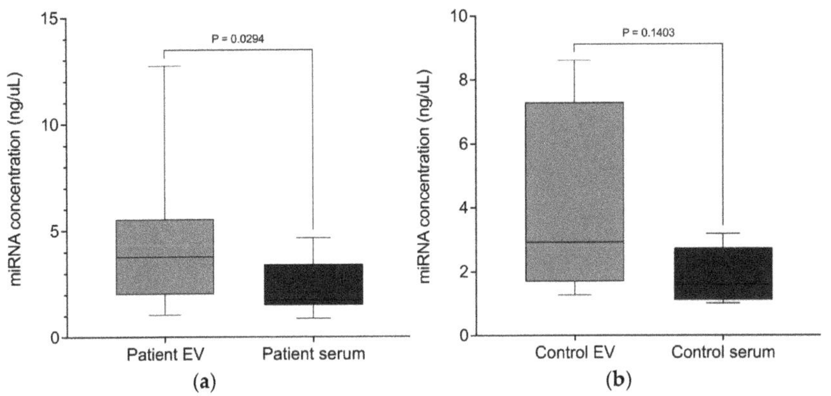

Figure 3. miRNAs are enriched in EVs after normalization to serum input volume. Box plots illustrate the distribution of normalized total miRNA concentrations in extracellular vesicles (EVs) and matched free-circulating serum fractions from lung cancer patients and healthy controls. miRNA concentrations were calculated based on original serum input volumes. Each plot shows the median with the interquartile range. (**a**) In lung cancer patients, EVs yielded significantly higher miRNA concentrations normalized to serum (mean: 4.71 ng/µL) than serum-derived free-circulating miRNA (2.39 ng/µL, $p = 0.0294$). (**b**) Among healthy controls, EV miRNA concentration (mean: 4.18 ng/µL) was also higher than in the serum (1.85 ng/µL), but the difference was not statistically significant ($p = 0.1403$).

3.5. Dysregulation of Several EVs miRNA and Circulating miRNA in Lung Cancer Patients

Previous studies have reported that multiple miRNAs show abnormal expression patterns in patients with lung cancer. Here, we conducted qRT-PCR for one tumor suppressor miRNA, Let-7a-5p, and one oncogenic miRNA, miR-21-3p, in EVs derived from 37 patients with lung cancer and compared them with 37 healthy individuals. miR-103a-3p was used as an endogenous control for normalization. In addition, we evaluated the circulating miRNAs in the serum of all patients and healthy individuals.

The results indicate, as shown in Table 3, that the expression levels of EVs Let-7a-5p (Figure 4a) was downregulated in lung cancer patients compared to the controls, while the expression of EVs miR-21-3p (Figure 4b) was significantly upregulated in lung cancer patients compared to the controls.

Table 3. EVs miRNAs differentially expressed in patients and healthy controls.

Groups	Patients EVs		Control EVs		*p* Value
	Mean	SD	Mean	SD	
hsa-let-7a-5p	0.76	0.35	1.96	0.46	0.0001
hsa-miR-21-3p	2.87	0.47	1.41	0.39	0.0001

Analysis of the circulating miRNA expression levels in serum (Table 4) was not able to detect the differences in Let-7a-5p expression between patients and HC as identified in EV miRNA. In total serum RNA, both groups maintained comparable expression of hsa-let-7a-5p, indicating that Let-7a-5p is efficiently targeted in EVs (Figure 5a). In contrast, the significantly elevated miR21-3p expression in patient serum is also observed when analyzing total serum RNA. (Figure 5b).

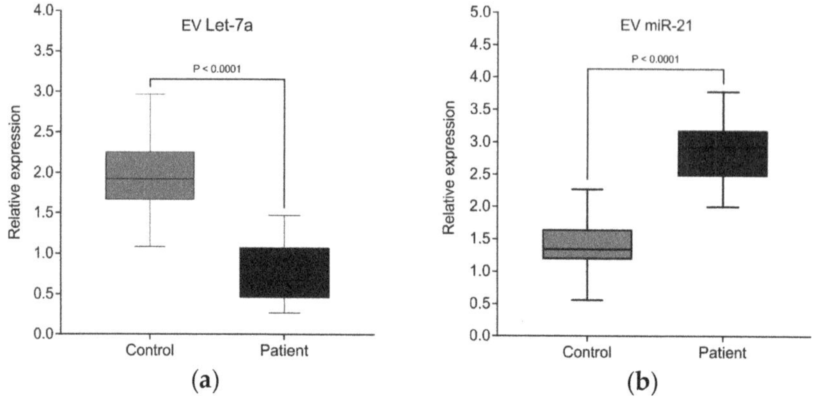

Figure 4. EVs miRNAs differentially expressed in lung cancer patients. Quantitative real-time PCR analysis of differentially expressed miRNAs in serum EVs from patients with lung cancer versus healthy controls. Let-7a-5p (**a**) and miR-21-3p (**b**) reached statistical significance.

Table 4. Circulating miRNAs differentially expressed in patients and healthy controls.

Groups	Patients Serum		Control Serum		p Value
	Mean	SD	Mean	SD	
hsa-let-7a-5p	1.21	0.41	1.40	0.72	0.16
hsa-miR-21-3p	3.29	0.51	1.92	0.91	0.0001

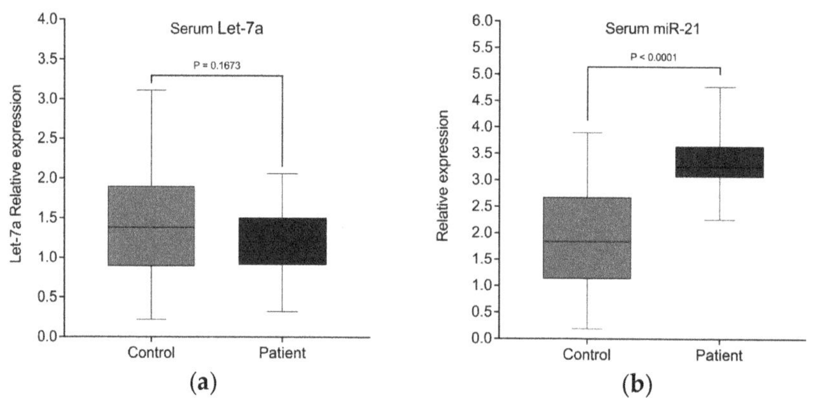

Figure 5. Circulating miRNAs differentially expressed in lung cancer patients. Quantitative real-time PCR analysis of differentially expressed miRNAs in serum EVs from patients with lung cancer versus healthy controls. Only hsa-miR-21-3p (**b**), but not hsa-Let-7a (**a**) reached statistical significance.

Interestingly, when comparing EV-associated and total serum miRNA levels within each group, we observed distinct distribution patterns for the two miRNAs. hsa-let-7a-5p was predominantly detected in the EV fraction, with minimal levels in the total serum in both patients and controls, indicating preferential encapsulation of this miRNA in EVs. In contrast, hsa-miR-21-3p was present in both EVs and total serum at comparable levels, suggesting that a substantial proportion of this miRNA circulates outside EVs as free miRNA, in addition to its EV-associated form.

3.6. Association of miRNA Expression with Clinicopathological Features

The expression levels of Let-7a-5p and miR-21-3p in EVs and the serum were analyzed with respect to different clinicopathological features of patients with lung cancer.

There was no statistically significant difference in the expression of Let-7a-5p (Table 5) in the EVs or serum of patients with lung cancer with respect to age group (<60 vs. ≥60 years) or gender (male vs. female subjects), with p-values > 0.05, as well as for healthy controls. Nevertheless, the expression levels of Let-7a-5p in EVs were downregulated in tumor patients at advanced stages (Stage III–IV) when compared with the expression levels found in early-stage patients (Stage I–II) ($p < 0.05$), though they remained unaltered in the serum. However, Let-7a-5p expression levels did not significantly differ between adenocarcinoma and squamous cell carcinoma ($p > 0.05$).

Table 5. Expression levels of Let-7a-5p in EVs and serum across clinicopathological features of lung cancer patients.

Clinicopathological Features	EVs (Mean ± SD)	*p* Value	Serum (Mean ± SD)	*p* Value
Age (<60 vs. ≥60)	0.72 ± 0.12	>0.05	1.12 ± 0.44	>0.05
Gender (Male vs. Female)	0.70 ± 0.13	>0.05	1.14 ± 0.46	>0.05
Smoking (Current Smokers vs. Non-smokers/ Former Smokers)	0.70 ± 0.14	>0.05	1.15 ± 0.42	>0.05
TNM Stages (Stage III–IV vs. Stage I–II)	0.67 ± 0.13	<0.05	1.16 ± 0.45	<0.05
Type of Cancer (AD vs. SCC)	0.71 ± 0.15	>0.05	1.13 ± 0.43	>0.05

Conversely, hsa-miR-21-3p (Table 6) was significantly upregulated in the EVs and serum from lung cancer patients in some clinicopathological features. Its expression in EVs was significantly higher in patients with advanced tumor stages (Stage III–IV) compared to patients with cancer in the early stages (Stage I–II) ($p < 0.01$). In addition, the levels of hsa-miR-21-3p were higher in adenocarcinoma patients compared to those with squamous cell carcinoma ($p < 0.05$). No significant associations between hsa-miR-21-3p expression levels and smoking status, age, or gender were detected ($p > 0.05$).

Table 6. Expression levels of miR-21-3p in EVs and serum across clinicopathological features of lung cancer patients.

Clinicopathological Features	EVs (Mean ± SD)	*p* Value	Serum (Mean ± SD)	*p* Value
Age (<60 vs. ≥60)	2.85 ± 0.35	>0.05	3.08 ± 0.41	>0.05
Gender (Male vs. Female)	2.80 ± 0.30	>0.05	3.12 ± 0.39	>0.05
Smoking (Current Smokers vs. Non-smokers/ Former Smokers)	2.70 ± 0.25	>0.05	3.10 ± 0.37	>0.05
TNM Stages (Stage III–IV vs. Stage I–II)	2.74 ± 0.33	<0.01	3.11 ± 0.43	<0.01
Type of Cancer (AD vs. SCC)	2.92 ± 0.32	<0.05	3.18 ± 0.33	<0.05

To specifically address the diagnostic utility of these two microRNAs at the early stages of lung cancer, we compared expression levels between early-stage NSCLC (Stage I–II) patients and healthy controls. No statistically significant differences were observed in either the serum or EVs.

4. Discussion

The majority of lung cancer patients are diagnosed at advanced stages, frequently leading to an unfavorable prognosis. This has driven researchers to develop biomarkers that can detect lung cancer at an early stage and improve the accuracy of diagnosis and treatment. In recent years, miRNAs have been discovered to play a crucial role in the pathogenesis and progression of lung cancer. Consequently, many research groups have focused on optimizing the potential of miRNAs as biomarkers for lung cancer [22].

Since miRNAs are involved in multiple cellular mechanisms that regulate tumor growth and progression, their use as biomarkers identified in blood has yielded very promising outcomes in the early detection of cancer. This is due to their relative stability against external factors such as pH alternation, storage, freezing, and thawing, as well as their resistance to degradation by endonucleases [23]. However, the results are sometimes contradictory, with variability in miRNA detection and inconsistent findings across different studies. This highlights the need for more reliable and consistent biomarkers for lung cancer detection.

To address these challenges, researchers are increasingly turning to EVs as an alternative source for miRNA as biomarkers. EVs are lipid bilayer nanovesicles that play a critical role in cell-to-cell communication by transporting bioactive molecules such as proteins, lipids, and nucleic acids, including miRNAs [24].

The miRNAs within EVs offer several advantages over free-circulating miRNAs. The miRNA within EVs is protected from degradation, thereby enhancing the stability and reliability of miRNA detection in bodily fluids. In addition, EVs are constantly released by living cells and are present in various body fluids, including the blood, urine, and saliva, making them accessible for non-invasive diagnostic tests. Most importantly, the miRNA profiles of EVs can reflect the molecular changes occurring within tumors, providing a more accurate snapshot of the disease state [6,18]. Despite this promising background, only a few studies have directly compared EVs and free circulating miRNAs in lung cancer.

In the present study, we isolated miRNAs from EVs and free-circulating miRNAs from serum in both lung cancer patients and healthy individuals. EV-derived miRNAs from lung cancer patients were obtained at an average of 471.2 ng per 100 μL serum, while the corresponding free-circulating fraction yielded 251.7 ng per 100 μL serum. Similarly, in healthy controls, EV-associated miRNAs were obtained at 417.7 ng per 100 μL serum, compared to 185.4 ng per 100 μL serum in the free-circulating component. These findings confirm a consistent enrichment of miRNAs in the EV compartment compared to free-circulating serum across both the cancer and control groups. This pattern aligns with previous studies [3]. For example, Dohmen et al. reported higher miRNA concentrations in exosomes versus serum in colorectal cancer patients (1504 ng/100 μL vs. 1024 ng/100 μL, respectively) [25]. Although the absolute concentrations in our lung cancer cohort are lower, the proportional enrichment in EVs is consistent, supporting the hypothesis that EVs provide a protective environment against serum RNase-mediated degradation.

The expression levels of miRNAs in cancer vary significantly, with both oncogenic and tumor-suppressive miRNAs being differentially regulated. Depending on the function of the miRNA, both variants can be beneficial for the tumor, inducing upregulation of miRNAs that act as proto-oncogenes, promoting tumor growth, and downregulation of miRNAs that act as tumor suppressors [26]. Based on this rationale, we analyzed an oncogenic and a tumor-suppressive miRNA in EVs derived from lung cancer patients, both previously reported as dysregulated in lung cancer patients [1].

In the present study, we found that the tumor suppressor miRNA Let-7a-5p is significantly downregulated in EVs derived from lung cancer patients compared to healthy individuals. In contrast, its abundance in free-circulating serum miRNA did not differ between groups. The downregulation of this miRNA in EVs isolated from lung cancer patients aligns with prior studies reporting reduced Let-7a-5p levels in EVs from lung [13], breast [27], and colorectal cancer [28].

However, the comparable expression levels of Let-7a-5p in the serum of both lung cancer patients and healthy controls in our present study contradicts previous findings that reported upregulation of this miRNA in the serum [29] of lung cancer patients. This discrepancy may be attributed to selective miRNA packaging mechanisms in EVs, which are regulated by specific RNA-binding proteins such as hnRNPA2B1 and YBX1 that recognize sequence motifs or secondary structures and direct miRNAs into EVs [30,31]. This selective encapsulation can lead to altered EV miRNA profiles independent of total serum miRNA levels. Furthermore, tumor cells may preferentially load tumor-suppressive miRNAs, such as let-7a, into EVs for secretion as a means of reducing their intracellular tumor-suppressive effects, while maintaining a balanced overall level in circulation contributed by non-tumor cells [32].

Multiple studies have reported the upregulation of miR-21-3p in various malignancies, both as free-circulating and EV-associated miRNA. Our data support these findings, demonstrating increased miR-21-3p levels in EVs isolated from the serum of patients with lung cancer [33] and free-circulating serum miR-21-3p [34]. Elevated miR-21 expression levels have been linked to tumor development, growth, and size through suppression of the tumor suppressor PTEN. This suggests the presence of miR-21 at early disease stages and thereby supports its potential utility in early detection.

Although previous studies have reported that both Let-7a-5p and miR-21-5p may serve as promising biomarkers for early-stage NSCLC detection due to their differential expression compared to healthy individuals [35,36], our findings did not reveal a statistically significant difference in the expression levels of these miRNAs between early-stage NSCLC patients (Stage I–II) and healthy controls. This lack of significance may be attributed to the limited number of Stage I patients in our cohort, reducing statistical power, as well as possible heterogeneity among early-stage disease presentations. Additionally, it is plausible that these two miRNAs alone are not sufficient for early detection, and a panel of multiple miRNAs or additional biomarkers might be required for improved sensitivity and specificity. Nevertheless, the overall trend of downregulation of Let-7a and upregulation of miR-21 in NSCLC patients relative to healthy controls aligns with previous reports and supports their utility in diagnosis and prognosis, particularly in more advanced stages [37,38].

Limitations

This study has some limitations. The cohort size was relatively small (n = 37 per group), which may limit the statistical power and generalizability of our findings. Furthermore, the absence of an independent validation cohort and the lack of blinded analysis restrict the extent to which the diagnostic potential of EV-associated hsa-miR-21-3p can be confirmed at this stage. Therefore, while our data suggest that EV-derived hsa-miR-21-3p is a promising biomarker for NSCLC detection, future studies with larger, independent, and blinded cohorts will be required to validate and extend these observations.

5. Conclusions

In conclusion, we were able to validate recent research findings regarding cancer miRNA enrichment in circulating EVs in contrast to the serum. EV levels of Let-7a-5p and miR-21-3p were significantly different in patients with lung cancer when compared with healthy controls. While free-circulating miR-21 levels were significantly increased in lung cancer patients compared to healthy controls, these differences were not observed for free-circulating Let-7a. Altogether, these findings support the potential of specific EV-miRNA cargo analysis as a minimally invasive approach in NSCLC detection and monitoring.

Author Contributions: D.J.S. and T.A.S., conceived and designed the study; D.J.S., K.S.R. and N.P.A. performed the experiments; D.J.S. wrote the paper; D.L., K.S.R., T.A.S., F.S., and G.H. reviewed and edited the manuscript. All authors have read and agreed to the published version of the manuscript.

Funding: This research received no external funding.

Institutional Review Board Statement: This study was conducted in accordance with the amended Declaration of Helsinki and was approved by the Ethics Committee of the University of Foggia, Italy (institutional review board approval number DDG N. 651 of 27 August 2022). Written informed consent was obtained from all participants prior to their inclusion in the study.

Informed Consent Statement: Written informed consent was obtained from all participants prior to their inclusion in the study.

Data Availability Statement: The datasets used and/or analyzed during the current study are available from the corresponding author on reasonable request.

Acknowledgments: The authors gratefully acknowledge the support of the Italian Ministry of Foreign Affairs and International Cooperation (MAECI) through a 2024–2025 research mobility grant, which supported a research stay in Italy under academic supervision.

Conflicts of Interest: The authors declare no conflicts of interest.

References

1. Farooq, M.; Herman, J.G. Noninvasive Diagnostics for Early Detection of Lung Cancer: Challenges and Potential with a Focus on Changes in DNA Methylation. *Cancer Epidemiol. Biomark. Prev.* **2020**, *29*, 2416–2422. [CrossRef] [PubMed]
2. Nooreldeen, R.; Bach, H. Current and Future Development in Lung Cancer Diagnosis. *Int. J. Mol. Sci.* **2021**, *22*, 8661. [CrossRef]
3. Tzaridis, T.; Reiners, K.S.; Weller, J.; Bachurski, D.; Schäfer, N.; Schaub, C.; Hallek, M.; Scheffler, B.; Glas, M.; Herrlinger, U.; et al. Analysis of Serum miRNA in Glioblastoma Patients: CD44-Based Enrichment of Extracellular Vesicles Enhances Specificity for the Prognostic Signature. *Int. J. Mol. Sci.* **2020**, *21*, 7211. [CrossRef]
4. Kumar, D.; Kumar, S.; Ayachit, G.; Bhairappanavar, S.; Ansari, A.; Sharma, P.; Soni, S.; Das, J. Cross-Kingdom Regulation of Putative miRNAs Derived from Happy Tree in Cancer Pathway: A Systems Biology Approach. *Int. J. Mol. Sci.* **2017**, *18*, 1191. [CrossRef]
5. Cekaite, L.; Eide, P.W.; Lind, G.E.; Skotheim, R.I.; Lothe, R.A. MicroRNAs as Growth Regulators, Their Function and Biomarker Status in Colorectal Cancer. *Oncotarget* **2016**, *7*, 6476–6505. [CrossRef]
6. Kinoshita, T.; Yip, K.W.; Spence, T.; Liu, F.-F. MicroRNAs in Extracellular Vesicles: Potential Cancer Biomarkers. *J. Hum. Genet.* **2017**, *62*, 67–74. [CrossRef]
7. Rodrigues, D.V.S.; Monteiro, V.V.S.; Navegantes-Lima, K.C.; Oliveira, A.L.; Gaspar, S.L.; Quadros, L.B.G.; Monteiro, M.C. MicroRNAs in Cell Cycle Progression and Proliferation: Molecular Mechanisms and Pathways. *Non-Coding RNA Investig.* **2018**, *2*, 28. [CrossRef]
8. Galagali, H.; Kim, J.K. The Multifaceted Roles of microRNAs in Differentiation. *Curr. Opin. Cell Biol.* **2020**, *67*, 118–140. [CrossRef] [PubMed]
9. Landskroner-Eiger, S.; Moneke, I.; Sessa, W.C. miRNAs as Modulators of Angiogenesis. *Cold Spring Harb. Perspect. Med.* **2013**, *3*, a006643. [CrossRef]
10. Pileczki, V.; Cojocneanu-Petric, R.; Maralani, M.; Berindan Neagoe, I.; Sandulescu, R. MicroRNAs as Regulators of Apoptosis Mechanisms in Cancer. *Med. Pharm. Rep.* **2016**, *89*, 50–55. [CrossRef] [PubMed]

11. Zhao, W.; Hu, J.; Hao, R.; Zhang, Q.; Guo, J.; Li, Y.; Xie, N.; Liu, L.; Wang, P.; Zhang, C.; et al. Induction of microRNA-let-7a Inhibits Lung Adenocarcinoma Cell Growth by Regulating cyclinD1. *Oncol. Rep.* **2018**, *40*, 1843–1854. [CrossRef]
12. Ma, W.; Ma, C.; Zhou, N.; Li, X.; Zhang, Y. Up-Regulation of miR-328-3p Sensitizes Non-Small Cell Lung Cancer to Radiotherapy. *Sci. Rep.* **2016**, *6*, 31651. [CrossRef] [PubMed]
13. Bai, J.; Shi, Z.; Wang, S.; Pan, H.; Zhang, T. MiR-21 and Let-7 Cooperation in the Regulation of Lung Cancer. *Front. Oncol.* **2022**, *12*, 950043. [CrossRef]
14. Lee, Y.S.; Dutta, A. The Tumor Suppressor microRNA *Let-7* Represses the HMGA2 Oncogene. *Genes Dev.* **2007**, *21*, 1025–1030. [CrossRef] [PubMed]
15. Xue, X.; Liu, Y.; Wang, Y.; Meng, M.; Wang, K.; Zang, X.; Zhao, S.; Sun, X.; Cui, L.; Pan, L.; et al. MiR-21 and MiR-155 Promote Non-Small Cell Lung Cancer Progression by Downregulating *SOCS1*, *SOCS6*, and *PTEN*. *Oncotarget* **2016**, *7*, 84508–84519. [CrossRef]
16. Shademan, B.; Karamad, V.; Nourazarian, A.; Masjedi, S.; Isazadeh, A.; Sogutlu, F.; Avcı, C.B. MicroRNAs as Targets for Cancer Diagnosis: Interests and Limitations. *Adv. Pharm. Bull.* **2023**, *13*, 435–445. [CrossRef] [PubMed]
17. Tzaridis, T.; Bachurski, D.; Liu, S.; Surmann, K.; Babatz, F.; Gesell Salazar, M.; Völker, U.; Hallek, M.; Herrlinger, U.; Vorberg, I.; et al. Extracellular Vesicle Separation Techniques Impact Results from Human Blood Samples: Considerations for Diagnostic Applications. *Int. J. Mol. Sci.* **2021**, *22*, 9211. [CrossRef]
18. Ko, S.Y.; Lee, W.; Naora, H. Harnessing microRNA-Enriched Extracellular Vesicles for Liquid Biopsy. *Front. Mol. Biosci.* **2024**, *11*, 1356780. [CrossRef]
19. Rabinowits, G.; Gerçel-Taylor, C.; Day, J.M.; Taylor, D.D.; Kloecker, G.H. Exosomal MicroRNA: A Diagnostic Marker for Lung Cancer. *Clin. Lung Cancer* **2009**, *10*, 42–46. [CrossRef]
20. Wu, H.; Zhou, J.; Mei, S.; Wu, D.; Mu, Z.; Chen, B.; Xie, Y.; Ye, Y.; Liu, J. Circulating Exosomal microRNA-96 Promotes Cell Proliferation, Migration and Drug Resistance by Targeting LMO7. *J. Cell. Mol. Med.* **2017**, *21*, 1228–1236. [CrossRef]
21. Welsh, J.A.; Goberdhan, D.C.I.; O'Driscoll, L.; Buzas, E.I.; Blenkiron, C.; Bussolati, B.; Cai, H.; Di Vizio, D.; Driedonks, T.A.P.; Erdbrügger, U.; et al. Minimal Information for Studies of Extracellular Vesicles (MISEV2023): From Basic to Advanced Approaches. *J. Extracell. Vesicle* **2024**, *13*, e12404. [CrossRef]
22. Wu, K.-L.; Tsai, Y.-M.; Lien, C.-T.; Kuo, P.-L.; Hung, J.-Y. The Roles of MicroRNA in Lung Cancer. *Int. J. Mol. Sci.* **2019**, *20*, 1611. [CrossRef] [PubMed]
23. Ishikawa, H.; Yamada, H.; Taromaru, N.; Kondo, K.; Nagura, A.; Yamazaki, M.; Ando, Y.; Munetsuna, E.; Suzuki, K.; Ohashi, K.; et al. Stability of Serum High-Density Lipoprotein-microRNAs for Preanalytical Conditions. *Ann. Clin. Biochem.* **2017**, *54*, 134–142. [CrossRef]
24. Duréndez-Sáez, E.; Torres-Martinez, S.; Calabuig-Fariñas, S.; Meri-Abad, M.; Ferrero-Gimeno, M.; Camps, C. Exosomal microRNAs in Non-Small Cell Lung Cancer. *Transl. Cancer Res. TCR* **2021**, *10*, 3128–3139. [CrossRef]
25. Dohmen, J.; Semaan, A.; Kobilay, M.; Zaleski, M.; Branchi, V.; Schlierf, A.; Hettwer, K.; Uhlig, S.; Hartmann, G.; Kalff, J.C.; et al. Diagnostic Potential of Exosomal microRNAs in Colorectal Cancer. *Diagnostics* **2022**, *12*, 1413. [CrossRef]
26. Ling, H.; Zhang, W.; Calin, G.A. Principles of microRNA Involvement in Human Cancers. *Chin. J. Cancer* **2011**, *30*, 739–748. [CrossRef]
27. Barone, I.; Gelsomino, L.; Accattatis, F.M.; Giordano, F.; Gyorffy, B.; Panza, S.; Giuliano, M.; Veneziani, B.M.; Arpino, G.; De Angelis, C.; et al. Analysis of Circulating Extracellular Vesicle Derived microRNAs in Breast Cancer Patients with Obesity: A Potential Role for Let-7a. *J. Transl. Med.* **2023**, *21*, 232. [CrossRef]
28. Mozammel, N.; Baghbani, E.; Amini, M.; Zaer, S.J.; Baghay Esfandyari, Y.; Tohidast, M.; Hosseini, S.S.; Rahmani, S.A.; Mokhtarzadeh, A.; Baradaran, B. The Simultaneous Effects of MIR-145-5p and Has-Let-7a-3p on Colorectal Tumorigenesis: In Vitro Evidence. *Adv. Pharm. Bull.* **2023**, *14*, 231–240. [CrossRef] [PubMed]
29. Pop-Bica, C.; Pintea, S.; Magdo, L.; Cojocneanu, R.; Gulei, D.; Ferracin, M.; Berindan-Neagoe, I. The Clinical Utility of miR-21 and Let-7 in Non-Small Cell Lung Cancer (NSCLC). A Systematic Review and Meta-Analysis. *Front. Oncol.* **2020**, *10*, 516850. [CrossRef]
30. Koppers-Lalic, D.; Hackenberg, M.; Bijnsdorp, I.V.; van Eijndhoven, M.A.J.; Sadek, P.; Sie, D.; Zini, N.; Middeldorp, J.M.; Ylstra, B.; de Menezes, R.X.; et al. Nontemplated Nucleotide Additions Distinguish the Small RNA Composition in Cells from Exosomes. *Cell Rep.* **2014**, *8*, 1649–1658. [CrossRef] [PubMed]
31. Shurtleff, M.J.; Temoche-Diaz, M.M.; Karfilis, K.V.; Ri, S.; Schekman, R. Y-Box Protein 1 Is Required to Sort microRNAs into Exosomes in Cells and in a Cell-Free Reaction. *eLife* **2016**, *5*, e19276. [CrossRef]
32. Villarroya-Beltri, C.; Gutiérrez-Vázquez, C.; Sánchez-Cabo, F.; Pérez-Hernández, D.; Vázquez, J.; Martin-Cofreces, N.; Martinez-Herrera, D.J.; Pascual-Montano, A.; Mittelbrunn, M.; Sánchez-Madrid, F. Sumoylated hnRNPA2B1 Controls the Sorting of miRNAs into Exosomes through Binding to Specific Motifs. *Nat. Commun.* **2013**, *4*, 2980. [CrossRef]

33. Lohajová Behulová, R.; Bugalová, A.; Bugala, J.; Struhárňanská, E.; Šafranek, M.; Juráš, I. Circulating Exosomal miRNAs as a Promising Diagnostic Biomarker in Cancer. *Physiol. Res.* **2023**, *72*, S193–S207. [CrossRef]
34. Zhou, Y.; Guo, D.; Zhang, Y. Association of MicroRNA-21 with P53 at Mutant Sites R175H and R248Q, Clinicopathological Features, and Prognosis of NSCLC. *Mol. Ther. Oncolytics* **2020**, *19*, 208–217. [CrossRef]
35. Zhang, W.-T.; Zhang, G.-X.; Gao, S.-S. The Potential Diagnostic Accuracy of Let-7 Family for Cancer: A Meta-Analysis. *Technol. Cancer Res. Treat.* **2021**, *20*, 15330338211033061. [CrossRef] [PubMed]
36. Wang, W.; Li, X.; Liu, C.; Zhang, X.; Wu, Y.; Diao, M.; Tan, S.; Huang, S.; Cheng, Y.; You, T. MicroRNA-21 as a Diagnostic and Prognostic Biomarker of Lung Cancer: A Systematic Review and Meta-Analysis. *Biosci. Rep.* **2022**, *42*, BSR20211653. [CrossRef] [PubMed]
37. Jeong, H.C.; Kim, E.K.; Lee, J.H.; Yoo, H.N.; Kim, J.K. Aberrant Expression of Let-7a miRNA in the Blood of Non-Small Cell Lung Cancer Patients. *Mol. Med. Rep.* **2011**, *4*, 383–387. [CrossRef] [PubMed]
38. Rai, S.; Garg, P.; Bhatt, S.; Latha, T.; Verma, A.; Banerjee, B.; Singh, M. The Diagnostic Role of microRNA 21 in Patients with Nonsmall Cell Lung Cancer: An Exploratory Study. *Lung India* **2020**, *37*, 501. [CrossRef]

biomedicines

MDPI

Article

Lyophilized Small Extracellular Vesicles (sEVs) Derived from Human Adipose Stem Cells Maintain Efficacy to Promote Healing in Neuronal Injuries

Brianna Jones [1,2], Rekha Patel [1], Bangmei Wang [1], Theresa Evans-Nguyen [2] and Niketa A. Patel [1,3,*]

[1] Research Service, J.A. Haley Veterans Hospital, Tampa, FL 33612, USA; brianna.jones2@va.gov (B.J.); niketa.patel@va.gov (N.A.P.); rekha.patel1@va.gov (R.P.); bangmei.wang@va.gov (B.W.)
[2] Department of Chemistry, College of Arts and Sciences, University of South Florida, Tampa, FL 33612, USA; bmjones1@usf.edu (B.J.); evansnguyen@usf.edu (T.E.-N.)
[3] Department of Molecular Medicine, Morsani College of Medicine, University of South Florida, Tampa, FL 33612, USA; niketa@usf.edu (N.A.P.)
* Correspondence: niketa.patel@va.gov

Abstract: Background: Traumatic brain injury (TBI) occurs in individuals of all ages, predominantly during sports, accidents, and in active military service members. Chronic consequences of TBI include declined cognitive and motor function, dementia, and emotional distress. Small extracellular vesicles (sEVs), previously referred to as exosomes, are nano-sized lipid vesicles that play a role in intercellular communication. Our prior research established the efficacy of sEVs derived from human adipose stem cells (hASC sEVs) in accelerating the healing of brain injuries. The hASC sEVs are a biologic therapeutic and need to be stored at −20 °C or −80 °C. This limits their use in translating to everyday use in clinics or their inclusion in first-aid kits for application immediately after injury. To address this, here we demonstrate that hASC sEVs can be stored at room temperature (RT) for two months post lyophilization. **Methods:** A transmission electron microscope (TEM) and nanoparticle tracking analysis (NTA) were used to validate the morphology of lyophilized RT sEVs. Using in vitro models of neuronal injury mimicking physical injury, inflammation, and oxidative stress, we demonstrate that lyophilized RT hASC sEVs are viable and promote the healing of neuronal injuries. **Results:** The lyophilized sEVs maintain their purity, size, and morphology upon rehydration. Lyophilized, RT stored sEVs showed better efficacy after two months compared with −80 °C stored sEVs. **Conclusions:** RT storage of lyophilized hASC sEVs maintains their efficacy to accelerate the healing of injuries in neuronal cells. This will advance the use of hASC sEVs, bringing them closer to use in clinics, home first-aid kits, and on battlefields by active service members.

Keywords: sEVs; exosomes; adipose stem cells; traumatic brain injury; TBI; hASC sEVs; lyophilization; NTA

1. Introduction

Traumatic brain injury (TBI) has exponentially increased in the last few years and affects nearly 50 million people globally. TBI is defined as a disruption or injury to brain function caused by an outside force, such as a blow or jolt to the head or an object entering the brain [1]. The effects from TBI can be either short- or long-term; the long-term effects are more severe and, in some cases, result in early death. Secondary injury, often tied to neuroinflammation, results from the primary brain injury and occurs over time, and it includes chemical, cellular, tissue, and blood vessel changes in the brain. Secondary injuries typically include ischemia, cerebral edema, hypoxia, and more [2]. These injuries can cause secondary cell death, resulting in a decrease in cell proliferation [3,4]. The development of treatments for these injuries is often difficult due to the complexity of progression. These complications stem from pathophysiological and prolonged development of secondary injuries. The most common treatments for secondary injury generally target neuroinflammation; however, there is a still a need for more effective treatments [5]. The impact of TBI may last for several years, and it can leave some individuals disabled or in need of rehospitalization even 10 years after the injury. Thus, the availability of robust treatment options in the hours following TBI is imperative [6,7].

One of the most widely affected demographics of TBI are active military service members and veterans. TBI is known to be the most impactful cause of disabilities related to combat [8]. TBI is a signature injury of the Global War on Terrorism (GWOT) conflicts, including post-9/11 conflicts, Operation Iraqi Freedom (OIF), Operation Enduring Freedom (OEF), and Operation New Dawn (OND) [9,10].

Recently, the definition and nomenclature of extracellular vesicles (EVs) have been updated according to the Information for Studies of Extracellular Vesicles (ISEV) [11]. Small extracellular vesicles (sEVs) are characterized as EVs that are lipid-membrane-bound particles less than 200 nm and released by cells. Exosomes are often identified through surface markers such as the tetraspanins CD9, CD63, CD81. However, research is still ongoing on whether these tetraspanins solely mark exosomes and no other intracellular multivesicular bodies.

Mesenchymal stem cells (MSCs) derived from adipose tissue have become a promising therapeutic for TBI due to their anti-inflammatory and regenerative properties [12]. However, since stem cells can differentiate into different phenotypes based on the stimuli, the secretome was evaluated. We have previously demonstrated that the secretome from human adipose stem cells (hASCs) contains large and small extracellular vesicles (EVs). We further characterized the sEV using the tetraspanin markers CD9, CD63, and CD81, which demonstrated that hASC sEVs (previously referred to as exosomes in our publications), contained long, noncoding RNA that was pivotal to driving the regeneration and repair post brain injury [4]. In this study, we used the hASCs from the same master hASC bank and collected its conditioned media to purify the sEVs and evaluate their efficacy upon lyophilization. Over the past decade, there has been an increased interest in the use of sEVs due to their important role in intercellular communication and drug-delivery applications. The sEVs carry cargo such as proteins, RNA, and DNA that can be transported from cell to cell and serve as biomarkers for disease progression and diagnosis [13]. The sEVs have also become a useful tool as a drug-delivery vehicle. Due to their low toxicity, biocompatibility, and ability to carry small molecules, these vesicles have also proven to be effective in delivering drugs [14,15].

There are various ways to isolate sEVs. The method of isolation can influence the purity, functionality, and performance of sEVs [16,17]. Some of the most common methods used include size exclusion-based methods and ultracentrifugation. Methods that include ultracentrifugation can harm the morphology of the sEVs due to the force and are often tedious. Size exclusion methods can remove larger EVs and contaminating particles that are not vesicles while keeping the sEVs intact [18]. More recently, size exclusion methods have been coupled with other methods such as ultrafiltration to facilitate more efficient removal of bigger particles. In this study, we investigated the efficiency of ExoSpin columns compared with qEV columns for sEV isolation.

The hASC sEVs have tremendous potential in treating TBI; however, there remains an issue with storage that limits their use in the clinic and battlefield. The sEVs stored at 4 °C show 100% efficacy up to 1 week. sEVs are usually stored long-term at −80 °C to preserve their size and cargo; however, several studies have reported that storage of EVs and sEVs at −80 °C can cause harm to their morphology and cargo over time, interfering with their performance [19,20]. In addition, rural clinics and battlefield clinics often do not have access to −80 °C ultra-low freezers. To address this issue, lyophilization has been proposed as a storage method at room temperature [21]. Lyophilization (freeze-drying) is a method that removes water from a sample using sublimation and desorption (Figure 1). There are three phases to the lyophilization process. The first phase is freezing, which involves cooling the material below its triple point. This can be achieved by rapidly freezing the sample in a −80 °C freezer for biological samples. The next phase is primary drying or sublimation. During sublimation, the pressure is lowered (↓) and the sample is heated (↑) to −20 °C so the water will sublimate and solidify while under vacuum [22]. The last phase is secondary drying or adsorption. During this phase, water-bound molecules are removed from the material by raising the temperature. During freezing and drying, the bilayer and cargo of the sEVs can be damaged due to the stresses they undergo during these processes. To combat this issue, cryoprotectants may be used [23].

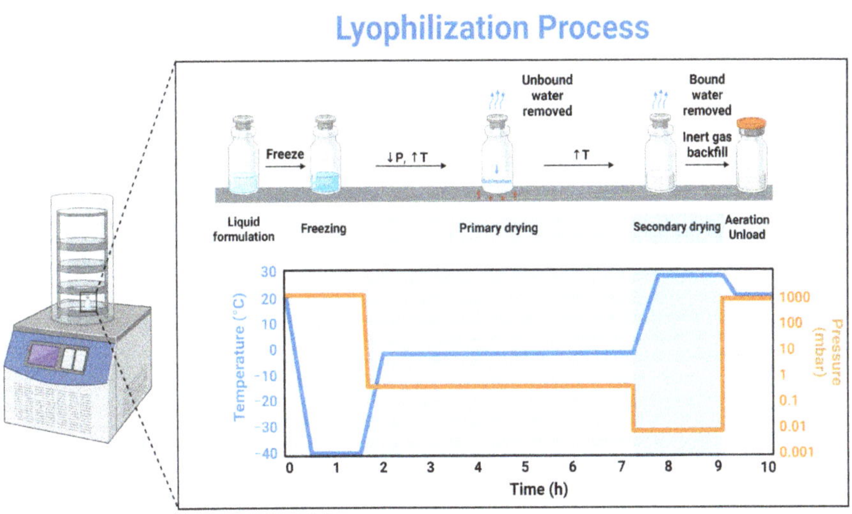

Figure 1. Schematic of the three processes that occur during lyophilization. The publication license can be found in Supplementary File S2 (Created in BioRender. Jones, B. (2024) https://BioRender.com/s06h883; accessed on 15 December 2024).

In this study, we used trehalose, a nonreducing disaccharide found in many organisms, to protect the hASC sEVs during lyophilization [24]. We investigated the sEVs' morphology, size, and concentration as well as protein concentrations post lyophilization and storage at room temperature. We then investigated the in vitro efficacy of the lyophilized hASC sEVs in models of neuronal injury mimicking TBI.

The aim of the study was to (1) compare two widely used EV isolation methods to establish an effective and reproducible isolation method for the extraction of sEVs from hASCs; (2) demonstrate that lyophilization with the addition of trehalose does not change the morphology or size of the sEVs; and (3) compare the efficacy of lyophilized RT stored sEVs with −80 °C stored sEVs using in vitro neuronal injury models.

2. Materials and Methods

2.1. Cell Culture

Studies were carried out using mouse hippocampal neuronal cell line (HT22) Dr. D.R. Schubert (Salk Institute, La Jolla, CA, USA). HT22 cells were cultured in DMEM (GibcoLifeTechnologies, Waltham, MA, USA: # 11,965–092), 10% FBS (Sigma, St. Louis, MO, USA; #F4135), and 1 × penicillin–streptomycin (Sigma #P4333) at 37 °C and 5% CO_2. The hASCs (ZenBio, Durham, NC, USA: #ASC-F-SL) were pooled from lean female subcutaneous depo with an average BMI of 27.9. All donors were non-smokers and non-diabetic. For collection of conditioned media (CM) from human adipose stem cells (hASCs), hASCs were grown to 90% confluence (8×10^6 hASCs) in T75 flasks, and then, cell medium was replaced with serum-free mesenchymal stem cell basal media with StemFlex medium kit (GibcoLifeTechnologies, Waltham, MA, USA, # A33494-01). The CM derived from hASCs was collected after 48 h.

2.2. sEV Isolation and Size Characterization

The CM (as described in Section 2.1) was then used to isolate sEVs. CM was centrifuged at 3000× *g* for 15 min to remove any hASC cell debris. The CM was then processed to isolate sEVs using 2 methods.

For hASC sEVs isolated using ExoSpin columns, ExoSpin™ (Cell Guidance systems, St. Louis, MO, USA: Catalog EX05) reagent was added to the CM and incubated for 20 min at room temperature. The mixture was centrifuged at 1500× *g* for 30 min to remove large EVs by precipitation, and the supernatant was added to the top of the ExoSpin column and centrifuged at 50× *g* for 60 s. The sEVs were eluted in PBS by centrifugation.

For sEVs isolated using qEV columns (35 nm from IZON, Bellaire, TX, USA), CM was concentrated using a 10 kDa molecular weight cut-off filter (MWCO) which retains the large EVS and allows only EVs smaller than 10 kDa to pass through the pores. qEV columns were prepared following the manufacturer's instructions using PBS as a buffer. The qEV column was mounted on the Automated Fraction Collector (AFC, from IZON, Bellaire, TX, USA), which enabled reproducible and exact collection of fractions by size exclusion chromatography. The concentrated CM was then added to the prepared qEV columns. The sEVs were eluted in PBS, and fractions were collected every 500 µL until a pink color was seen eluting from the column (end of sample collection). Nanoparticle tracking analysis (NTA3.1, Build 3.1.46 RRID SCR-014239) was used to analyze size and concentration of sEVs in each fraction. The fractions containing a single peak of sEV particles within 35–200 nm size were identified and used in the TEM to image the morphology and in the experimental setups.

2.3. Transmission Electron Microscopy (TEM)

For the hASC sEVs, 4 µL at a concentration of 1×10^8 particles/mL was placed on a carbon-filled coated copper mesh grid. The sample was then incubated for 10 min at room temperature. The excess liquid was then removed from the grid using filter paper. One drop of 0.2 micron filtered, boiled distilled water was placed on the grid and removed three times to rinse off PBS. Sample was left to dry overnight. Samples were then imaged using a JEOL 1400 transmission electron microscope at 100 k× magnification. All TEM images are the original images. To select which TEM images would be used, the following criteria were followed: (1) The low-magnification image should show two or more sEVs in the field or include minimal debris from the sEV; (2) the size of the particles present should be between 30 and 150 nm and have a spherical or cup shape with a distinct, well-defined border; (3) the image should have good contrast to show the membrane of the vesicle; and (4) the particles present should have electron-dense areas inside of the defined border to indicate the cargo is present [25].

2.4. Lyophilization

A total of 500 μL of isolated sEVs at a concentration of 4.5×10^8 particles/mL was buffer exchanged to 50 mM trehalose in water using 50 kDa MWCO filters. The buffer-exchanged samples were aliquoted into ten 50 μL samples, and then rapidly frozen. Samples were lyophilized overnight using a FreeZone 4.5 liter Console Freeze Dry System from Labconco Corporation, Kansas City, MO, USA and stored at room temperature for 2–8 weeks. Before use, lyophilized samples were rehydrated with PBS to their original volume and used in the experiments. For lyophilized sEVs without trehalose, sEV samples were buffer-exchanged to water and rapidly frozen, and then lyophilized overnight.

2.5. Protein Concentrations

To determine protein concentrations of −80 °C sEVs and lyophilized hASC sEVs, a nanodrop spectrophotometer was used. A 1 μL amount of sample was placed on the nanodrop and measured at an absorbance of 280 nm. Measurements were conducted thrice for each sample.

2.6. Scratch Assay

To evaluate the hASC sEVs for wound-healing efficacy, a scratch assay was performed using HT22 cells. HT22 cells were grown to confluency in a 12-well plate, and a scratch was created using a p10 pipet tip. The CM was replaced and 2 μg/mL of hASC sEVs or lyophilized hASC sEVs was added to the cells. Cell migration was imaged on a Keyence BZ-X810 microscope from Keyence Corporation, Tampa, FL, 33607) at 0, 16, and 24 h at 4× magnification.

2.7. DiD-Labeled sEV Uptake

HT22 cells were grown to confluency in an 8-well chamber plate and used to assess exosomal uptake. The hASC sEVs were incubated with 100 nM DiD, prepared according to manufacturer's instructions in EtOH, for 30 min. Then, 2 μg/mL of labeled hASC sEVs were added to HT22 cells stained with 4′,6-diamidino-2-phenylindole (DAPI) and imaged using a Keyence BZ-X810 microscope after 24 h at 40× magnification. At the 24 h mark, the fluorescence intensity was measured and assessed using the Keyence software (v 1.1.1.8), Keyence Corporation, Tampa, FL, 33607. One window was used to measure the fluorescence intensity. A window was chosen if it had (1) a high concentration of sEVs present and (2) a wide spread of cells present with little to no clumping.

2.8. In Vitro Inflammation Model

HT22 cells were plated in an 8-well chamber plate and grown to confluency. Cells were treated with 5 ng/mL of LPS for six hours. Medium was changed, and 2 μg/mL of sEVs was added for 18 h. Immunochemistry was performed as described below.

2.9. In Vitro Oxidative Stress Model

HT22 cells were plated in an 8-well chamber plate and grown to confluency. Cells were treated with 1:1000 H_2O_2 for 1 h. Medium was changed, and 2 μg/mL of sEVs was added for 18 h. Immunochemistry was performed as described below.

2.10. Immunochemistry

HT22 cells were plated in an 8-well chamber plate and grown to confluency. Medium was then removed, and cells were washed 3 times with PBS and fixed with 4% paraformaldehyde for 30 min. Cells were rinsed with PBS and blocked with 1% bovine serum albumin for 30 min at room temperature. Cells were washed 3 times with PBS and then incubated with primary antibodies for Ki-67 overnight at 4 °C. Cells were rinsed with PBS 3 times and incubated in secondary fluorescent antibody for 1 h at room temperature. Cells were stained with 4′,6-diamidino-2-phenylindole (DAPI) for 15 min at room temperature to visualize the nucleus. Samples were imaged at 20× using a Keyence microscope.

2.11. Statistical Analysis Methods

Statistical analyses were performed using GraphPad Prism SPSS Analysis Software V.10.0.2 (GraphPad PRISM™ Software (v 10.0.0), IBM SPSS Inc., Boston, MA, USA). Comparisons of the means were made between groups using unpaired Student's t-tests or ANOVA analysis. The significance of the results is indicated by the (*) symbol with the corresponding p-values: * $p < 0.05$, ** $p < 0.01$, *** $p < 0.001$, **** $p < 0.0001$.

3. Results

3.1. Optimal Method of hASC sEV Preparation

Kits using reagents to precipitate EVs from hASC conditioned media (CM) sometimes result in impurities in the final sEV preparation. Hence, we sought to compare two widely used methods to determine the method yielding pure sEVs (size 35–200 nm). The hASC cells were plated in T-25 flasks, and conditioned media (CM) was collected. The sEVs were isolated from the CM as described in the Methods section. The NTA data revealed that the qEV columns demonstrated cleaner particle size distribution peaks compared with the ExoSpin columns. The particle size distribution peak from the ExoSpin column had a sharp peak at 56 nm, but the tailing of the peak showed various other sizes (Figure 2A). The peak from the qEV isolation showed a sharp peak at 145 nm and one smaller peak at 213 nm (Figure 2B). These data established that the qEV column combined with ultrafiltration produces pure particle size distributions compared with the ExoSpin Columns. From here on, the qEV method was used to prepare and purify the hASC sEVs for the experiments. To establish the morphology of the hASC sEVs, transmission electron microscopy was used to image the sEVs after extraction (Figure 2C). The TEM images show round-shaped sEVs at a size of 141 nm at 40 k× and 80 k× magnification.

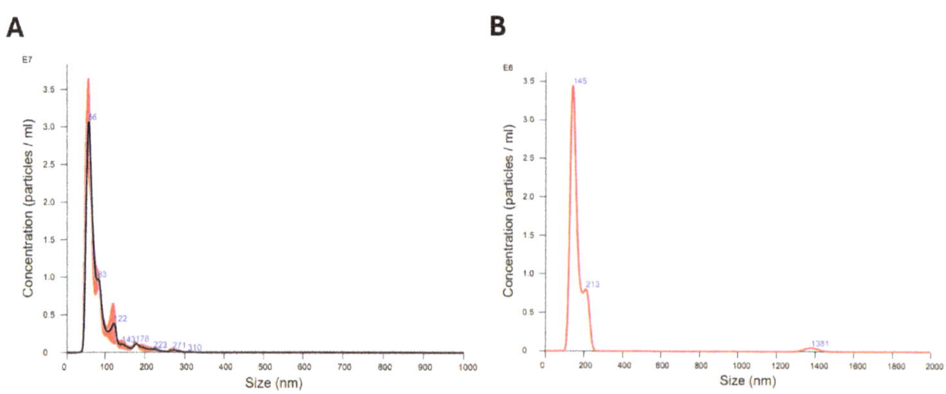

Figure 2. *Cont.*

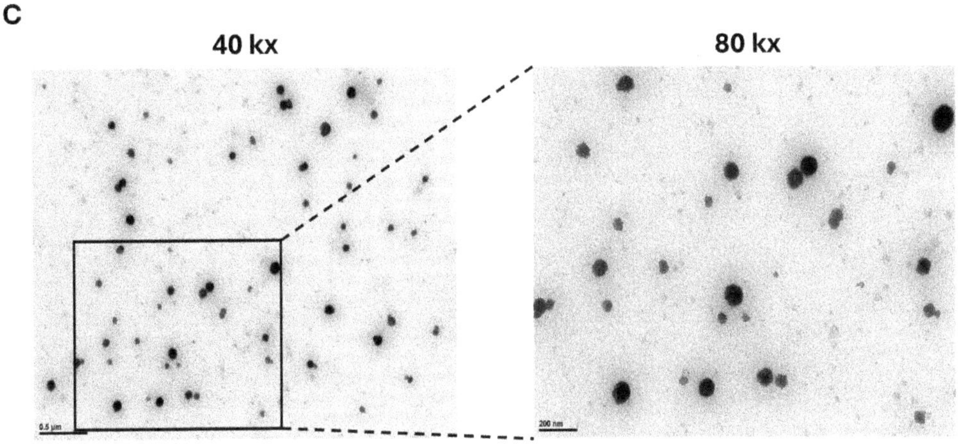

Figure 2. NTA and TEM data showing the sizes and concentrations of sEVs isolated from hASCs. (**A**) sEV elution from ExoSpin column showing an average size of 80.3 nm and concentration of 9.84×10^8 particles/mL. (**B**) sEV elution from qEV column showing a peak size of 145 nm and concentration of 9.20×10^7 particles/mL. Measurements in triplicate for each sample. (**C**) TEM image showing hASC sEVs extracted from a qEV column at 40 k× and 80 k× magnification. Scale bar = 500 nm and 200 nm, respectively.

3.2. Lyophilization Has No Effect on Concentration or Morphology of hASC sEVs

The hASC sEVs were purified using qEV columns and divided into two aliquots. One aliquot was stored at −80 °C, and the other aliquot was lyophilized. The hASC sEVs were lyophilized, stored at room temperature (RT), and analyzed after 2 weeks and compared with the sEVs stored at −80 °C. At the 2-week mark, the −80 °C stored exosome and the lyophilized RT samples with trehalose had protein concentrations of approximately 2 µg/mL. This was also observed at the 1- and 2-month marks. All protein concentrations were within 1% of each other (Table 1) between the −80 °C stored sEVs and the lyophilized RT samples with trehalose (Table 1). For lyophilized sEVs without trehalose, there was a decrease in protein concentration of almost 50% seen at the 2-week mark.

Table 1. Protein and particle concentrations of −80 °C sEVs and lyophilized room temperature sEVs. All measurements were performed in triplicate. Statistical analysis was performed by two-tailed Student's *t*-test or ANOVA analysis.

Storage Time	Sample	Protein Concentration (µg/mL)	*p*-Value	Size (nm)	*p*-Value	Concentration (particles/mL)	*p*-Value
2 Weeks	−80 °C sEV Lyophilized sEV + trehalose Lyophilized sEV—trehalose	2.047 ± 0.036 2.039 ± 0.037 1.163 ± 0.027	0.0014	157 ± 32 157 ± 17 182 ± 159	0.1840	2.59×10^7 2.42×10^7 1.74×10^6	0.2535
1 Month	−80 °C sEV Lyophilized sEV	2.122 ± 0.015 2.158 ± 0.025	0.8468	159 ± 39 131 ± 23	0.0782	5.03×10^7 1.44×10^7	0.1454
2 Months	−80 °C sEV Lyophilized sEV	2.003 ± 0.024 2.022 ± 0.017	0.9135	155 ± 56 151 ± 64	0.7649	2.12×10^7 1.03×10^7	0.3788

To evaluate the morphology, hASC sEVs were imaged using TEM. At two weeks, both the −80 °C sEVs and the lyophilized RT with trehalose sEVs showed intact spherical morphology shapes (Figure 3D). The sizes of the sEVs were within 10% compared with the freshly extracted sEVs based on NTA data (Figure 3A). The lyophilized RT sEVs without trehalose did not show intact morphology, and a change in size was observed based on TEM images and NTA data (Figure 3G). There were also signs of aggregation and loss of protein observed. Due to these changes, lyophilized sEVs without trehalose were not evaluated after 2 weeks. The sizes of the sEV samples at 1 and 2 months, stored either at −80 °C or lyophilized and stored at room temperature, remained within 10% of each other (Figure 3B,C). There were no changes observed in morphology after 1 month in both the sEVs stored at −80 °C and sEVs lyophilized and stored at RT. After 2 months of storage, the morphology of the sEV samples was still spherical for both lyophilized sEVs stored at room temperature and sEVs stored at −80 °C (Figure 3E,F). However, samples stored at −80 °C showed signs of aggregation in the TEM images and NTA data. Loss of protein was also observed in the TEM images for the −80 °C sEVs.

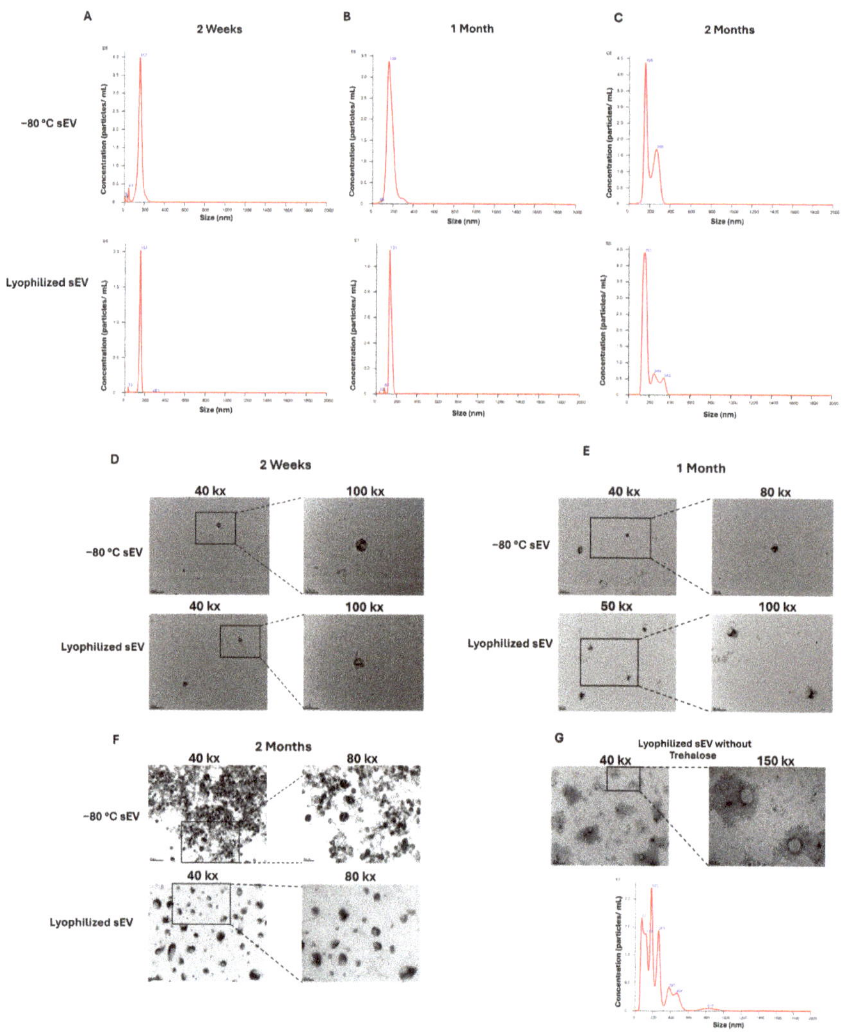

Figure 3. TEM images of −80 °C sEVs and lyophilized sEVs at low and high magnifications and NTA data showing the sizes of the −80 °C sEVs and lyophilized sEVs after 2 weeks, 1 month, and

2 months. (**A**) NTA data showing sizes of hASC sEVs after 2 weeks of storage. (**B**) NTA data showing sizes of hASC sEVs after 1 month of storage. (**C**) NTA data showing sizes of hASC sEVs after 2 months of storage. (**D**) TEM images of sEVs after 2 weeks of storage. (**E**) TEM images of sEVs after 1 month of storage. (**F**) TEM images of sEVs after 2 months of storage. (**G**) NTA data and TEMs of lyophilized sEVs without trehalose after 2 weeks of storage. For 40 k× images, the scale bar = 500 nm. For 50 k×, 80 k×, and 100 k× images, the scale bar = 200 nm. For 150 k× images, the scale bar = 100 nm.

3.3. Lyophilized sEVs Stored at Room Temperature Promote Wound Healing in Neuronal Cells

To assess cellular uptake of the hASC sEVs in HT22 cells, 2 μg/mL of DiD-labeled sEVs were applied to the cells and monitored for 24 h. The sEVs were incubated in DiD at a concentration of 100 nM for 30 min and centrifuged to remove excess dye, and then added to the cells. After 24 h, DAPI stain was added and used to visualize the nuclei of the cells in this experiment. We first evaluated the staining effects of DiD alone on the cells. DiD without the sEVs stained the cell membrane of the cells, whereas the labeled sEVs can be seen as small circles in the nucleus and cytoplasm. The fluorescence intensity of the DiD was about 17,000 (Figure 4A). Both −80 °C stored sEVs and lyophilized hASC sEVs with trehalose were taken up efficiently by the HT22 cells. The fluorescence intensity for the −80 °C stored sEVs and lyophilized RT sEVs was about 27,000 and 26,000, respectively; however, for the lyophilized sEVs without trehalose, the intensity was about 20,000 (Figure 4B).

We then evaluated the efficacy of the lyophilized hASC sEVs for treating wounds using the in vitro scratch assay, which creates cell-free gaps in the cell culture mimicking wounds. HT22 cells were wounded by creating a scratch (described in Methods). Then, 2 μg/mL of sEVs stored at −80 °C and a lyophilized sEV sample stored at room temperature was applied to the HT22 cells. Wound closure was assessed for 24 h and compared with a control without sEVs (Figure 4C). The wound closure percentages of the −80 °C stored sEVs and the lyophilized RT sEVs with trehalose at the 24 h mark were comparable, at 95% for both samples. The lyophilized RT sEVs without trehalose showed a wound closure of only 68%. Due to this low wound closure percentage and uptake, lyophilized sEVs without trehalose were not used in further studies. The rate of migration of HT22 cells to close the wound was also similar between the −80 °C stored sEVs and the lyophilized RT sEVs with trehalose (Figure 4D). We also assessed the effects of trehalose on its own in the cells. A wound closure of 59% was observed, a 5% difference from the control.

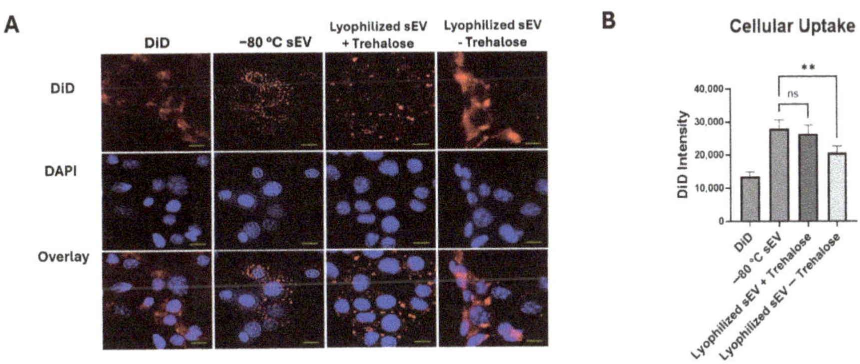

Figure 4. *Cont.*

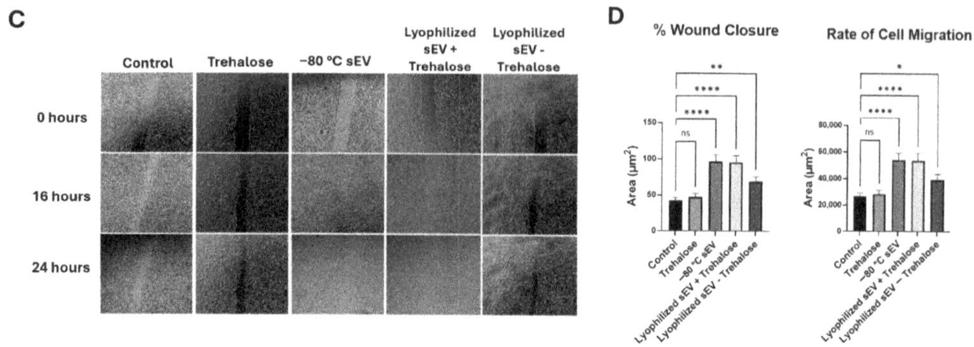

Figure 4. Cellular uptake and wound closure comparison of −80 °C sEVs and lyophilized RT sEVs at two weeks in HT22 cells. (**A**) Cellular uptake of DiD and DiD-labeled sEVs over 24 h, imaged at 40× (scale bar = 25 μm). (**B**) Graphical comparison of DiD intensity. The images for DiD, DAPI, and the overlay are all images of the same section of cells. DiD is being used to stain the sEVs in this study, while DAPI stains the nuclei of the cells. The overlay shows both DiD and DAPI in one image together to visualize how well the DiD-labeled sEVs are taken up by the cells. A high cell colocalization with sEV indicates that a higher number of sEVs are making their way into the cells. Statistical analysis was performed by ANOVA analysis, with no significant differences between −80 °C stored sEVs compared with lyophilized RT sEVs with trehalose. (**C**) Scratch assay over 24 h, imaged at 4×. (**D**) Comparison of % wound closure and rate of cell migration between samples. The images in each column shown in the figure demonstrate a scratch in the HT22 cells at different time intervals. The scratch shown at each time interval is the same scratch in the same section of cells to demonstrate how each treatment affects the ability of the cells to close the wound gap. A high % wound closure indicates how well the sEVs are repairing the damage to the cells. Statistical analysis was performed by ANOVA analysis (* $p < 0.05$, ** $p < 0.01$, and **** $p \leq 0.0001$, no significance (ns)).

3.4. Lyophilized sEVs Promote Wound Healing Efficiently After 1 Month at Room Temperature

The cellular uptake was also assessed for 1 month, and no significant changes were observed between the lyophilized RT and the −80 °C stored sEVs (Figure 5A). The fluorescence intensities for the −80 °C stored sEVs and the lyophilized RT sEVs were about 27,000 and 25,000, respectively (Figure 5B). Next, we evaluated the efficacy of the lyophilized hASC sEVs stored at room temperature for one month. Scratch assay was performed in HT22 cells followed by treatment with −80 °C stored sEVs and lyophilized (room temperature for 1 month) hASC sEVs (Figure 5C). There was no change in the efficacy of the lyophilized RT sEVs. Both the −80 °C sEVs and the lyophilized RT samples showed a 100% wound closure at 24 h. The wound treated with lyophilized, RT sEVs had a higher rate of cell migration to fill the wound gap (Figure 5D).

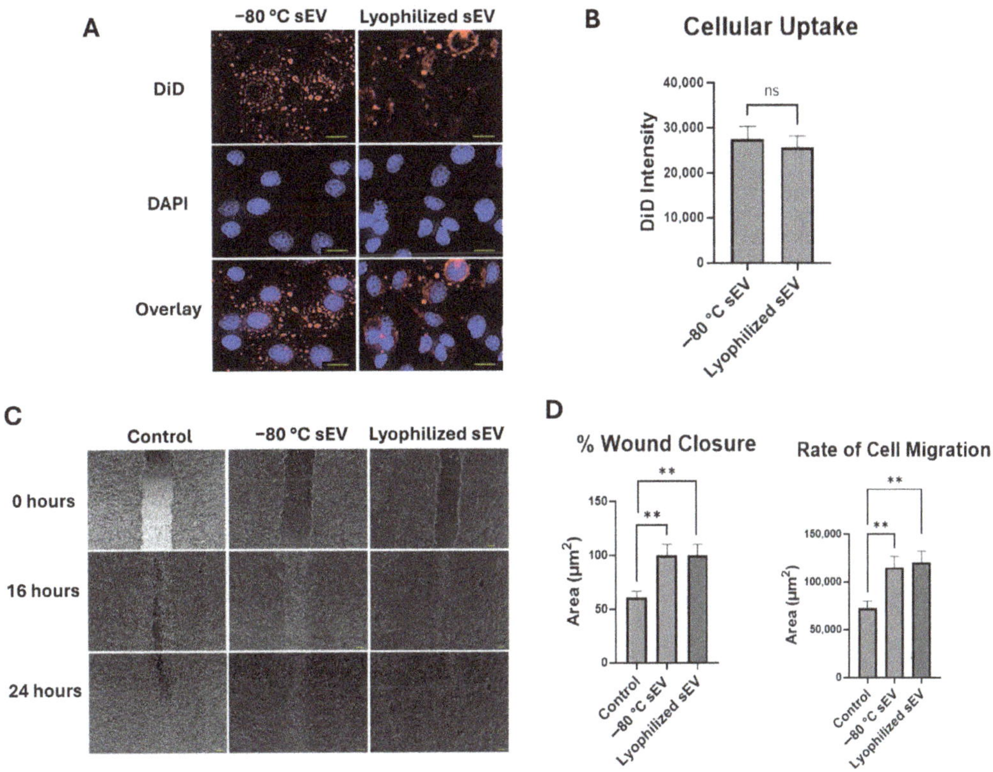

Figure 5. Cellular uptake and wound closure comparison of −80 °C sEVs and lyophilized RT sEVs at one month in HT22 cells. (**A**) Cellular uptake of DiD-labeled sEVs over 24 h, imaged at 40× (scale bar = 25 μm). (**B**) Graphical comparison of DiD intensity. The images for DiD, DAPI, and the overlay are all images of the same section of cells. DiD is being used to stain the sEVs in this study, while DAPI stains the nuclei of the cells. The overlay shows both DiD and DAPI in one image together to help visualize how well the DiD-labeled sEVs are taken up by the cells. A high cell colocalization with sEVs indicates that a higher number of sEVs are making their way into the cells. Statistical analysis was performed by two-tailed Student's *t*-test, no significance (ns). (**C**) Scratch assay over 24 h, imaged at 4×. (**D**) Comparison of % wound closure and rate of cell migration between samples. The images in each column shown in the figure demonstrate a scratch in the HT22 cells at different time intervals. The scratch shown at each time interval is the same scratch in the same section of cells to demonstrate how each treatment affects the ability of the cells to close the wound gap. A high % wound closure indicates how well the sEVs are repairing the damage to the cells. Statistical analysis was performed by ANOVA analysis ** $p < 0.01$).

3.5. Lyophilized sEVs Promote Wound Healing Efficiently After 2 Months at Room Temperature

Cellular uptake and wound healing were assessed after 2 months of storage at room temperature following lyophilization. Both samples of sEVs displayed similar DiD intensity values over a 24 h period (Figure 6A,B). We then investigated the efficacy of the lyophilized hASC sEVs (stored at room temperature for 2 months) in HT22 cells using a scratch assay over 24 h (Figure 6C). At the 16 h mark, the −80 °C sEVs showed a significant difference in wound closure compared with the lyophilized RT sEVs. The −80 °C sEVs were at 74%, while the lyophilized sEVs were at 87% wound closure (Figure 6D). The lyophilized RT sEVs also demonstrated better efficacy, showing a wound closure of 100%, compared with the −80 °C sEVs, which showed a closure of 92% at the 24 h mark (Figure 6E).

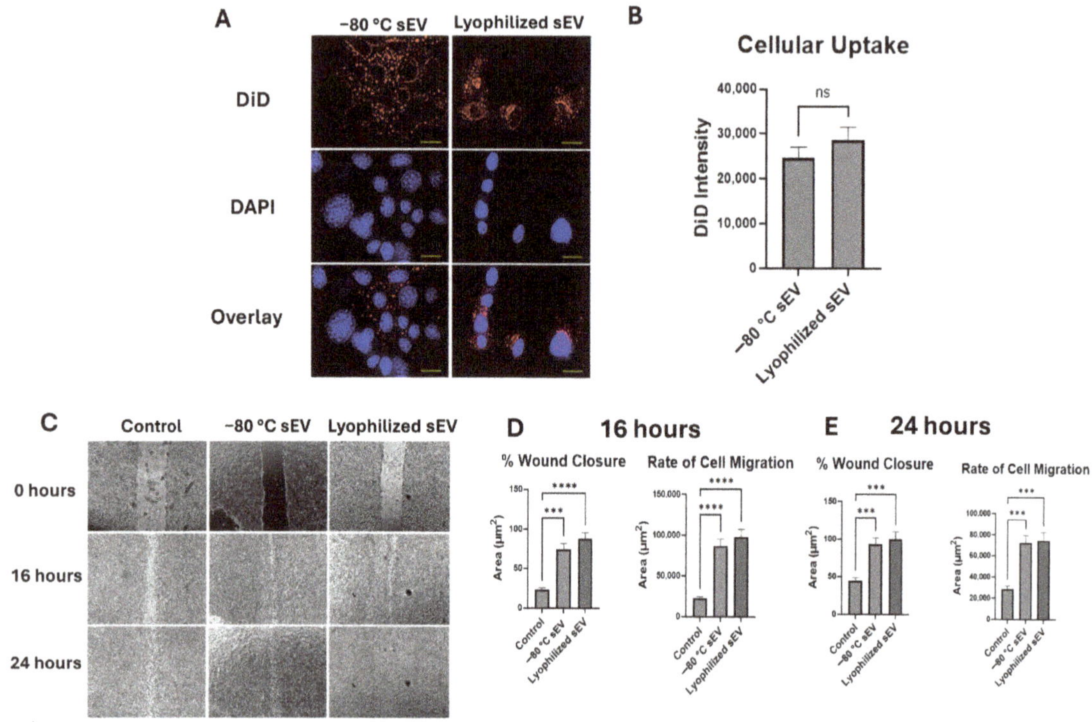

Figure 6. Cellular uptake and wound closure comparison of −80 °C sEVs and lyophilized RT sEVs at two months in HT22 cells. (**A**) Cellular uptake of DiD-labeled sEVs over 24 h, imaged at 40× (scale bar = 25 µm). (**B**) Graphical comparison of DiD intensity. The images for DiD, DAPI, and the overlay are all images of the same section of cells. DiD is being used to stain the sEVs in this study, while DAPI stains the nuclei of the cells. The overlay shows both DiD and DAPI in one image together to help visualize how well the DiD-labeled sEVs are taken up by the cells. A high cell colocalization with sEV indicates that a higher number of sEVs are making their way into the cells. Statistical analysis was performed by two-tailed Student's *t*-test, no significance (ns). (**C**) Scratch assay over 24 h, imaged at 4×. (**D**) Comparison of % wound closure and rate of cell migration between samples after 16 h. Statistical analysis was performed by two-tailed Student's *t*-test. (**E**) Comparison of % wound closure and rate of cell migration between samples after 24 h. The images in each column shown in the figure demonstrate a scratch in the HT22 cells at different time intervals. The scratch shown at each time interval is the same scratch in the same section of cells to demonstrate how each treatment affects the ability of the cells to close the wound gap. A high % wound closure indicates how well the sEVs are repairing the damage to the cells. Statistical analysis was performed by ANOVA analysis *** $p < 0.001$, and **** $p \leq 0.0001$.

3.6. Lyophilized sEVs Rescue Cell Proliferation in Neuronal Cells with Underlying Inflammation In Vitro

The efficacy of the lyophilized hASC sEVs was investigated using a cell proliferation assay in an inflammation model. HT22 cells were exposed to lipopolysaccharide (LPS) to mimic underlying inflammation and treated with 2 µg/mL lyophilized RT hASC sEVs (stored at room temperature for one or two months) for 24 h. The cells were then stained with Ki-67, a marker for proliferation, and imaged on a Keyence microscope (Figure 7A,B). After exposure to LPS, cell proliferation decreased dramatically, which was rescued by treatment with the lyophilized RT hASC sEVs.

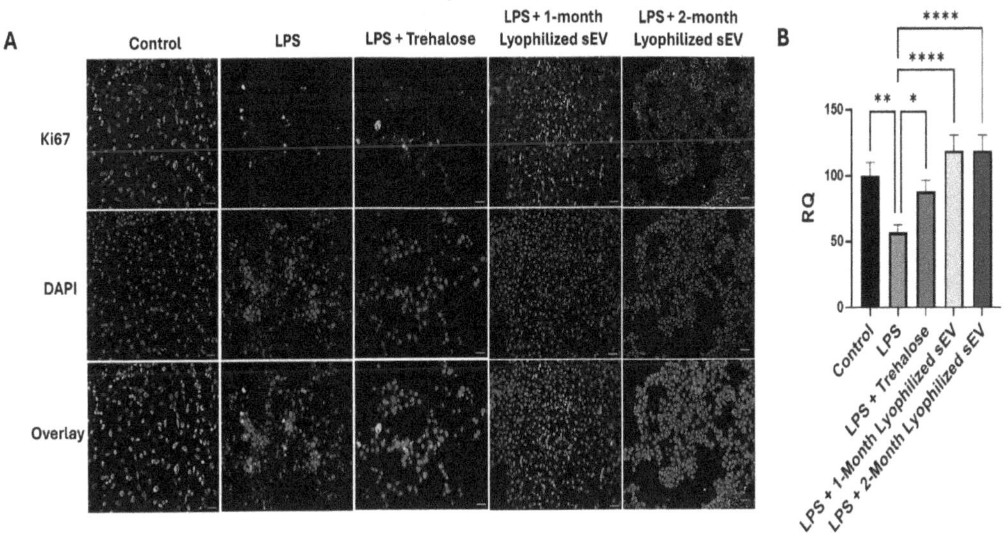

Figure 7. Immunochemistry assay of HT22 cells treated with 5 ng/mL LPS for 6 h, after which the medium was changed, and the cells were treated with 2 µg of sEVs for 18 h. (**A**) Cells were stained using Ki-67 as a marker for proliferation and DAPI as a nucleus stain and imaged with a Keyence BZx-810 microscope at 20× (scale bar = 50 µm). (**B**) Determination of colocalization of Ki-67 and DAPI was determined using the Keyence software. The images for Ki67, DAPI, and the overlay are all images of the same section of cells. Ki67 stains proliferating cells, while the DAPI stains the nuclei of the cells. The overlay shows both the Ki67 and DAPI in one image together to visualize cell proliferation occurring from each treatment. Statistical analysis was performed by ANOVA analysis (* $p < 0.05$, ** $p < 0.01$, and **** $p \leq 0.0001$).

After treatment with the hASC sEVs, proliferation increased, which is what was observed during this study. Cells without any treatment were used as a control, and the percent of Ki-67 was 51%. Cells that were treated with LPS showed a decrease in proliferation. Cells that were treated with LPS followed by lyophilized sEVs showed a rescue of cell proliferation. We also looked at the effects of trehalose and observed a slight increase in proliferation, but it was significantly lower compared with the rescue by sEVs.

3.7. Lyophilized sEVs Decrease Oxidative Stress in Neuronal Cells

Neuronal cells were treated with hydrogen peroxide (H_2O_2) to mimic oxidative stress for one hour, and the efficacy of lyophilized sEVs for rescuing proliferation was assessed over 18 h (Figure 8A). After treatment with sEVs post oxidative stress, an increase in proliferation was observed in each type of sEV. Results showed an increase of 107% for one-month lyophilized samples and 102% for two-month lyophilized sEVs (Figure 8B). This demonstrates that the lyophilized sEVs, stored up to two months at room temperature, are efficient at decreasing oxidative stress in neuronal cells. Trehalose treatment did not rescue oxidative stress induced by peroxide.

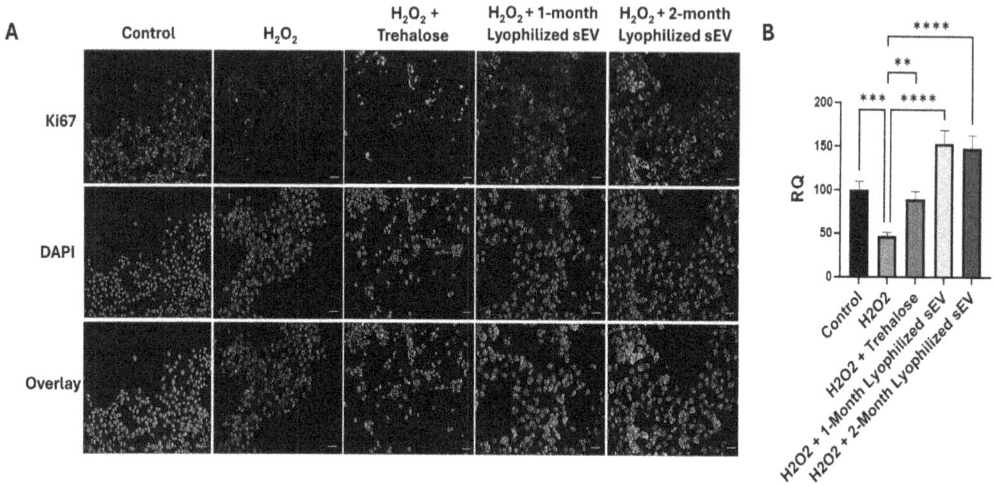

Figure 8. Immunochemistry assay of HT22 cells treated with 1:1000 hydrogen peroxide for 1 h, after which the medium was changed, and the cells were treated with 2 µg of lyophilized sEVs for 18 h. (**A**) Cells were stained using Ki-67 as a marker for proliferation and DAPI as a nucleus stain and imaged with a Keyence BZx-810 microscope at 20× (scale bar = 50 µm). (**B**) Determination of colocalization of Ki-67 and DAPI was determined using the Keyence software. The image for Ki67, DAPI, and the overlay are all images of the same section of cells. Ki67 stains proliferating cells, while the DAPI stains the nuclei of the cells. The overlay shows both the Ki67 and DAPI in one image together to visualize cell proliferation occurring from each treatment. Statistical analysis was performed by ANOVA analysis (** $p < 0.01$, *** $p < 0.001$, **** $p \leq 0.0001$).

4. Discussion

In this study, we have established that qEV columns are a better isolation method than ExoSpin kits. We also established that lyophilization with the addition of trehalose preserves the size and morphology of hASCs sEVs. We were then able to test if the lyophilized sEVs performed equally to the −80 °C sEVs after being stored at RT using several in vitro assays of neuronal injury that mimic TBI. We found that the lyophilized RT sEVs were significantly better at promoting wound healing than the −80 °C stored sEVs. This was demonstrated through physical injury, inflammation, and oxidative stress.

We previously demonstrated the efficacy of hASC sEVs in promoting repair and regeneration in traumatic brain injury in vivo [4,26,27]. The lyophilized hASC sEVs will be used in a similar setup. Other groups have also utilized sEVs derived from ASC and showed that they have immunoregulatory properties [28,29]. To address the limitations of room temperature storage and viability of hASC sEVs, we undertook this systematic evaluation. First, we evaluated the effect on the purity of sEVs using two different size exclusion techniques. Comparisons of size and concentration were evaluated using NTA data. In accordance with previous studies, the qEV size exclusion column coupled with ultrafiltration produced pure sEVs efficiently [30,31]. Our previous studies used CD9, CD63, and CD81 markers to verify that the sEVs described here contain exosomes [4,26,27].

The hASC sEVs have a tremendous potential in wound healing. However, storage remains an issue for translation to clinics. In this study, the use of lyophilization as a storage method for sEVs was explored. In previous studies, lyophilization has been investigated as a storage method for sEVs using trehalose. It was reported that sEVs can be stored at room temperature for one week after lyophilization with the addition of trehalose [21].

Without trehalose, aggregation and a change in morphology can occur, which we have demonstrated. Here, we sought to evaluate the efficacy of lyophilized hASC sEVs on neuronal wound healing potential after storage at room temperature for two months, which has not been demonstrated so far. To evaluate the effects of lyophilization, the morphology, size, and functionality of the hASC sEVs were evaluated after two, four, and eight weeks of storage at room temperature. Our data demonstrate that lyophilization is an effective long-term storage method, and we further establish that the protein concentration and size were unchanged between the lyophilized samples with trehalose. During the lyophilization process, trehalose can form a protective layer around the bilayer of the sEV. Trehalose can form hydrogen bond interactions with the polar head groups of the bilayer, effectively keeping the bilayer and cargo inside the sEVs safe from damage [32]. It was also demonstrated that the morphology and size of the lyophilized sEVs after two months did not show a difference between samples. It is also worth noting that the lyophilized samples showed a smaller size distribution than the sEVs stored at −80 °C.

Our results have demonstrated that sEVs are efficiently being taken up by HT22 cells. In some cases, aggregation of the sEVs can be seen, which could be due to their low zeta potential [33]. We have initiated studies to investigate the mechanism underlying the aggregation of the sEVs. It is reported that smaller extracellular vesicles such as sEVs have faster cellular uptake [34]. The uptake demonstrated by each sEV sample in this study supports this notion, as each sample is relatively in the same size range. Our results also demonstrate that the sEVs are present in the cytoplasm and nucleus of the HT22 cells, showing efficient internalization of sEVs. There was also no change observed in the efficiency of the sEVs' cellular uptake post lyophilization. hASC sEVs have shown regenerative capabilities due to the biological material secreted inside of their sEVs. We have previously shown that these hASC sEVs can be used for wound healing in vitro and in vivo in TBI models [4,26,27].

Finally, we also evaluated the effects of lyophilization on the efficacy of hASC sEVs using in vitro neuronal injury models mimicking physical injury, inflammation, and oxidative stress. We have shown that hASC sEVs have regenerative capabilities and can be used to increase cell proliferation in neuronal cells in vitro [26]. In this study, we used lyophilized sEVs to assess the efficacy of the lyophilization of sEVs stored at room temperature, and the results demonstrate that the efficacy of sEVs to promote wound healing is maintained. TBI is an injury that affects many people every year, and it is known to cause secondary injuries that damage neuronal cells. LPS, which was used to mimic underlying inflammation caused by TBI in vitro, and hydrogen peroxide, which mimics oxidative stress caused by TBI, were used to assess the lyophilized sEVs' efficacy to rescue the cell proliferation. It was also important to evaluate the effects of trehalose under oxidative stress, as it has been reported that trehalose can increase proliferation under oxidative stress in high concentrations. These data further support the assertion that lyophilization can be used as a storage method for sEVs at room temperature for two months and can be effectively used to treat neuronal injury seen in TBI.

The lyophilization of sEVs could also be applied to engineered EVs. EVs have regularly been used as therapeutics in the past few years by loading them with mRNA, proteins, peptides, and more. Long-term storage of the engineered vesicles would still require storage temperatures of −20 °C or −80 °C, causing a potential issue in clinical settings. Lyophilization could be proposed as a solution to this issue. In a previous study, sEVs loaded with Gaussia luciferase showed a little change in the pharmacokinetics of the engineered sEVs before and after lyophilization, suggesting that lyophilization can be used for engineered EVs [21]. To our knowledge, this is the only study that has shown lyophilization of engineered EVs. There is still much more research that should be performed regarding the lyophilization of engineered EVs.

In summary, we have demonstrated that lyophilization can be used as an effective room temperature storage of hASC sEVs for two months without any harmful effects on morphology, concentration, cell migration, and cellular uptake. We have also established that the efficacy of lyophilized sEVs for wound healing is comparable to sEVs stored at −80 °C up to 4 weeks, and is better than the sEVs stored at −80 °C after 8 weeks, based on in vitro assays used to mimic TBI injuries. We have initiated in vivo studies using lyophilized, room temperature stored sEVs in rodent models of TBI. In the previous study, we demonstrated the intranasal route of delivery of hASC sEVs post TBI, and we have undertaken a similar intranasal delivery of lyophilized sEVs. The in vivo study will provide information on genomic changes by RNAseq, which can be compared with our previously published results using freshly prepared sEVs. Here, we successfully demonstrated the viability and efficacy of lyophilized sEVs stored at room temperature, thereby enabling the initiation of in vivo studies using lyophilized RT sEVs. The hASC sEVs are applied topically for dermal wounds [35] or administered intranasally for TBI [27], and they do not need any carrier, thus adding to the advantage of hASC sEVs in accelerating the healing of wounds.

5. Conclusions

In conclusion, we have shown that qEV produces clean size-distribution peaks. The sEVs extracted from qEV columns showed cleaner peaks based on the NTA results. Lyophilization can be used as a storage method for sEVs at room temperature for two months with the addition of trehalose without any damage to performance or structure. This method does not inhibit the performance of the hASC sEVs, as demonstrated by neuronal in vitro injury models such as scratch assay, LPS-induced inflammation, and hydrogen peroxide-induced oxidative stress. Thus, lyophilized sEVs stored at room temperature can be incorporated into first-aid kits in the future, which will advance their translation to clinic and routine use by all individuals.

Supplementary Materials: The following supporting information can be downloaded at: https://www.mdpi.com/article/10.3390/biomedicines13020275/s1. Table S1: The raw data for Figures 4–8; File S1: The original images for Figures 4–8; File S2: BioRender publication permission for schematic of lyophilization process; File S3: BioRender publication permission for schematic of graphical abstract.

Author Contributions: Conceptualization, N.A.P.; methodology, B.J., R.P., B.W.; validation, T.E.-N., N.A.P.; formal analysis, B.J.; investigation, B.J., R.P.; resources, T.E.-N., N.A.P.; writing—original draft preparation, B.J.; writing—review and editing, B.J., N.A.P.; visualization, B.J.; supervision, T.E.-N., N.A.P.; project administration, N.A.P.; funding acquisition, N.A.P. All authors have read and agreed to the published version of the manuscript.

Funding: This work was supported by the Department of Veterans Affairs, VA Merit Award I0 BX005591 (N.A.P.) and VA Research Career Scientist Award IK6BX005387 (N.A.P.). This work does not reflect the views or opinions of the James A. Haley VA Hospital or the US Government.

Institutional Review Board Statement: Not applicable.

Informed Consent Statement: Not applicable.

Data Availability Statement: The original contributions presented in the study are included in the article; further inquiries can be directed to the corresponding author.

Acknowledgments: The authors acknowledge the University of South Florida Chemical, Purification, Analysis and Screening facility for the use of the lyophilizer. The authors also acknowledge the NSF Bridge to the Doctorate Program, Alfred P. Sloan Foundation, and the McKnight Fellowship Program as funding sources for Brianna Jones. The authors acknowledge Amanda Garces from the University of South Florida Health Core Facility for the use of TEM.

Conflicts of Interest: The authors declare no conflicts of interest.

References

1. Mollayeva, T.; Mollayeva, S.; Colantonio, A. Traumatic brain injury: Sex, gender and intersecting vulnerabilities. *Nat. Rev. Neurol.* **2018**, *14*, 711–722. [CrossRef] [PubMed]
2. McKee, A.C.; Daneshvar, D.H. The neuropathology of traumatic brain injury. In *Handbook of Clinical Neurology*; Elsevier: Amsterdam, The Netherlands, 2015; Volume 127, pp. 45–66. [CrossRef]
3. Acosta, S.A.; Tajiri, N.; Shinozuka, K.; Ishikawa, H.; Grimmig, B.; Diamond, D.M.; Sanberg, P.R.; Bickford, P.C.; Kaneko, Y.; Borlongan, C.V. Long-term upregulation of inflammation and suppression of cell proliferation in the brain of adult rats exposed to traumatic brain injury using the controlled cortical impact model. *PLoS ONE* **2013**, *8*, e53376. [CrossRef]
4. Patel, N.A.; Moss, L.D.; Lee, J.Y.; Tajiri, N.; Acosta, S.; Hudson, C.; Parag, S.; Cooper, D.R.; Borlongan, C.V.; Bickford, P.C. Long noncoding RNA MALAT1 in exosomes drives regenerative function and modulates inflammation-linked networks following traumatic brain injury. *J. Neuroinflamm.* **2018**, *15*, 204. [CrossRef] [PubMed]
5. Brett, B.L.; Gardner, R.C.; Godbout, J.; Dams-O'Connor, K.; Keene, C.D. Traumatic Brain Injury and Risk of Neurodegenerative Disorder. *Biol. Psychiatry* **2022**, *91*, 498–507. [CrossRef]
6. Dams-O'Connor, K.; Juengst, S.B.; Bogner, J.; Chiaravalloti, N.D.; Corrigan, J.D.; Giacino, J.T.; Harrison-Felix, C.L.; Hoffman, J.M.; Ketchum, J.M.; Lequerica, A.H.; et al. Traumatic brain injury as a chronic disease: Insights from the United States Traumatic Brain Injury Model Systems Research Program. *Lancet Neurol.* **2023**, *22*, 517–528. [CrossRef]
7. Jiang, J.Y.; Gao, G.Y.; Feng, J.F.; Mao, Q.; Chen, L.G.; Yang, X.F.; Liu, J.F.; Wang, Y.H.; Qiu, B.H.; Huang, X.J. Traumatic brain injury in China. *Lancet Neurol.* **2019**, *18*, 286–295. [CrossRef]
8. Elder, G.A. Update on TBI and Cognitive Impairment in Military Veterans. *Curr. Neurol. Neurosci. Rep.* **2015**, *15*, 68. [CrossRef]
9. Lazarus, R.; Helmick, K.; Malik, S.; Gregory, E.; Agimi, Y.; Marion, D. Continuum of the United States military's traumatic brain injury care: Adjusting to the changing battlefield. *Neurosurg. Focus.* **2018**, *45*, E15. [CrossRef]
10. Yamamoto, S.; DeWitt, D.S.; Prough, D.S. Impact & Blast Traumatic Brain Injury: Implications for Therapy. *Molecules* **2018**, *23*, 245. [CrossRef]
11. Welsh, J.A.; Goberdhan, D.C.I.; O'Driscoll, L.; Buzas, E.I.; Blenkiron, C.; Bussolati, B.; Cai, H.; Di Vizio, D.; Driedonks, T.A.P.; Erdbrugger, U.; et al. Minimal information for studies of extracellular vesicles (MISEV2023): From basic to advanced approaches. *J. Extracell. Vesicles* **2024**, *13*, e12404. [CrossRef]
12. Syzdykbayev, M.; Kazymov, M.; Aubakirov, M.; Kurmangazina, A.; Kairkhanov, E.; Kazangapov, R.; Bryzhakhina, Z.; Imangazinova, S.; Sheinin, A. A Modern Approach to the Treatment of Traumatic Brain Injury. *Medicines* **2024**, *11*, 10. [CrossRef] [PubMed]
13. Mathew, B.; Mansuri, M.S.; Williams, K.R.; Nairn, A.C. Exosomes as Emerging Biomarker Tools in Neurodegenerative and Neuropsychiatric Disorders-A Proteomics Perspective. *Brain Sci.* **2021**, *11*, 258. [CrossRef] [PubMed]
14. Ha, D.; Yang, N.; Nadithe, V. Exosomes as therapeutic drug carriers and delivery vehicles across biological membranes: Current perspectives and future challenges. *Acta Pharm. Sin. B* **2016**, *6*, 287–296. [CrossRef] [PubMed]
15. Zhang, H.; Wang, S.; Sun, M.; Cui, Y.; Xing, J.; Teng, L.; Xi, Z.; Yang, Z. Exosomes as smart drug delivery vehicles for cancer immunotherapy. *Front. Immunol.* **2022**, *13*, 1093607. [CrossRef] [PubMed]
16. Gao, J.; Li, A.; Hu, J.; Feng, L.; Liu, L.; Shen, Z. Recent developments in isolating methods for exosomes. *Front. Bioeng. Biotechnol.* **2022**, *10*, 1100892. [CrossRef]
17. Langevin, S.M.; Kuhnell, D.; Orr-Asman, M.A.; Biesiada, J.; Zhang, X.; Medvedovic, M.; Thomas, H.E. Balancing yield, purity and practicality: A modified differential ultracentrifugation protocol for efficient isolation of small extracellular vesicles from human serum. *RNA Biol.* **2019**, *16*, 5–12. [CrossRef]
18. Gamez-Valero, A.; Monguio-Tortajada, M.; Carreras-Planella, L.; Franquesa, M.; Beyer, K.; Borras, F.E. Size-Exclusion Chromatography-based isolation minimally alters Extracellular Vesicles' characteristics compared to precipitating agents. *Sci. Rep.* **2016**, *6*, 33641. [CrossRef]
19. Jeyaram, A.; Jay, S.M. Preservation and Storage Stability of Extracellular Vesicles for Therapeutic Applications. *AAPS J.* **2017**, *20*, 1. [CrossRef]

20. Kusuma, G.D.; Barabadi, M.; Tan, J.L.; Morton, D.A.V.; Frith, J.E.; Lim, R. To Protect and to Preserve: Novel Preservation Strategies for Extracellular Vesicles. *Front. Pharmacol.* **2018**, *9*, 1199. [CrossRef]
21. Charoenviriyakul, C.; Takahashi, Y.; Nishikawa, M.; Takakura, Y. Preservation of exosomes at room temperature using lyophilization. *Int. J. Pharm.* **2018**, *553*, 1–7. [CrossRef]
22. Bahr, M.M.; Amer, M.S.; Abo-El-Sooud, K.; Abdallah, A.N.; El-Tookhy, O.S. Preservation techniques of stem cells extracellular vesicles: A gate for manufacturing of clinical grade therapeutic extracellular vesicles and long-term clinical trials. *Int. J. Vet. Sci. Med.* **2020**, *8*, 1–8. [CrossRef]
23. Guan, T.; Miao, Y.; Xu, L.; Yang, S.; Wang, J.; He, H.; Tang, X.; Cai, C.; Xu, H. Injectable nimodipine-loaded nanoliposomes: Preparation, lyophilization and characteristics. *Int. J. Pharm.* **2011**, *410*, 180–187. [CrossRef] [PubMed]
24. Kundu, A.K.; Chandra, P.K.; Hazari, S.; Ledet, G.; Pramar, Y.V.; Dash, S.; Mandal, T.K. Stability of lyophilized siRNA nanosome formulations. *Int. J. Pharm.* **2012**, *423*, 525–534. [CrossRef] [PubMed]
25. Pascucci, L.; Scattini, G. Imaging extracelluar vesicles by transmission electron microscopy: Coping with technical hurdles and morphological interpretation. *Biochim. Biophys. Acta Gen. Subj.* **2021**, *1865*, 129648. [CrossRef]
26. El Bassit, G.; Patel, R.S.; Carter, G.; Shibu, V.; Patel, A.A.; Song, S.; Murr, M.; Cooper, D.R.; Bickford, P.C.; Patel, N.A. MALAT1 in Human Adipose Stem Cells Modulates Survival and Alternative Splicing of PKCdeltaII in HT22 Cells. *Endocrinology* **2017**, *158*, 183–195. [CrossRef]
27. Moss, L.D.; Sode, D.; Patel, R.; Lui, A.; Hudson, C.; Patel, N.A.; Bickford, P.C. Intranasal delivery of exosomes from human adipose derived stem cells at forty-eight hours post injury reduces motor and cognitive impairments following traumatic brain injury. *Neurochem. Int.* **2021**, *150*, 105173. [CrossRef]
28. Chen, Y.; Li, J.; Ma, B.; Li, N.; Wang, S.; Sun, Z.; Xue, C.; Han, Q.; Wei, J.; Zhao, R.C. MSC-derived exosomes promote recovery from traumatic brain injury via microglia/macrophages in rat. *Aging* **2020**, *12*, 18274–18296. [CrossRef]
29. Tang, L.; Xu, Y.; Wang, L.; Pan, J. Adipose-derived stem cell exosomes ameliorate traumatic brain injury through the NLRP3 signaling pathway. *Neuroreport* **2023**, *34*, 677–684. [CrossRef]
30. Franco, C.; Ghirardello, A.; Bertazza, L.; Gasparotto, M.; Zanatta, E.; Iaccarino, L.; Valadi, H.; Doria, A.; Gatto, M. Size-Exclusion Chromatography Combined with Ultrafiltration Efficiently Isolates Extracellular Vesicles from Human Blood Samples in Health and Disease. *Int. J. Mol. Sci.* **2023**, *24*, 3663. [CrossRef]
31. Veerman, R.E.; Teeuwen, L.; Czarnewski, P.; Gucluler Akpinar, G.; Sandberg, A.; Cao, X.; Pernemalm, M.; Orre, L.M.; Gabrielsson, S.; Eldh, M. Molecular evaluation of five different isolation methods for extracellular vesicles reveals different clinical applicability and subcellular origin. *J. Extracell. Vesicles* **2021**, *10*, e12128. [CrossRef]
32. Sivanantham, A.; Jin, Y. Impact of Storage Conditions on EV Integrity/Surface Markers and Cargos. *Life* **2022**, *12*, 697. [CrossRef] [PubMed]
33. Wang, Y.; Zhang, L.; Li, Y.; Chen, L.; Wang, X.; Guo, W.; Zhang, X.; Qin, G.; He, S.H.; Zimmerman, A.; et al. Exosomes/microvesicles from induced pluripotent stem cells deliver cardioprotective miRNAs and prevent cardiomyocyte apoptosis in the ischemic myocardium. *Int. J. Cardiol.* **2015**, *192*, 61–69. [CrossRef]
34. Caponnetto, F.; Manini, I.; Skrap, M.; Palmai-Pallag, T.; Di Loreto, C.; Beltrami, A.P.; Cesselli, D.; Ferrari, E. Size-dependent cellular uptake of exosomes. *Nanomedicine* **2017**, *13*, 1011–1020. [CrossRef] [PubMed]
35. Patel, R.S.; Impreso, S.; Lui, A.; Vidyarthi, G.; Albear, P.; Patel, N.A. Long Noncoding RNA GAS5 Contained in Exosomes Derived from Human Adipose Stem Cells Promotes Repair and Modulates Inflammation in a Chronic Dermal Wound Healing Model. *Biology* **2022**, *11*, 426. [CrossRef] [PubMed]

biomedicines

MDPI

Article

Grapefruit-Derived Vesicles Loaded with Recombinant HSP70 Activate Antitumor Immunity in Colon Cancer In Vitro and In Vivo

Luiza Garaeva [1,†], Elena Komarova [2,†], Svetlana Emelianova [1], Elena Putevich [1], Andrey L. Konevega [1], Boris Margulis [2], Irina Guzhova [2,*] and Tatiana Shtam [1,2,*]

1 St. Petersburg Nuclear Physics Institute Named by B.P. Konstantinov of National Research Centre «Kurchatov Institute», Orlova roshcha 1, Gatchina 188300, Russia; garaeva_laa@pnpi.nrcki.ru (L.G.); emelyanova_ss@pnpi.nrcki.ru (S.E.); putevich_ed@pnpi.nrcki.ru (E.P.); konevega_al@pnpi.nrcki.ru (A.L.K.)

2 Institute of Cytology of Russian Academy of Sciences, Tikhoretsky Ave. 4, St. Petersburg 194064, Russia; elpouta@yahoo.com (E.K.); margulis@incras.ru (B.M.)

* Correspondence: irina.guzh@gmail.com (I.G.); shtam_ta@pnpi.nrcki.ru (T.S.); Tel.: +7-921-974-44-34 (T.S.)

† These authors contributed equally to this work.

Abstract: Background/Objectives: Stress protein HSP70 administered exogenously has demonstrated high potential as an efficient adjuvant in antitumor immune response. To enhance the antigen-presenting activity, bioavailability, and stability of exogenous recombinant human HSP70, we propose incorporating it into plant extracellular vesicles. Earlier, we found that grapefruit-derived extracellular vesicles (GEV) were able to store the protein with no loss of its major function, chaperone activity. **Methods**: In this study, we tested whether HSP70 loaded into GEV (GEV-HSP70) could elicit an antitumor immune response in cellular and animal models of colorectal cancer. **Results:** To test the hypothesis in vitro, human and mouse colorectal cancer cell lines were used. We have shown that the addition of HSP70, either in free form or as part of GEVs, increases the sensitivity of human (HCT-116, DLD1) or mouse (CT-26) colon cancer cells to mouse cytotoxic lymphocytes and human NK-92 cells. Moreover, the amount of protein in the form of GEV-HSP70 required to cause the same activation of antitumor immunity was 20 times less than when HSP70 was added in free form. In a colon carcinoma model in vivo, GEV-HSP70 were inoculated subcutaneously into BALB/c mice together with CT-26 cells to form a tumor node. As compared with the control groups, we observed an increase in the lifespan of animals and a decrease in the tumor size, as well as a decrease in the level of TGFB1 IL-10 factors in the blood plasma. In vitro analysis of the immunomodulatory activity of GEV-HSP70 showed that antitumor response in GEV-HSP70-treated mice was associated with the accumulation of CD8+ cells. **Conclusions**: These results demonstrate the high feasibility and efficacy of the new technique based on HSP70 encapsulated in plant vesicles in activation of the specific response to colon tumors.

Keywords: HSP70; extracellular vesicles; plant-derived extracellular vesicles; drug delivery systems; antitumor immunity; colon cancer

1. Introduction

Immunotherapy is now the method of choice for a great number of cancers, and almost all the techniques employ the ability of specific molecules to enhance the antitumor response of a patient. Some of such molecules serve as adjuvants that are able to recognize tumor-associated antigens and participate in their presentation by dendritic cells. This function is typical for HSP70 molecular chaperone that was convincingly proven to elicit antigen-presenting activity leading to the activation of both innate and adaptive immune response [1,2]. It is well established that HSP70 or its particular peptides linked to tumor antigens work efficiently in numerous anti-cancer vaccine constructs whose efficacy has been established in pre-clinical and clinical trials [3–11]. Notably, pure recombinant HSP70 alone was employed in cell and animal tumor models and demonstrated the ability to generate a powerful immune response towards melanoma tumors [12,13]. In our studies, human recombinant HSP70 was also employed to increase the recognizability of C6 glioblastoma cells in vitro and in vivo [14], which was probably related to the ability of the chaperone to bind the phosphatidylserine component of the plasma membrane and penetrate living cells [15,16]. It was found that HSP70 entering melanoma and colon cancer cells displaced its intracellular counterpart and expulsed the latter being soluble or embodied in exosomes; in the latter form, HSP70 demonstrated greater immunogenic and antitumor activity [17–19]. Thus, delivery of pure HSP70 to a tumor could potentially lead to activation of both adaptive and innate antitumor immune responses.

The use of extracellular vesicles as carriers is a promising approach for the delivery of therapeutic biomolecules. Given that the use of animal-derived exosomes is hampered by ethical and manufacturing restrictions, plant-derived vesicles have been increasingly considered as effective delivery vehicles for exogenous therapeutic biomolecules in recent years [20–22]. Plant-derived extracellular vesicles are nanosized particles secreted by plant cells, surrounded by a lipid bilayer, and containing proteins, lipids, and nucleic acids. It is believed that plant vesicles mainly mediate the response of plant cells to abiotic stress and pathogen infection [20–22]. A few studies have successfully attempted to use intact plant vesicles from cabbage and ginger to deliver therapeutic biomolecules [23–25], including ours, which showed that grapefruit vesicles can effectively deliver exogenous recombinant HSP70 to cultured mammalian cells while maintaining its functional activity [26]. The data prompted us to use the HSP70 protein inserted in plant vesicles obtained from grapefruit which were demonstrated to hold considerable amounts of the active chaperone [26]. Thus, the aim of this work was to test the possibility of using grapefruit vesicles to deliver exogenous HSP70 to colon tumor cells in vivo with subsequent analysis of the activation of antitumor immunity.

2. Materials and Methods

2.1. Recombinant HSP70 Preparation

Synthesis of human recombinant HSP70 protein was carried out in *E. coli* bacteria transfected with pMS-Hsp70 plasmid (presented by Prof. R. Morimoto, Evanston, IL, USA). The obtained BL21 DE3 bacterial strain was grown on LB medium at 37 °C to OD = 0.5. HSP70 expression was induced by 1 mM IPTG followed by co-incubation for two hours, after which the bacteria were harvested and lysed at −80 °C freezing after 30 min incubation at room temperature in a buffer: 0.5 mM ethylenediaminetetetraacetic acid (EDTA), 50 mM Na_3PO_4, pH 8.5 with 1 mg/mL lysozyme. The protein was purified by sequential two-step chromatography. Bacterial lysates were passed through a DEAE-Sepharose column (GE Healthcare UK Ltd., Little Chalfont, UK) equilibrated with buffer A [20 mM NaCl, 20 mM Tris-HCl, 0.1 mM EDTA, pH 7.5], after which bound proteins containing Hsp70 were eluted from the column with buffer A containing 0.5 M NaCl. The eluate was dissolved in buffer B [20 mM Tris-HCl, 2 mM MgCl2, pH 7.5] and passed through ATP-agarose (Sigma-Aldrich, St Louis, MO, USA). HSP70 was eluted with 15 mM ATP, added up to 5 mM EDTA, and precipitated with ammonium sulfate followed by centrifugation. The precipitate was dissolved in phosphate buffer (PBS) and subjected to dialysis using Pierce Slide-a-Lyser cassettes (Pierce, Rockford, IL, USA). The resulting HSP70 solution was further purified by incubation with polymyxin B-agarose gel (Sigma-Aldrich, St Louis, MO, USA) and sterilized by passing through a 0.2 mm pore diameter filter (Millipore, Burlington, MA, USA). Protein concentration was measured according to the Bradford method.

2.2. Isolation of Vesicles from Fruit Parts of Citrus × Paradisi (Grapefruits) and Loading of Grapefruit-Derived Vesicles with Proteins

For the isolation of grapefruit-derived extracellular vesicles (GEV), the sequential ultracentrifugation method was applied, as described earlier [26]. The juice was obtained using a household citrus juicer from supermarket-purchased grapefruits. The obtained juice was successively centrifuged (JA-10 rotor, Avanti J-25I Centrifugation, Beckman Coulter, Brea, CA, USA) at 1500× *g*, 3000× *g*, 16,000× *g*, and 10,000× *g* for 30 min, three times for 20 min, 1 h and 15 h, respectively, after which the supernatant was ultracentrifuged (Ti45 rotor, Optima L-90K Ultracentrifuge, Beckman Coulter, Brea, CA, USA) at 4 °C at 150,000× *g* for 2 h, followed by resuspension of the gel pellet in PBS overnight at 4 °C. The pellets were then broken mechanically with a pipette, diluted with PBS, and centrifuged at 16,000× *g* for 1 h (SW55 rotor, Optima L-90K Ultracentrifuge, Beckman Coulter, Brea, CA, USA) for additional purification. The collected supernatant was again ultracentrifuged for 2 h at 150,000× *g* (SW55 rotor, Optima L-90K Ultracentrifuge Beckman Coulter, Brea, CA, USA) to concentrate the vesicles. The resulting transparent pellets were diluted with PBS and incubated overnight at 4 °C. The resulting grapefruit vesicle preparations were then flash-frozen in liquid nitrogen and stored at −80 °C for further experiments.

The size of GEVs and their concentration in suspensions were determined by Nanoparticle Tracking Analysis (NTA) using the NanoSight LM10 (Malvern Instruments, Worcestershire, UK) analyzer, equipped with a blue laser (45 mW at 405 nm) and a C11440-5B camera (Hamamatsu Photonics K.K., Fukuoka City, Japan). Recording and data analysis were performed using the NTA software 2.3. The following parameters were evaluated during the analysis of recordings monitored for 60 s: the average hydrodynamic diameter, the mode of distribution, the standard deviation, and the concentration of vesicles in the suspension.

A combination of passive and active cargo loading was used. Recombinant human HSP70 protein at a final concentration of 0.1 mg/mL was mixed with suspension of GEVs at a final concentration of ~3×10^{12} particles/mL and incubated overnight at 4 °C. Then, the mixture was sonicated at a frequency of 35 kHz for 15 min at RT by the Bandelin SONOREX SUPER ultrasonic bath (Bandelin Electronic GmbH & Co. KG, Berlin, Germany) at room temperature and incubated for an additional 90 min at 4 °C. To remove the excess free protein, the vesicles were purified using ultrafiltration through a 100-kDa filter (Amicon, Millipore, Temecula, CA, USA) ten times with washing by PBS. The obtained suspension of HSP70-loaded grapefruit vesicles (GEV-HSP70) was adjusted to the starting volume of the initial suspension of GEVs with PBS and sterilized by filtration through a 0.22 µm filter (Millipore, Temecula, CA, USA). The final concentration of loaded GEVs was established by NTA.

2.3. Evaluation of the Efficiency of the GEV Loading by Western-Blotting

The HSP70 protein amount in the samples of GEV-HSP70 was determined by western blotting. The purified samples of GEV-HSP70 were incubated at 4 °C for 30 min with 20 µL of lysis buffer (7M urea, 2M thiourea, 4% CHAPS, 1% DTT). The same number (2×10^{11}) of vesicles isolated from grapefruit (without loading procedure) was analyzed in parallel. Recombinant HSP70 at 0.2, 0.5, 1.0, and 2.0 µg per lane was also analyzed by Western blotting. The protein samples were diluted in Laemmli buffer (BioRad, Hercules, CA, USA), subjected to 10% SDS-PAGE containing 0.1% SDS, and transferred to the PVDF membrane (Thermo Scientific, Waltham, MA, USA) using the Trans-Blot Turbo Transfer System (BioRad, Hercules, CA, USA). Immunoblotting was performed according to the Blue Dry Western protocol [27]. Mouse monoclonal antibodies to HSP70 (clone 8D1, patent # Ru2722398) were used as primary antibodies at 1:500 dilution. Horseradish peroxidase-conjugated rabbit anti-mouse polyclonal antibodyies (Cloud-Clone Corp., Wuhan, China) were used as secondary antibodies at 1:5000 dilution. Chemiluminescent detection of the protein bands was performed with Clarity Western ECL Blotting Substrate (Bio-Rad, Hercules, CA, USA) and ChemiDoc System (BioRad, Hercules, CA, USA). Aliquots of the recombinant HSP70 (0.2 to 2 μg per lane) were used in densitometry for subsequent evaluation of the amount of protein loaded into GEV-HSP70.

2.4. Cryo-Electron Microscopy Evaluation of the Efficiency of the GEV Loading Using Western-Blotting

Direct visualization of the grapefruit-derived vesicles and loaded GEVs was performed by Cryo-EM as described previously [26,28]. The aqueous solution of the sample was applied on a glow-discharged lacey carbon EM grid, which was then plunge-frozen into the precooled liquid ethane with Vitrobot Mark IV (ThermoFisher Scientific, Waltham, MA, USA). The samples were studied using a cryo-electron microscope Titan Krios 60-300 TEM/STEM (ThermoFisher Scientific, Waltham, MA, USA), equipped with TEM direct electron detector Falcon II (ThermoFisher Scientific, Waltham, MA, USA) and Cs image corrector (CEOS, Heidelberg, Germany) at accelerating voltage of 300 kV. To minimize radiation damage during image acquisition, low-dose mode in EPU software (ThermoFisher Scientific, Waltham, MA, USA) was used. The resulting micrographs of GEVs were analyzed using the open-source image analysis and processing program ImageJ 1.54g (National Institutes of Health, Bethesda, MD, USA).

2.5. Cells

HCT116 and DLD1 human colon cancer cells were obtained from the Cell Culture Collection, Institute of Cytology of the RAS (St. Petersburg, Russia). Mouse colon carcinoma CT-26 cells were kindly provided by Prof. G. Multhoff (Technical University of Munchen, Germany). Cultured CT-26 cells were stably transfected with pHIV-iRFP720-E2A-Luc plasmid as previously described [17]. The resulting $CT26_{iRFP720\text{-}E2A\text{-}Luc}$ cells expressed near far-red fluorescent protein (ex. 698 nm/em. 720 nm) and luciferase. To assess the activation of the antitumor immune response in vitro, a culture of natural killer (NK) cells was used. NK-92 cells were kindly provided by Dr. Elena Kovalenko (Shemyakin-Ovchinnikov Institute of Bioorganic Chemistry, RAS (Moscow, Russia).

HCT116 and DLD1 cells were cultured in DMEM-F12 (BioLot, St. Petersburg, Russia) containing 10% heat inactivated fetal bovine serum (FBS) and CT-26 or $CT\text{-}26_{iRFP720\text{-}E2A\text{-}Luc}$ cells were grown in RPMI-1640 media supplemented with 10% FBS (HyClone, Logan, UT, USA), 2 mM L-glutamine, 100 U/mL penicillin and 0.1 mg/mL streptomycin (PanEco, Moscow, Russia) in a 5% CO_2 atmosphere with 90% humidity. The number and viability of cells were estimated on a LUNA-II™ Automated Cell Counter (Logos Biosystems, Dongan-gu, Republic of Korea) after mixing the cell suspension with trypan blue (1:1).

2.6. Cytotoxicity Assay

The cytotoxicity assay was performed with the xCELLigence RTCA system (Agilent, Santa Clara, CA, USA). This impedance-based assay carries out label-free, real-time, high-throughput analysis of cell growth and lymphocyte-mediated cytotoxicity [29]. Since NK cells and other lymphocytes are non-adhesive, they do not possess impedance [29]; therefore, a change in electrical signal relates only to adherent tumor cells. To evaluate the sensitivity of cancer cells (incubated with soluble recombinant HSP70 or HSP70 in the composition of GEVs) to cytotoxic lymphocytes, intact CT-26 mouse colon cancer cells and HCT116 or DLD1 human colon cancer cell were seeded in the wells of an E-plate at concentrations of 5×10^3 cells/well and incubated during 18 h at standard condition. Then HSP70 (50 μg/mL or 5 μg/mL), or the GEVs loaded with recombinant HSP70 (0.5×10^{12} GEVs/mL, concentration of loaded HSP70 ~2.5 μg/mL), or GEVs without loading (0.5×10^{12} GEVs/mL), were added. 18 h later, effector cells isolated from the spleen of C3HA mice (3×10^5 cells/well) or human NK-92 cells (1×10^6 cells/well) were added with the exchange of culture medium, and recording was carried out over the next 48 h. Each experimental point was duplicated within one experiment. All experiments were performed in triplicate.

2.7. Animal Experiments

All in vivo experiments were carried out following the requirements of the Institute of Cytology of the Russian Academy of Sciences Ethic Committee (Identification number F18-00380). Male C3HA mice were obtained from the Scientific and Production Enterprise "Nursery of Laboratory Animals" of the Institute of Bioorganic Chemistry of the Russian Academy of Sciences (Pushchino, Russia). BALB/c mice were purchased from the Biomedical Technology Research Center (Nizhniy Novgorod, Russia).

Male BALB/c mice were used for subcutaneous CT-26 tumor formation. The mice were divided into 4 groups (18 animal/group) and subcutaneously injected with 2×10^5 $CT26_{iRFP720\text{-}E2A\text{-}Luc}$ cells (hereafter referred to as CT-26) per mouse. The cells were previously mixed with: (i) cultural medium ("Untreated" group); (ii) HSP70 (50 µg/mouse, "HSP70" group); (iii) GEVs loaded with HSP70 (4×10^{11} loaded vesicles/mouse, quantity of loaded HSP70 ~2 µg/mouse, "GEV-HSP70" group); (iiii) GEVs (4×10^{11} vesicles/mouse, "GEV" group).

Tumor formation in animals of the experimental groups was assessed every 3 days starting from the eighth day after the injection of CT-26 cells using direct measurement of the tumor node with a caliper. The tumor volume was estimated using the formula $V = L \times D \times \frac{D}{2}$, where L is the length of the largest dimension, and D is the width or the smallest dimension.

Tumor growth rate was also estimated by weighing tumors taken from 8 control and treated animals on day 21 after engrafting; blood and spleens were collected on the same day. Tumors were photographed and weighed. Blood plasma was frozen at −80 °C before cytokine measurement by ELISA, while spleens were used immediately. Five random $CT26_{iRFP720\text{-}E2A\text{-}Luc}$-injected mice from each group were subjected to bioimaging with the use of the IVIS Spectrum imaging system (Perkin-Elmer, Beaconsfield, UK) on day 21.

The lifespan of four experimental groups of animals, each consisting of 10 mice, was assessed daily for 3 months, with the fact of death of each animal recorded. Survival curves were established according to the method of Kaplan-Meier and compared using a Mantel-Cox method.

To estimate the specific cytotoxic activity, the splenocytes of mice from all experimental groups were used. For the precise analysis of the total or specific CD8+ cell response, we first isolated spleen cells from animals belonging to appropriate treatment groups and further divided each into two groups. One group was incubated with Dynabeads FlowComp™ Mouse CD8 (Invitrogen, Carlsbad, CA, USA) to isolate CD8+ cells, and the other comprised the total lymphocyte fraction. These cell populations were used as effector cells, which were added to CT-26 cells at a ratio of 100:1. Cell viability was analyzed using the xCELLigence equipment as described above.

The collected blood of 5 animals from each group was centrifuged for 1 h at 3000× g at +4 °C to obtain blood plasma. The level of cytokines TGFB-1 and IL-10 in the blood plasma of experimental animals was assessed using the ELISA Kit for Transforming Growth Factor Beta 1 (TGFb1) (Cloud-Clone Corp., Wuhan, China) and ELISA Kit for Interleukin 10 (IL10) (Cloud-Clone Corp., Wuhan, China) according to the manufacturer's instructions. All the probes were triplicated.

2.8. Statistics

Visualization and analysis of the obtained data were carried out in GraphPad Prism 9.5.1 software. For multiple comparisons of group means, one-way ANOVA with Tukey's test was used. To process data on the survival of experimental animals, the Kaplan-Meier estimate was used. Analysis of the results of western blotting and Cryo-EM was carried out using the freely available software ImageJ 1.54g. Data are presented as mean ± SD.

3. Results

3.1. Characterization of Native and HSP70-Loaded GEVs

First, we analyzed the particle concentration and size of GEVs as well as their morphology and integrity before and after the loading procedure. Using NTA method, we showed that there were no significant changes in the median particle size after loading. The particles had a median size of 58 ± 7 nm before and 56 ± 6 nm after the loading (Figure 1A,B), but the concentration of particles decreased by a factor of 1.5–2 times.

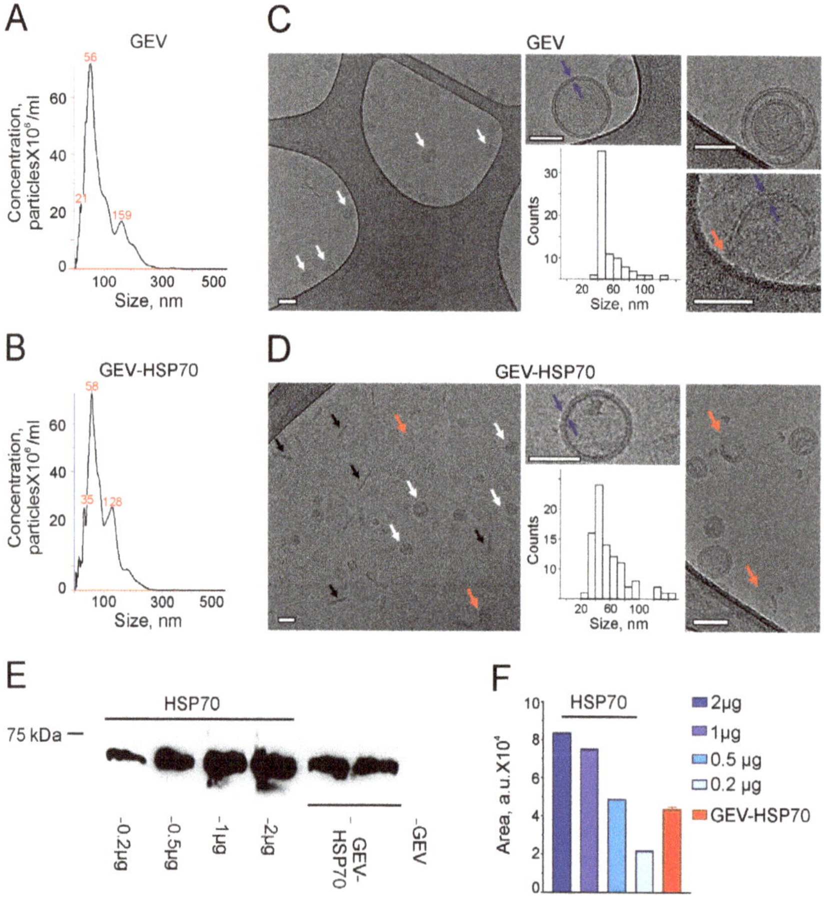

Figure 1. Size, concentration, and morphology of grapefruit-derived vesicles before (GEV) and after loading procedure (GEV-HSP70). (**A**,**B**) Typical examples of nanoparticle tracking analysis (NTA) of the sample of isolated GEV (**A**) and GEV-HSP70 (**B**). (**C**,**D**) Cryo-EM images of GEV (**C**) or GEV-HSP70 (**D**). White arrows indicate vesicles with intact membrane, red arrows indicate vesicles with broken membrane, and black arrows—debris in the sample. The blue arrows depict a lipid bilayer membrane of the vesicle. Scale bars are 50 nm. Inset–size distribution histogram. A total of 100 particles were analyzed. (**E**,**F**) Loading efficiency of GEV with HSP70 protein: (**E**) Example of Western blot (WB) of HSP70 in the initial GEV (line 7) and GEV-HSP70 (lines 5,6) in an amount of 10^{11} particles per line. Recombinant HSP70 in an amount from 0.2 µg to 2 µg per line (lines 1–4). (**F**) Cumulative quantification of HSP70 loaded into GEV obtained from WB.

The study using Cryo-EM demonstrated that native GEVs have a predominantly spherical shape, surrounded by a lipid bilayer with an average particle size of 53 ± 20 nm. Double vesicles and particles with impaired membrane integrity were occasionally encountered (Figure 1C). The GEV-HSP70 showed the appearance of some contaminant debris in the sample, as well as an increase in the number of vesicles with impaired integrity. At the same time, the average size of the analyzed particles did not change and was 55 ± 18 nm (Figure 1D). Thus, using the NTA and Cryo-EM methods, it was shown that the loading procedure does not significantly change the overall morphology and size of GEVs.

The loading efficiency of human recombinant HSP70 into GEVs was quantified using WB with anti-HSP70 antibodies (Figure 1E,F). Lysed GEV-HSP70 in an amount of 10^{11} particles/lane was applied to the WB, as well as rHSP70 in an amount from 0.2 μg to 2 μg per lane. Using ImageJ software, we established a linear standard curve (R = 0.92), according to the equation of which it was found that 10^{11} particles contain approximately 0.5 μg of protein. Thus, in all animal experiments, the administered 4×10^{11} GEV-HSP70-corresponded to about 2 μg of recombinant HSP70 per dose, and in vitro experiments used approximately 0.5 μg/well but not more than 1 μg/well of the protein.

3.2. *Recombinant HSP70 Loaded into GEVs Effectively Stimulates Immune Cell Activity In Vitro*

Recently, we have demonstrated that mouse exosomal HSP70, as well as a soluble HSP70, were able to pull out intracellular chaperones on cancer cell surfaces and activate the cytotoxic response of natural killer (NK) cells [12]. In this study, we tested the immunomodulatory activity of GEV-HSP70 in several colon cancer models.

At first, to test whether GEV-HSP70 is also capable of sensitizing cancer cells to cytotoxic cells, we used two human colon carcinoma cells, HCT-116 and DLD1, incubated with GEV-HSP70, in cytotoxic T lymphocyte (CTL) assay using xCELLigence technique. It is shown that the pre-incubation of human colon cancer cells with GEV-HSP70 resulted in a 2-3-fold reduction of cell index, which indicated an increase in the sensitivity of tumor cells to cytotoxic NK-92 cells (Figure 2A,B).

Then, we compared the immunomodulatory activity of GEV-HSP70 and HSP70 in mouse CT-26 colon carcinoma cells in vitro. CT-26 cells were preincubated with rHSP70 (10 μg/well), as well as with GEV-HSP70 (10^{11} particles/well, containing about 0.5 μg of rHSP70), then naïve lymphocytes obtained from the spleens of C3HA mice (Figure 2C) or NK-92 cells (Figure 2D) were added and cytotoxic activity was monitored in real-time using the xCELLigence technique. We observed an increase in the toxic effect of CTL both to cells incubated with HSP70 in free form or GEV-HSP70 (Figure 2C,E). Of note, the effect was equal for cells that were co-incubated with free HSP70 (10 μg), the amount of which was 20 times higher than in GEV-HSP70 (about 0.5 μg of HSP70). A similar result was obtained when NK-92cells were used. The effect of natural killer cells was observed after 10 h of co-incubation, and cell survival decreased by 50% (Figure 2D,F). To test the assumption that accumulation of rHSP70 in mouse cells is more efficient when the protein is encapsulated in vesicles, free rHSP70 was also previously added to the cells in an amount of 1 μg, which approximately corresponds to its content in GEV-HSP70 samples. It was shown that the amount of free HSP70 comparable to that loaded in GEVs does not lead to NK cell activation, as do unloaded GEVs (Figure 2D,F).

Thus, we have shown that the addition of HSP70 in free form and as part of GEVs increases the sensitivity of human (HCT-116, DLD1) or mouse (CT-26) colon cancer cells to mouse cytotoxic lymphocytes and human NK-92 cells. Moreover, as part of GEVs, HSP70 caused activation of antitumor immunity when the amount of protein was 20 times less as compared to the protein added in free form.

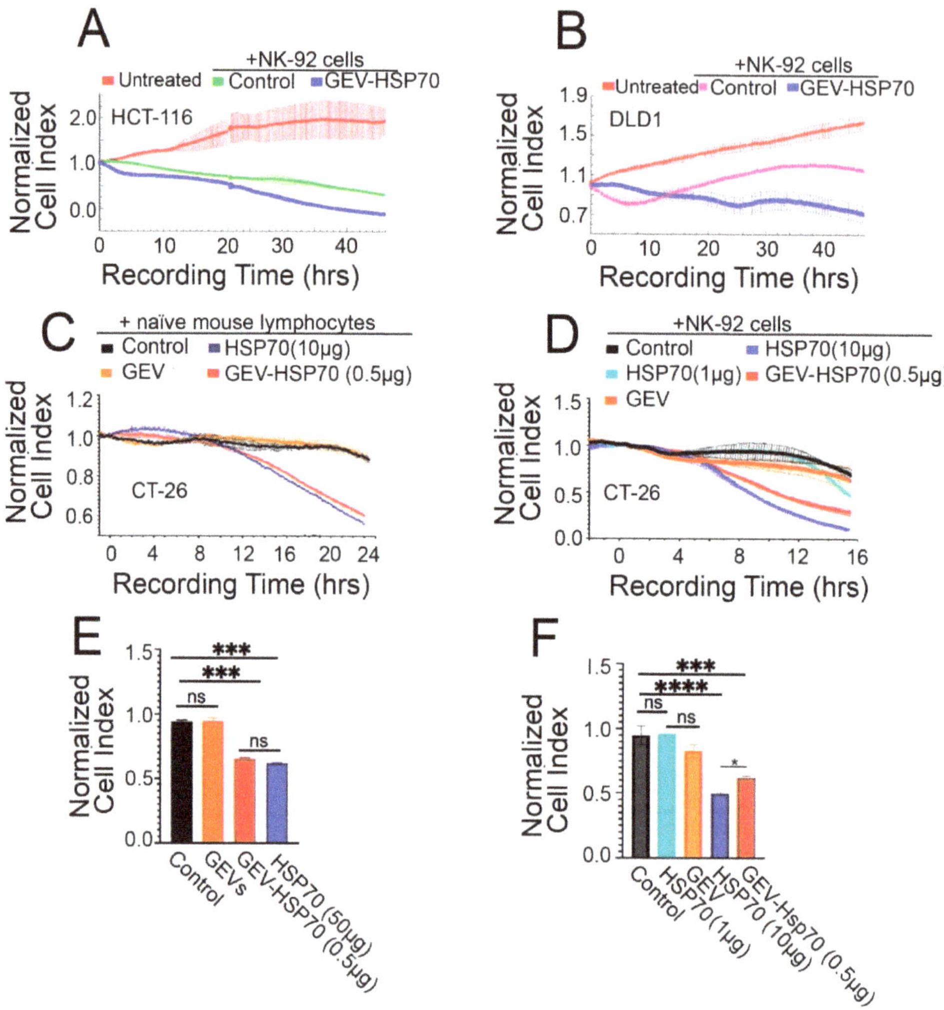

Figure 2. Effect of free HSP70 and GEV-HSP70 on the proliferative activity of human and murine colon cancer cells when attacked by cytotoxic lymphocytes (CTL) from naïve C3HA mice or human NK-92 cells. (**A**,**B**) GEV-HSP70 increases the sensitivity of human colon cancer cells to the NK cells action: HCT-116 (**A**) and DLD1 (**B**) cells were seeded to wells of E-plate and incubated or not with GEV-HSP70 for 24 h, and then NK-92 cells were added into wells. Recoding on xCELLigence equipment lasted 45 h. (**C**–**F**) Effect of free and GEV-loaded HSP70 on the proliferative activity of CT-26 cells when attacked by CTL from naïve C3HA mice or human NK-92 cells. (**C**,**E**) Proliferative activity of CT-26 cells preincubated with HSP70 (10 μg), GEV (0 μg HSP70), and GEV-HSP70 (about 0.5 μg HSP70) when exposed to the CTL. (F,H). Proliferative activity of CT-26 cells preincubated with HSP70 (10 μg or 1 μg), GEV (0 μg HSP70), and GEV-HSP70 (about 0.5 μg HSP70) upon exposure to NK-92 cells. Addition of rHSP70, GEV-HSP70, and naïve GEVs at 24 h of incubation, addition of effector cells at 40 h of incubation. For the (**E**,**F**) panels, the last observation time point was chosen for analysis. In panels (**A**–**D**), the normalization point for the proliferation curves is chosen to correspond to the time point of effector cells. Pairwise multiple comparisons were performed using ANOVA with Tukey's posterior test. A statistically significant difference between the is indicated as **** for $p < 0.0001$, *** for $p \leq 0.0005$, * for $p < 0.05$, ns—not statistically significant.

3.3. Antitumor Effect of HSP70 and GEV-HSP70 in a Mouse Model of Colorectal Cancer

Next, we analyzed the effect of GEV-HSP70 on the tumor growth of CT-26 cells in vivo. A single administration of the GEV, GEV-HSP70 (2 μg HSP70/dose), and HSP70 (50 μg) were used at the same time as tumor cells were inoculated subcutaneously to male Babl/c mice.

For three weeks after inoculation of tumor cells, either intact or in the presence of GEV, HSP70, or GEV-HSP70, we measured the volume of growing tumors. We observed a delay in tumor growth in the "HSP70" and 'GEV-HSP70' groups; their average size on the last day of measurement was significantly lower than the size in the "Untreated" group or in the "GEV" group (2.0 ± 0.2 for "GEV-HSP70" or 1.0 ± 0.4 for "HSP70" groups vs 3.4 ± 0.6 and 2.7 ± 0.4 cm^3 for "Untreated" and "GEV" groups respectively) (Figure 3A).

Then, tumors from eight animals from each group were isolated (Figure 3B) and weighed (Figure 3C). Again, the weight of tumors from the "Untreated" group or from the "GEV" group varied significantly from the "HSP70" and "GEV-HSP70" groups (0.5 ± 0.3 and 0.5 ± 0.2 g for "GEV-HSP70" and "HSP70" respectively vs. 1.1 ± 0.4 and 0.9 ± 0.3 g for "Untreated" and "GEV" groups respectively). It was also shown that the average tumor luminescence in "GEV-HSP70" was 4.0-fold less than in the "Untreated" group and 5.8-fold less than in the "GEV" group. The luminescence of tumors from the "HSP70" group was not statistically different from that in the "GEV-HSP70" group (Figure 3D,E).

Animal survival of ten remaining mice in each group was monitored over a 90-day period, which showed a 3-fold increase in lifespan for animals in the "HSP70" and "GEV-HSP70" groups compared to the control groups (Figure 3F). The average life span in the two control groups, "Untreated" and "GEV", was 32.3 ± 5.4 and 29.8 ± 4.8 days, respectively, while in the "GEV-HSP70" and "HSP70" groups, 3 mice in each group survived the observation time (90 days), and the remaining had average lifespan 42.2 ± 9.6 and 45.9 ± 9.0 days.

The data obtained indicate that the delivery of HSP70 into CT-26 tumor cells as part of grapefruit vesicles leads to a decrease in the tumor growth as well as, tumor weight, or size, as well as an increase in the life expectancy of experimental animals compared to the control group with the same efficiency, as free rHSP70 in 25-fold exceeding quantities.

3.4. Activation of a Specific Immune Response in Animals Received HSP70 and GEV-HSP70 in a Mouse Model of Colon Carcinoma

To analyze if the immune response was possibly stimulated in animals by HSP70 administration, blood samples were collected on the 21 days of tumor growth, followed by ELISA assay for TGFβ-1 and IL10. It was shown that in the blood of mice of the "HSP70" and "GEV-HSP70" groups, there was a significant reduction in the levels of IL-10 and TGFβ-1 compared to the "Untreated" group (Figure 4A,B). It is also worth noting that in the "GEV" group, we observed a 2-fold decrease in the level of pro-inflammatory IL-10 in the blood.

In order to further verify that the observed in vivo antitumor effects are related to the activation of a specific immune response, the proliferative activity of CT-26 cells was assessed during their co-incubation with the total fraction of lymphocytes obtained from the spleens of mice of experimental and control groups, as well as during co-cultivation of CT-26 cells with a fraction of cytotoxic CD8+ T lymphocytes obtained from the total lymphocyte fraction using the DynabeadsFlowComp™ Mouse CD8 kit. Cell viability and proliferative activity were assessed using the xCellLigence system. It was shown that after the addition of total lymphocytes or CD8+ T cells obtained from HSP70 or GEV-HSP70 groups of mice, CT-26 cell viability was reduced by 30% and 20%, respectively (Figure 4C,E). Lymphocyte fractions depleted of CD8+ cells, for which no stimulatory or cytotoxic effect was observed, were also used as a control (Figure 4D). The data obtained indicate that specific CD8+ cytotoxic T lymphocytes are involved in the observed in vivo antitumor effect of HSP70, both in free form and loaded into GEVs.

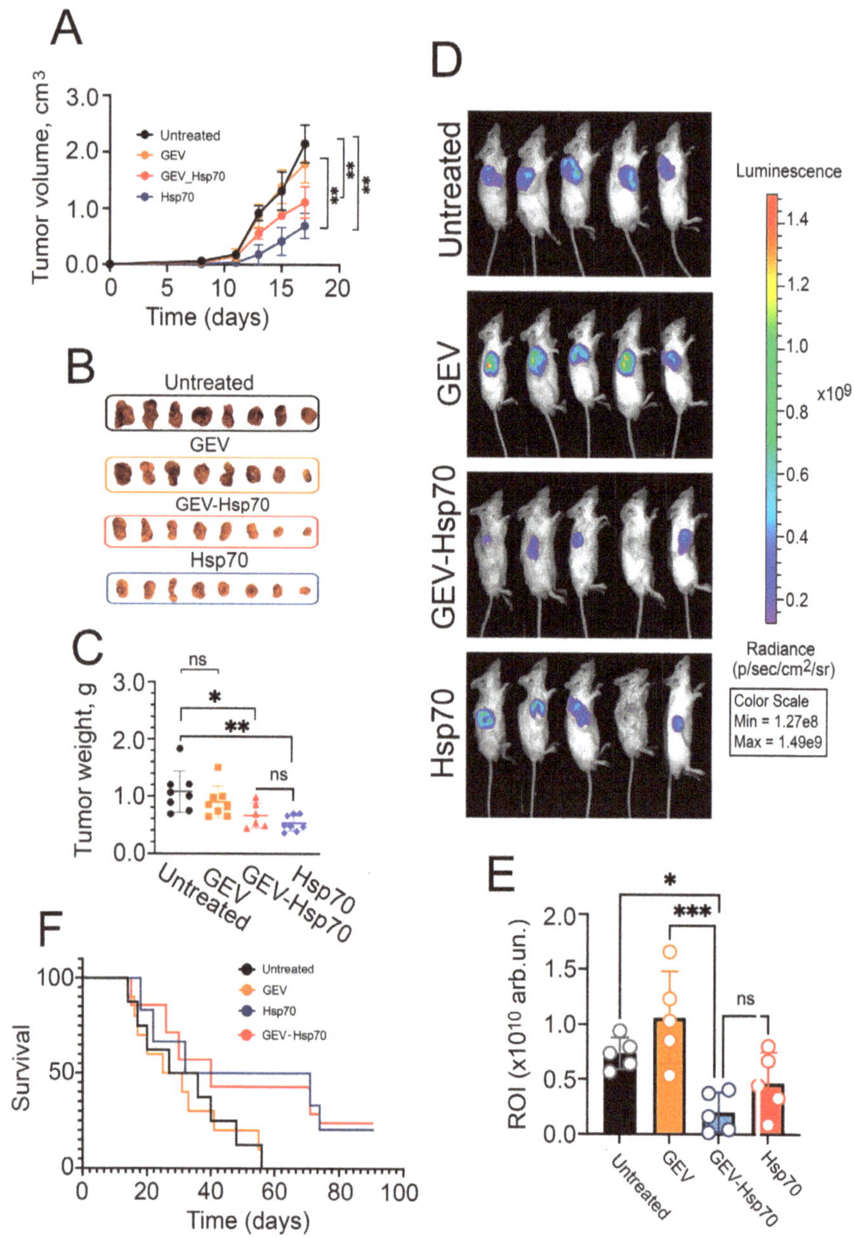

Figure 3. Antitumor effect of HSP70 and GEV-HSP70 in a mouse model of colorectal carcinoma. (**A**) Analysis of the growth rate of the tumor node during the 21st day of observation in 4 groups of animals after inoculation of CT-26 cells (Untreated) or CT-26 cells mixed with GEV, GEV-HSP70 (2 µg HSP70/dose), and with HSP70 (50 µg/dose) (N = 8) (**B**,**C**) Twenty-one days after CT-26 cells inoculation tumors were isolated, photographed (**B**) and weighed (**C**) (N = 8). (**D**,**E**) Analysis of the tumor size by the intravital luminescence imaging system (N = 5). (**F**) Life expectancy of animals in control and experimental groups (N = 10). Legend *** for $p \leq 0.0005$, ** for $p \leq 0.005$, * for $p < 0.05$, ns—not statistically significant.

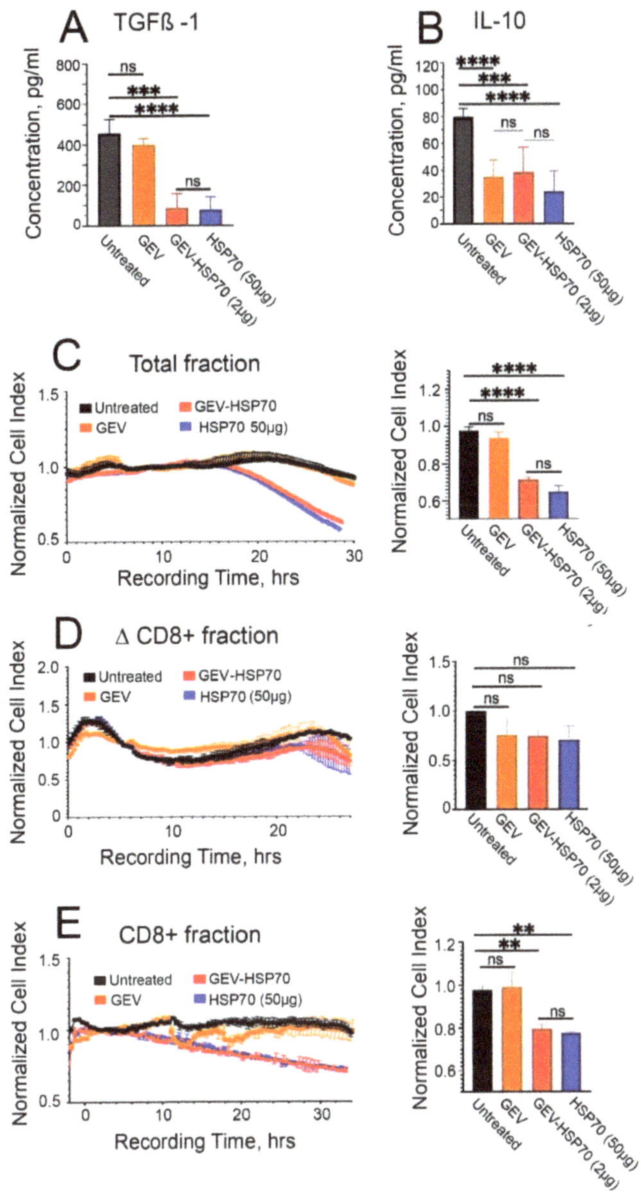

Figure 4. GEV-HSP70 and free HSP70 induce a specific antitumor immune response in the CT-26 mouse model of colorectal carcinoma. (**A**,**B**) Assessment of the concentration of cytokines IL-10 and TGFB-1 in the blood plasma of mice 21 days after inoculation with CT-26 cells (Untreated), CT-26 cells mixed with GEV, GEV-HSP70 (about 2 μg HSP70/dose) or HSP70 (50 μg/dose) (N = 5). (**C**) Proliferative activity of CT-26 cells when exposed to the total fraction of lymphocytes isolated from the spleens of mice of experimental and control groups. (**D**) The influence of the lymphocyte fraction depleted of CD8+ T-lymphocytes on the proliferative activity of CT-26 cells. (**E**) Cytostatic effect of CD8+ T lymphocytes from mice from experimental and control groups on the proliferation of CT-26 cells (N = 5). Pairwise multiple comparisons were performed using ANOVA with Tukey's posterior test. $p < 0.0001$ = ****, $p \leq 0.0005$ = ***, $p \leq 0.005$ = **, ns—not statistically significant.

4. Discussion

Multifaceted function of HSP70 chaperone in tumor growth and immune response to cancer is well established, and there are hundreds of publications dedicated to this topic [30]. In addition to its protective activity, HSP70 was shown to leave cancer cells or enter them; when occurring exogenously, HSP70, by binding tumor antigens or a variety of other polypeptides, is able to regulate immune response to cancer cells by triggering the mechanisms of innate and adaptive immunity [2].

HSP70 is released from tumor cells in free form or within extracellular vesicles (EV) [2,31]. HSP70-containing EVs or exosomes strongly affect tumor progression by promoting the activity of Tregs or inducing myeloid-derived suppressor cells, which help the tumor avoid immune surveillance [32,33]. On the other hand, HSP70-containing EVs from heat-treated CT-26 and B16 melanoma cells exhibited antitumor activity, which seemed to be associated with the enhancement of a strong Th1 immune response [4]. Exosomes from mouse colon carcinoma MC38 cells also showed strong antitumor effects associated with the conversion of regulatory T cells into Th17 cells [34]. Our earlier data demonstrated that EVs from tumor cells loaded with HSP70 caused high antitumor immune responses in mouse B16 melanoma and CT-26 colon carcinoma-bearing mice, activating CD8+ dependent immune response [17]. Taking into account that tumor exosomes may be dangerous to apply as a therapeutic agent, we loaded grapefruit vesicles with pure HSP70 and found that they efficiently activated innate pro-tumor immunity to colorectal cancer cells in vitro slowed down tumor growth and increased the survival rate in the animal model in vivo, stimulating specific antitumor CD8+ dependent immunity, which was accompanied by a reduction in the amount of pro-tumor cytokines, TGFβ-1 and IL-10.

5. Conclusions

Summarizing the results, we can conclude that the HSP70 protein activates the antitumor immune response in the models of colorectal cancer, both in vitro and in vivo. Recombinant HSP70 protein can be loaded into grapefruit vesicles while maintaining its functionality. Moreover, in both cell and animal models, HSP70 in the composition of GEVs has the same antitumor effect as a 20-fold greater amount of the free form of the chaperone.

Author Contributions: Methodology, L.G., E.K. and B.M.; validation, L.G. and E.K.; formal analysis, L.G.; investigation, L.G., E.K., S.E. and E.P.; writing—Original Draft, L.G., I.G. and T.S.; data curation, E.K.; visualization, S.E.; supervision, A.L.K., B.M., I.G. and T.S.; funding acquisition, A.L.K. and T.S.; conceptualization, B.M., I.G. and T.S.; writing—review and editing, B.M., I.G. and T.S.; project administration, I.G. and T.S. All authors have read and agreed to the published version of the manuscript.

Funding: The study was supported by the Russian Science Foundation project 19-74-20146-p (cryo-EM, NTA, cell culture experiments). This work was partially (animal experiments) supported by the Ministry of Science and Higher Education of the RF (Project 075-15-2021-1360).

Institutional Review Board Statement: All in vivo experiments were carried out following the requirements of the Institute of Cytology of the Russian Academy of Sciences Ethic Committee (Identification number F18-00380).

Informed Consent Statement: Not applicable.

Data Availability Statement: No additional data available.

Acknowledgments: We thank Eugeniy Yastremskiy and Roman Kamyshinsky for assistance with cryo-EM experiments. We also thank Anastasia Nikitina for her assistance in conducting experiments using laboratory animals. The authors acknowledge the support and the use of facilities of the Resource Center for Probe and Electron Microscopy at the NRC "Kurchatov Institute".

Conflicts of Interest: The authors declare no competing interests.

References

1. Cuzzubbo, S.; Mangsbo, S.; Nagarajan, D.; Habra, K.; Pockley, A.G.; McArdle, S.E.B. Cancer Vaccines: Adjuvant Potency, Importance of Age, Lifestyle, and Treatments. *Front. Immunol.* **2021**, *11*, 615240. [CrossRef] [PubMed]
2. Hu, B.; Liu, G.; Zhao, K.; Zhang, G. Diversity of extracellular HSP70 in cancer: Advancing from a molecular biomarker to a novel therapeutic target. *Front. Oncol.* **2024**, *14*, 1388999. [CrossRef] [PubMed]
3. Noessner, E.; Gastpar, R.; Milani, V.; Brandl, A.; Hutzler, P.J.S.; Kuppner, M.C.; Roos, M.; Kremmer, E.; Asea, A.; Calderwood, S.K.; et al. Tumor-Derived Heat Shock Protein 70 Peptide Complexes Are Cross-Presented by Human Dendritic Cells. *J. Immunol.* **2002**, *169*, 5424–5432. [CrossRef] [PubMed]
4. Cho, J.; Lee, Y.-S.; Kim, S.-H.; Ko, J.-K.; Kim, C.-W. MHC independent anti-tumor immune responses induced by Hsp70-enriched exosomes generate tumor regression in murine models. *Cancer Lett.* **2009**, *275*, 256–265. [CrossRef] [PubMed]
5. Huang, C.; Zhao, J.; Li, Z.; Li, D.; Xia, D.; Wang, Q.; Jin, H. Multi-chaperone-peptide-rich mixture from colo-carcinoma cells elicits potent anticancer immunity. *Cancer Epidemiol.* **2010**, *34*, 494–500. [CrossRef]
6. Albakova, Z.; Armeev, G.A.; Kanevskiy, L.M.; Kovalenko, E.I.; Sapozhnikov, A.M. HSP70 Multi-Functionality in Cancer. *Cells* **2020**, *9*, 587. [CrossRef]
7. Asghari Vostakolaei, M.; Abdolalizadeh, J.; Hejazi, M.S.; Kordi, S.; Molavi, O. Hsp70 in Cancer: Partner or Traitor to Immune System. *Iran. J. Allergy Asthma Immunol.* **2020**, *18*, 589–604. [CrossRef]
8. Zhao, K.; Zhou, G.; Liu, Y.; Zhang, J.; Chen, Y.; Liu, L.; Zhang, G. HSP70 Family in Cancer: Signaling Mechanisms and Therapeutic Advances. *Biomolecules* **2023**, *13*, 601. [CrossRef]
9. Das, J.K.; Xiong, X.; Ren, X.; Yang, J.-M.; Song, J. Heat Shock Proteins in Cancer Immunotherapy. *J. Oncol.* **2019**, *2019*, 3267207. [CrossRef]
10. Zhang, X.; Huang, Y.; Li, X.; Wang, Y.; Yuan, Y.; Li, M. Preparation of a new combination nanoemulsion-encapsulated MAGE1-MAGE3-MAGEn/HSP70 vaccine and study of its immunotherapeutic effect. *Pathol. Res. Pract.* **2020**, *216*, 152954. [CrossRef]
11. Weng, D.; Calderwood, S.K.; Gong, J. A Novel Heat Shock Protein 70-Based Vaccine Prepared from DC Tumor Fusion Cells: An Update. In *Chaperones. Methods in Molecular Biology*; Humana: New York, NY, USA, 2023; pp. 209–219.
12. Ito, A.; Matsuoka, F.; Honda, H.; Kobayashi, T. Antitumor effects of combined therapy of recombinant heat shock protein 70 and hyperthermia using magnetic nanoparticles in an experimental subcutaneous murine melanoma. *Cancer Immunol. Immunother.* **2004**, *53*, 26–32. [CrossRef] [PubMed]
13. Geng, H.; Zhang, G.; Xiao, H.; Yuan, Y.; Li, D.; Zhang, H.; Qiu, H.; He, Y.; Feng, Z. HSP70 vaccine in combination with gene therapy with plasmid DNA encoding sPD-1 overcomes immune resistance and suppresses the progression of pulmonary metastatic melanoma. *Int. J. Cancer* **2006**, *118*, 2657–2664. [CrossRef] [PubMed]
14. Shevtsov, M.A.; Pozdnyakov, A.V.; Mikhrina, A.L.; Yakovleva, L.Y.; Nikolaev, B.P.; Dobrodumov, A.V.; Komarova, E.Y.; Meshalkina, D.A.; Ischenko, A.M.; Pitkin, E.; et al. Effective immunotherapy of rat glioblastoma with prolonged intratumoral delivery of exogenous heat shock protein Hsp70. *Int. J. Cancer* **2014**, *135*, 2118–2128. [CrossRef] [PubMed]
15. Schilling, D.; Gehrmann, M.; Steinem, C.; De Maio, A.; Pockley, A.G.; Abend, M.; Molls, M.; Multhoff, G. Binding of heat shock protein 70 to extracellular phosphatidylserine promotes killing of normoxic and hypoxic tumor cells. *FASEB J.* **2009**, *23*, 2467–2477. [CrossRef]
16. Abkin, S.V.; Pankratova, K.M.; Komarova, E.Y.; Guzhova, I.V.; Margulis, B.A. Hsp70 chaperone-based gel composition as a novel immunotherapeutic anti-tumor tool. *Cell Stress Chaperones* **2013**, *18*, 391–396. [CrossRef]
17. Komarova, E.Y.; Suezov, R.V.; Nikotina, A.D.; Aksenov, N.D.; Garaeva, L.A.; Shtam, T.A.; Zhakhov, A.V.; Martynova, M.G.; Bystrova, O.A.; Istomina, M.S.; et al. Hsp70-containing extracellular vesicles are capable of activating of adaptive immunity in models of mouse melanoma and colon carcinoma. *Sci. Rep.* **2021**, *11*, 21314. [CrossRef]
18. Shevtsov, M.A.; Komarova, E.Y.; Meshalkina, D.A.; Bychkova, N.V.; Aksenov, N.D.; Abkin, S.V.; Margulis, B.A.; Guzhova, I.V. Exogenously delivered heat shock protein 70 displaces its endogenous analogue and sensitizes cancer cells to lymphocytes-mediated cytotoxicity. *Oncotarget* **2014**, *5*, 3101–3114. [CrossRef]
19. Gonzalez-Melero, L.; Hernandez, R.M.; Santos-Vizcaino, E.; Igartua, M. Tumour-derived extracellular vesicle based vaccines for melanoma treatment. *Drug Deliv. Transl. Res.* **2023**, *13*, 1520–1542. [CrossRef]
20. Cui, Y.; Gao, J.; He, Y.; Jiang, L. Plant extracellular vesicles. *Protoplasma* **2020**, *257*, 3–12. [CrossRef]
21. Feng, H.; Yue, Y.; Zhang, Y.; Liang, J.; Liu, L.; Wang, Q.; Feng, Q.; Zhao, H. Plant-Derived Exosome-Like Nanoparticles: Emerging Nanosystems for Enhanced Tissue Engineering. *Int. J. Nanomed.* **2024**, *19*, 1189–1204. [CrossRef]
22. Akuma, P.; Okagu, O.D.; Udenigwe, C.C. Naturally. Occurring Exosome Vesicles as Potential Delivery Vehicle for Bioactive Compounds. *Front. Sustain. Food Syst.* **2019**, *3*, 23. [CrossRef]
23. Li, Z.; Wang, H.; Yin, H.; Bennett, C.; Zhang, H.; Guo, P. Arrowtail RNA for Ligand Display on Ginger Exosome-like Nanovesicles to Systemic Deliver siRNA for Cancer Suppression. *Sci. Rep.* **2018**, *8*, 14644. [CrossRef] [PubMed]
24. You, J.Y.; Kang, S.J.; Rhee, W.J. Isolation of cabbage exosome-like nanovesicles and investigation of their biological activities in human cells. *Bioact. Mater.* **2021**, *6*, 4321–4332. [CrossRef] [PubMed]
25. Feng, W.; Teng, Y.; Zhong, Q.; Zhang, Y.; Zhang, J.; Zhao, P.; Chen, G.; Wang, C.; Liang, X.-J.; Ou, C. Biomimetic Grapefruit-Derived Extracellular Vesicles for Safe and Targeted Delivery of Sodium Thiosulfate against Vascular Calcification. *ACS Nano* **2023**, *17*, 24773–24789. [CrossRef] [PubMed]

26. Garaeva, L.; Kamyshinsky, R.; Kil, Y.; Varfolomeeva, E.; Verlov, N.; Komarova, E.; Garmay, Y.; Landa, S.; Burdakov, V.; Myasnikov, A.; et al. Delivery of functional exogenous proteins by plant-derived vesicles to human cells in vitro. *Sci. Rep.* **2021**, *11*, 6489. [CrossRef]
27. Naryzhny, S.N. Blue Dry Western: Simple, economic, informative, and fast way of immunodetection. *Anal. Biochem.* **2009**, *392*, 90–95. [CrossRef]
28. Emelyanov, A.; Shtam, T.; Kamyshinsky, R.; Garaeva, L.; Verlov, N.; Miliukhina, I.; Kudrevatykh, A.; Gavrilov, G.; Zabrodskaya, Y.; Pchelina, S.; et al. Cryo-electron microscopy of extracellular vesicles from cerebrospinal fluid. *PLoS ONE* **2020**, *15*, e0227949. [CrossRef]
29. Peper, J.K.; Schuster, H.; Löffler, M.W.; Schmid-Horch, B.; Rammensee, H.-G.; Stevanović, S. An impedance-based cytotoxicity assay for real-time and label-free assessment of T-cell-mediated killing of adherent cells. *J. Immunol. Methods* **2014**, *405*, 192–198. [CrossRef]
30. Mazurakova, A.; Solarova, Z.; Koklesova, L.; Caprnda, M.; Prosecky, R.; Khakymov, A.; Baranenko, D.; Kubatka, P.; Mirossay, L.; Kruzliak, P.; et al. Heat shock proteins in cancer—Known but always being rediscovered: Their perspectives in cancer immunotherapy. *Adv. Med. Sci.* **2023**, *68*, 464–473. [CrossRef]
31. Elmallah, M.I.Y.; Cordonnier, M.; Vautrot, V.; Chanteloup, G.; Garrido, C.; Gobbo, J. Membrane-anchored heat-shock protein 70 (Hsp70) in cancer. *Cancer Lett.* **2020**, *469*, 134–141. [CrossRef]
32. Chalmin, F.; Ladoire, S.; Mignot, G.; Vincent, J.; Bruchard, M.; Remy-Martin, J.-P.; Boireau, W.; Rouleau, A.; Simon, B.; Lanneau, D.; et al. Membrane-associated Hsp72 from tumor-derived exosomes mediates STAT3-dependent immunosuppressive function of mouse and human myeloid-derived suppressor cells. *J. Clin. Invest.* **2010**, *120*, 457–471. [CrossRef] [PubMed]
33. Diao, J.; Yang, X.; Song, X.; Chen, S.; He, Y.; Wang, Q.; Chen, G.; Luo, C.; Wu, X.; Zhang, Y. Exosomal Hsp70 mediates immunosuppressive activity of the myeloid-derived suppressor cells via phosphorylation of Stat3. *Med. Oncol.* **2015**, *32*, 35. [CrossRef] [PubMed]
34. Guo, D.; Chen, Y.; Wang, S.; Yu, L.; Shen, Y.; Zhong, H.; Yang, Y. Exosomes from heat-stressed tumour cells inhibit tumour growth by converting regulatory T cells to Th17 cells via IL-6. *Immunology* **2018**, *154*, 132–143. [CrossRef] [PubMed]

biomedicines

MDPI

Article

Artificial Extracellular Vesicles Generated from T Cells Using Different Induction Techniques

Ekaterina A. Zmievskaya [1,*], Sabir A. Mukhametshin [1], Irina A. Ganeeva [1], Elvina M. Gilyazova [1], Elvira T. Siraeva [1], Marianna P. Kutyreva [2], Artur A. Khannanov [2], Youyong Yuan [3] and Emil R. Bulatov [1,4]

1 Institute of Fundamental Medicine and Biology, Kazan Federal University, 420008 Kazan, Russia
2 A.M. Butlerov Institute of Chemistry, Kazan Federal University, 420008 Kazan, Russia
3 School of Biomedical Sciences and Engineering, South China University of Technology, Guangzhou International Campus, Guangzhou 511442, China
4 Shemyakin-Ovchinnikov Institute of Bioorganic Chemistry, Russian Academy of Sciences, 117997 Moscow, Russia
* Correspondence: chembio.kazan@gmail.com

Abstract: Cell therapy is at the forefront of biomedicine in oncology and regenerative medicine. However, there are still significant challenges to their wider clinical application such as limited efficacy, side effects, and logistical difficulties. One of the potential approaches that could overcome these problems is based on extracellular vesicles (EVs) as a cell-free therapy modality. One of the major obstacles in the translation of EVs into practice is their low yield of production, which is insufficient to achieve therapeutic amounts. Here, we evaluated two primary approaches of artificial vesicle induction in primary T cells and the SupT1 cell line—cytochalasin B as a chemical inducer and ultrasonication as a physical inducer. We found that both methods are capable of producing artificial vesicles, but cytochalasin B induction leads to vesicle yield compared to natural secretion, while ultrasonication leads to a three-fold increase in particle yield. Cytochalasin B induces the formation of vesicles full of cytoplasmic compartments without nuclear fraction, while ultrasonication induces the formation of particles rich in membranes and membrane-related components such as CD3 or HLAII proteins. The most effective approach for T-cell induction in terms of the number of vesicles seems to be the combination of anti-CD3/CD28 antibody activation with ultrasonication, which leads to a seven-fold yield increase in particles with a high content of functionally important proteins (CD3, granzyme B, and HLA II).

Keywords: T cells; extracellular vesicles; artificial vesicles; vesicle induction; ultrasonication

1. Introduction

T cell-based immunotherapy, including CAR-T, TILs, Tregs, and many others, represents one of the most promising types of modern cell therapy in the fields of oncology and autoimmune diseases. Despite its success, this type of therapy has some drawbacks—live cells are difficult to store, transport, and dose, and in the majority of cases, they have to be autologous for each patient. These challenges may limit the availability and accessibility of this therapy for patients. However, ongoing research and development are focused on overcoming these obstacles and improving the feasibility and efficacy of T cell-based immunotherapies.

One potential approach to address these issues is the use of artificial extracellular vesicles (EVs). EVs are a heterogeneous group of nano-sized lipid vesicles of cellular origin. They are typically classified into three types based on their size and mechanism of formation: exosomes, microvesicles, and apoptotic bodies. The biochemical composition and functional properties of EVs are determined by the parental cell type and physiological state, making them a cell-free analog of cell therapy. Artificial vesicles (AVs) are designed to mimic the biological properties of EVs and can be produced in a scalable and standardized manner to achieve more convenient storage, transportation, and dosage than for live cells [1].

The secretion of EVs by T cells is a natural process, particularly in response to TCR-specific activation. T cell-secreted EVs are known to carry a variety of effector proteins such as CD3, MHC-I and MHC-II, CD2, LFA-1, CXCR4, and FasL, as well as small RNAs [2]. Functionally, EVs derived from $CD8^+$ T cells have been shown to possess immune-activating and antitumor properties, while EVs from Tregs have been shown to have immunomodulatory effects [1].

Overall, EVs represent a promising therapeutic agent due to their stability, biosafety, and capability to target specific tissues with better penetration than cells [3]. Some reports claim that they also have the potential to cross biological barriers such as the blood–brain barrier [4]. EVs can also be used as drug delivery vehicles and have advantages over other nanoscale delivery approaches, including better biocompatibility, longer half-life, and lower immunogenicity and toxicity. By combining the natural properties of EVs with therapeutic small molecules, the overall therapeutic efficacy can be significantly enhanced [5].

The main obstacle to EV technology becoming a viable treatment option is the difficulty of large-scale production. Natural EVs have a very low yield, sufficient for academic research but insufficient for industrial or clinical use. Up to a 500 L high-density perfusion bioreactor may need to be used to manufacture the required amount of EVs for clinical use [6].

As a result, several approaches are being investigated to increase EV production yield. The strategies include dynamic culture, hypoxia, starvation, low pH, chemical stimulation (vesiculation buffer, cytochalasin B, and sulfhydryl blocking agents), physical stimulation (shear stress, high-frequency ultrasonication (US), and irradiation), cell membrane disruption (extrusion, nitrogen cavitation, and low-frequency ultrasonication) [7].

In this study, we aimed to investigate and compare two main approaches for the generation of artificial extracellular vesicles from T cells: chemical stimulation (cytochalasin B) and cell membrane disruption (low-frequency ultrasonication). The detailed study design is presented in Figure 1.

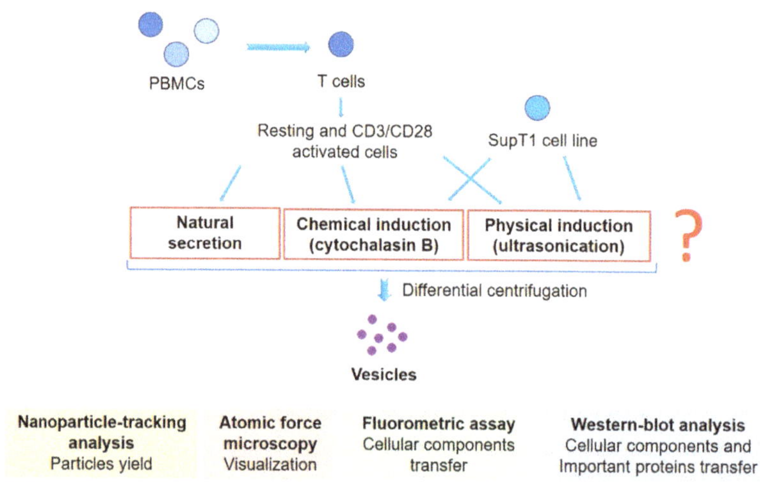

Figure 1. The scheme of the experiment includes the induction of artificial vesicles from primary T lymphocytes and SupT1 cell line with two methods under investigation and further comprehensive study of obtained vesicles.

2. Materials and Methods

2.1. T Cells' Isolation and Expansion

Peripheral blood mononuclear cells (PBMCs) were obtained from the whole blood of a healthy donor (according to ethics approval and written informed consent) by Ficoll (Paneco, Moscow, Russia) density centrifugation at 800× g for 30 min. The buffy coat was collected and washed twice with Dulbecco's phosphate-buffered saline, and the cells were seeded in 10% RPMI with L-glutamine and penicillin–streptomycin (Paneco, Moscow Russia). T cells were activated with T-cell TransAct (Miltenyi, Bergisch Gladbach, Germany) according to the manufacturer's protocol, and IL-2 (Prospec, Rehovot, Israel) was added at a concentration of 300 IU/mL. T cells were counted every two days, and a fresh medium containing IL-2 was added to maintain a cell density of approximately 1×10^6 cells/mL. After 14 days of expansion, cell populations were phenotyped by flow cytometry for CD3, CD4, and CD8 markers (Figure S1, Supplementary Materials).

2.2. SupT1 Cell Culture and Transduction

SupT1 (ATCC CRL-1942, mycoplasma free) cells were cultured in 10% RPMI supplemented with penicillin–streptomycin and L-glutamine. To obtain AVs, the cells were washed twice with DPBS and resuspended in serum-free RPMI. To obtain SupT1(Kat+) cells, SupT1 expressing red fluorescent protein Katushka2S, lentiviral transduction was performed using second-generation lentivirus harvested from HEK293FT culture and concentrated using Amicon 15 (Merck, Darmstadt, Germany). Transduction was performed with protamine sulfate at a concentration of 50 µg/mL for 16 h. The medium was then replaced, and a selective antibiotic (blasticidine) was added after 48 h. The selection of SupT1(Kat+) continued for 1 week. The efficacy of Katushka2S transduction was determined by flow cytometry (Figure S2, Supplementary Materials).

2.3. MV Induction and Collection

To obtain microvesicles from primary T cells, the cells were harvested on day 14, washed twice with DPBS, and seeded at a density of 1×10^6 cells/mL in a serum-free AIM-V medium (Thermo Fisher, Waltham, MA, USA) containing 300 IU/mL IL-2. The cells were then divided into two parts. One portion was left in a CO_2 incubator (ESCO, Seoul, Republic of Korea) to allow for resting T-cell culture, while the other was reactivated using T-cell TransAct (Miltenyi, Auburn, CA, USA). After 48 h of incubation, the supernatants were obtained by centrifugation to separate natural microvesicles (MVs), while the cell pellets were washed twice with DPBS, resuspended in serum-free media, and subsequently induced to generate AVs.

2.4. AV Induction

To obtain AVs, the cells were washed twice with DPBS and resuspended in serum-free media. AVs were then induced using either cytochalasin B or ultrasonication. For cytochalasin B induction, cytochalasin B (ChB) was added at a concentration of 10 µg/mL, and the cells were incubated in a CO_2 incubator (ESCO, Seoul, South Korea) for 30 min. The cells were then gently vortexed for 30 s. For ultrasonication induction, the cells were subjected to ultrasonication impact using a Bandelin Sonopuls HD2200 (Bandelin, Berlin, Germany) homogenizer at cycle 5 and 20% power for 1 min.

2.5. MV and AV Isolation

The isolation of MVs and AVs was performed by differential centrifugation. First, the cell pellet was obtained by centrifugation at 300× g for 10 min, followed by centrifugation of the supernatant at 2000× g for 10 min to remove debris and apoptotic bodies. Finally, the vesicles were sedimented by centrifugation at 15,000× g for 20 min. After separation, the samples were washed twice with DPBS.

2.6. Nanoparticle Tracking Analysis

Nanoparticle tracking analysis (NTA) was performed using NanoSight LM-10 (Malvern Instruments, Malvern, UK). The detector was a C11440-50B CMOS camera with an FL-280 image capture sensor from Hamamatsu Photonics (Shizuoka, Japan). Measurements were performed in a special cuvette for aqueous solutions equipped with a 405 nm laser (CD version, S/N 2990491) and a sealing ring made of Kalrez material. The temperature was recorded for all measurements using an OMEGA HH804 contact thermometer (Engineering Inc., Chicago, IL, USA). Samples for analysis were collected and injected into the measuring cell using a 1 mL two-part glass syringe (tuberculin) through the Luer (Hamilton Company, Reno, NV, USA). To increase the statistical dose, the sample was pumped through the measuring chamber using a piezoelectric dispenser. Each sample was acquired six times sequentially; the acquisition time was sequential and was 60 s. The NanoSight images were processed using NTA 2.3 software applications (build 0033), as previously described [8]. The detailed work is currently presented in the "Principle of Operation" by B. Carr and A. Malloy [9]. The hydrodynamic diameter was calculated using the two-dimensional Einstein–Stokes equation [10].

2.7. Atomic Force Microscopy

For atomic force microscopy (AFM), the vesicle samples were washed twice and resuspended in sodium phosphate buffer (pH 7.4). A drop of the suspension was placed on a coverslip and dried in a vacuum oven for 30 min. AFM was then performed using Dimension FastScan (Bruker, Billerica, MA, USA). AFM images were obtained in the PeakForceQNM mode (quantitative nanomechanical mapping) using standard silicon cantilevers ScanAsyst-Fluid+ (Bruker, Billerica, MA, USA) with a curvature of 2 nm and stiffness of 0.7 N/m. PeakForceQNM is a non-resonant, discontinuous contact method of AFM measurement. The probe moved vertically in a sinusoidal manner.

2.8. Total Protein Assay

MVs and cell pellets were lysed using a RIPA buffer (Thermo Fisher, Waltham, MA, USA) with the addition of Halt Protease Inhibitor Cocktail (Thermo Fisher, Waltham, MA, USA) to prevent protein degradation. Lysates were incubated for 30 min at 4 °C and then centrifuged at 16,000× g for 30 min at 4 °C. The supernatant was collected and aliquoted for storage at −80 °C. The total protein concentration in the samples was determined using a Pierce BCA Protein Assay Kit (Thermo Fisher, Waltham, MA, USA) according to the manufacturer's instructions. Optical density (OD) measurements were performed at 562 nm using an Infinite 200 Pro microplate reader (Tecan, Männedorf, Switzerland).

2.9. Western Blot Analysis

For immunoblotting, samples were subjected to SDS-PAGE electrophoresis in TGX FastCast 12% gel (Bio-Rad, Hercules, CA, USA) at 70 V and 180 V. Briefly, 1 μg of total protein per well was loaded for primary T-cell samples, and 2 μg of protein per well for SupT1 cell samples. Western C protein ruler (Bio-Rad, Hercules, CA, USA) was used for size estimation. The SDS-PAGE gels were transferred to 0.45 μm PVDF membranes (Bio-Rad, Hercules, CA, USA) using a Mini Trans-Blot Cell (Bio-Rad, Hercules, CA, USA) at a constant voltage of 17 V for 30 min using Turbo Transfer Buffer (Bio-Rad, Hercules, CA, USA). The membrane was blocked with 5.0% nonfat dry milk in PBS-Tween for 1.5 h at room temperature. The β-actin antibody (A00730, GenScript, Piscataway, NJ, USA) was used at a dilution of 1:2000 in 5% milk-PBS-Tween for staining for 1.5 h at room temperature. The membranes were then washed with PBST-Tween for 4 × 15 min. The primary antibody to the protein of interest was used overnight at 4 °C at the recommended dilution with slow mixing. The membranes were washed with PBS-Tween for 4 × 15 min. HRP-conjugated secondary antibody was then added at the recommended dilution in 5% milk-PBS-Tween and incubated for 1 h at room temperature, followed by washing with PBS-Tween for 4 × 15 min. Then, 1.2 mL Pierce ECL Western Blotting Substrate (Bio-Rad,

Hercules, CA, USA) was added, and the membranes were incubated for 2–5 min. Images of the membranes were obtained using the ChemiDoc XRS+ system (Bio-Rad, Hercules, CA, USA). The images were processed densitometrically in ImageJ (1.53k) software for relative protein amount estimation and β-actin normalization.

List of antibodies used: CD3 (ab699, Abcam, Waltham, MA, USA), granzyme B (ab134933, Abcam, Waltham, MA, USA), MHCII (ab180779, Abcam, Waltham, MA, USA), calnexin (MAA280Hu22, Cloud-Clone, Wuhan, China), HSP-70 (AF5466, Affinity, Darlinghurst, Australia), Lamin B1 (PAF548Mi01, Cloud-Clone, Wuhan, China), anti-rabbit HRP-conjugated antibody (ab9751, Abcam, Waltham, MA, USA), anti-mouse HRP-conjugated antibody (ab205729, Abcam, Waltham, MA, USA).

2.10. Fluorometric Assay

The fluorometric assay was performed using a VarioSkan microplate reader (Thermo Fisher, Waltham, MA, USA) in a black 96-well plate. For the DiI (Thermo Fisher, Waltham, MA, USA) and Calcein AM (Abcam, Waltham, MA, USA) assays, cells were pre-stained prior to obtaining vesicles. Cells were washed twice with DPBS, stained with the dyes for 20 min in a CO_2 incubator, washed twice to remove the dyes, and then used for AV induction. A suspension of vesicles from stained cells in DPBS was used for the fluorometric assay. For Hoechst 33258 (Abcam, USA), AVs were first obtained and then stained with Hoechst 33258 for 20 min.

2.11. Flow Cytometry

For flow cytometry, 3×10^5 cells were harvested, washed twice with DPBS, and stained with antibodies for 20 min. Cells were then washed twice to remove antibodies, and flow cytometry analysis was performed using FACS Aria III (BD Biosciences, Fremont, CA, USA). List of antibodies used: CD3-FITC (344804, Biolegend, San Diego, CA, USA), CD4-APC (354408, Biolegend, San Diego, CA, USA), and CD8-PE (344706, Biolegend, San Diego, CA, USA).

2.12. Statistical Analysis

Kruskal–Wallis test with Dunn's post hoc test was used for atomic force microscopy data. One-way ANOVA with Tukey post hoc test was used for fluorometric and total protein data, except for the Hoechst33258 assay, for which a *t*-test was used. Data analysis was performed using GraphPad Prism 5. In the graphs, p-value < 0.05 is marked *, $p < 0.01$ is marked **, and $p < 0.001$ is marked ***.

3. Results

3.1. Cytochalasin B and Ultrasonication Result in T-Cell AVs with Different Yield, Size Distribution, and Mechanical Properties

Our aim was to investigate the ability of cytochalasin B (ChB) and ultrasonication (US) to induce the generation of AVs from T cells and to assess their yield and size. To achieve this, we first isolated PBMCs, which were then activated with CD3/CD28 antibodies and expanded for two weeks in media containing IL-2. The cells were then washed twice with DPBS, split in half, and placed in optimized serum-free media. One half was left to incubate, while the other was first reactivated with CD3/CD28 antibodies and then incubated. After 48 h, the supernatants were collected as a source of natural T cell-derived MVs. The cells were then washed twice with DPBS and used to obtain AVs. All samples were processed in parallel by differential centrifugation (see list of samples in Table 1 and scheme in Figure 2).

The obtained samples were analyzed using nanoparticle tracking analysis (Figure 3). The particle concentration was measured and used to calculate the microvesicle yield per parent cell (Figure 4A). In general, AVs generated with ChB or US showed a lower mean and mode size than natural MVs (Figure 4B). For natural MVs, the yield was equal to 1858 particles per cell, whereas after activation, this number increased three-fold. Cytochalasin B allowed us to obtain AVs with a yield comparable to that of natural MVs. Ultrasonication alone produced AVs at a level similar to activation (4978 AVs US per T cell vs. 5437 aMVs per activated T cell), and ultrasonication combined with activation led to a seven-fold increase in the yield of AVs compared to natural MVs. Using a similar ultrasonication induction method, Wang et al. reported an 18.5-fold increase in AV yield from mesenchymal stem cells (MSCs) compared to natural MVs [11]. Interestingly, cytochalasin B-induced AVs from renal carcinoma cell lines (786-O, ACHN) showed only a 1.8–3.7-fold increase in yield compared to natural MVs [12].

Table 1. List of sample abbreviations and methods of induction.

Cell Source	Method of Induction	Sample Abbreviation
Resting T cells	No (natural secretion)	MVs (naturally secreted microvesicles)
Resting T cells (or SupT1 cells)	Cytochalasin B at 10 μg/mL for 30 min, with vortex	AVs ChB (artificial vesicles generated with cytochalasin B)
Resting T cells (or SupT1 cells)	Ultrasonication 20 kHz, amplitude 36 μm, 1 min (0.5 s sonication, 0.5 s pause)	AVs US (artificial vesicles generated with ultrasonication)
Activated T cells	No (natural secretion)	aMVs (natural microvesicles from activated T cells)
Activated T cells	Cytochalasin B at 10 μg/mL for 30 min, with vortex	AVs aChB (artificial vesicles from activated T cells generated with cytochalasin B)
Activated T cells	Ultrasonication 20 kHz, amplitude 36 μm, 1 min (0.5 s sonication, 0.5 s pause)	AVs aUS (artificial vesicles generated from activated T cells with ultrasonication)

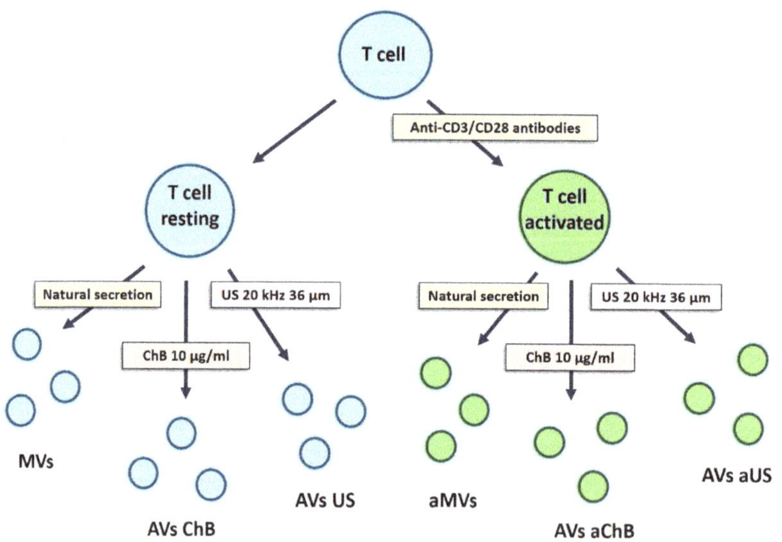

Figure 2. Scheme of experiments with primary T cells. Two types of cell sources were used—resting and activated T cells. Additionally, two types of induction were tested—chemical induction with cytochalasin B and physical induction with ultrasonication. Naturally secreted vesicles were used as a control.

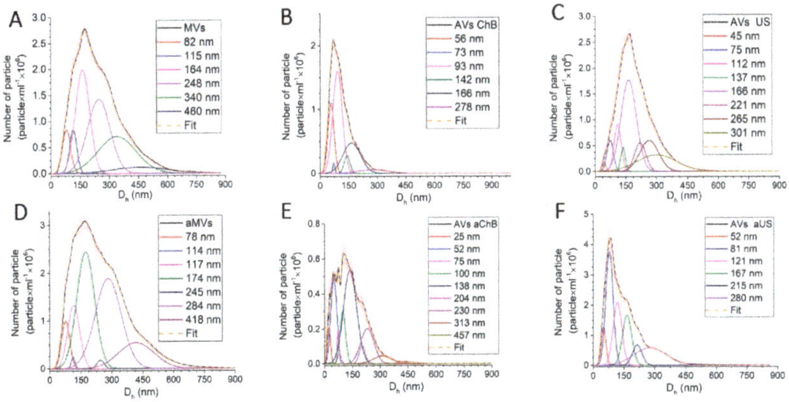

Figure 3. Size distribution measured by nanoparticle tracking analysis of vesicle samples generated from T cells: (**A**) MVs (naturally secreted from resting T cells); (**B**) AVs ChB (artificial vesicles generated with cytochalasin B from resting T cells); (**C**) AVs US (artificial vesicles generated with ultrasonication from resting T cells); (**D**) aMVs (MVs secreted by activated T cells); (**E**) AVs aChB (artificial vesicles generated with cytochalasin B from activated T cells); (**F**) AVs aUS (artificial vesicles generated with ultrasonication from activated T cells).

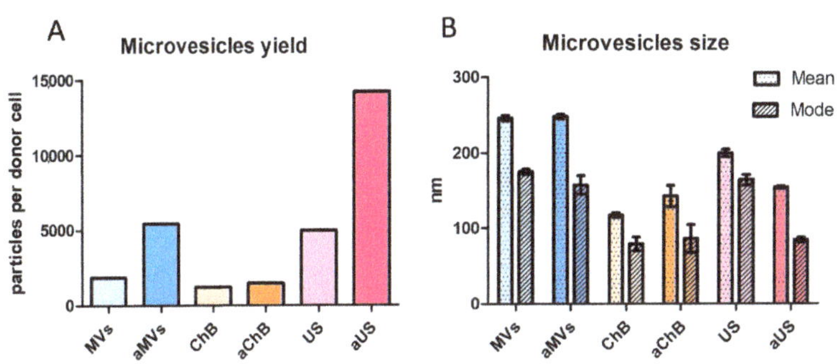

Figure 4. Comparison of yields and sizes of microvesicles generated using different induction techniques: (**A**) calculated microvesicle yields (number) per donor primary T cell (calculation is based on concentration measured by nanoparticle tracking analysis); (**B**) mean and mode microvesicle sizes measured by nanoparticle tracking analysis. MVs (naturally secreted from resting T cells); AVs ChB (artificial vesicles generated with cytochalasin B from resting T cells); AVs US (artificial vesicles generated with ultrasonication from resting T cells); aMVs (MVs secreted by activated T cells); AVs aChB (artificial vesicles generated with cytochalasin B from activated T cells); AVs aUS (artificial vesicles generated with ultrasonication from activated T cells). All samples were analyzed in five repetitions.

In terms of particle size distribution, we found that both chemical (ChB) and physical (US) induction methods resulted in more uniform MVs with lower dispersion and smaller average size than natural MVs in general (Figure 3). Functional analysis revealed interesting patterns, suggesting that irrespective of the type of induction, a population of vesicles with a size of 77 ± 3 nm was present in all samples. Another population of small vesicles 114–115 nm in size was also observed (Figure 3A,D). We assume that both 77 ± 3 nm and 114–115 nm particles represent exosomes that are characteristic of natural vesicles from resting and activated T cells. The next well-differentiated population of natural MVs is 169 ± 5 nm in size, while other larger fractions potentially can be attributed to smaller vesicle associates, as observed in a recent study [8]. Cytochalasin B-induced membrane vesicles demonstrated lower polydispersity with a significant population of small particles 51 ± 5 nm in size (Figure 3B,E). At the same time, vesicles generated with ChB from activated T cells contained many larger particle clusters, consistent with AFM data (Figure 5). Ultrasonication-induced vesicles showed a similar set of clusters but with the opposite correlation between resting and activated T cells; vesicles from activated T cells were predominantly represented by a 45–52 nm population with smaller mean size and polydispersity (Figure 3C,F). These observations were also consistent with AFM data (Figure 5C,F).

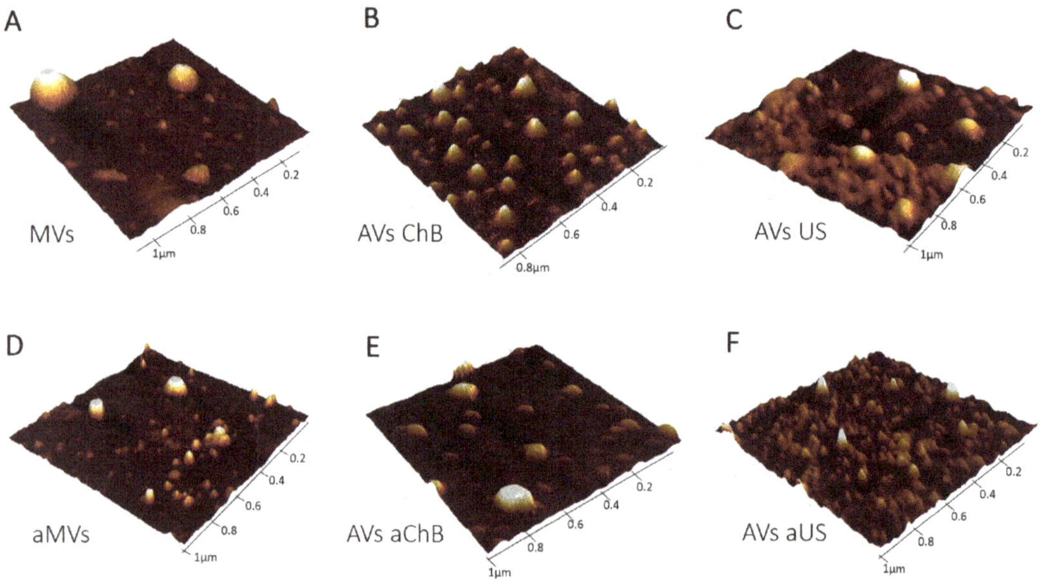

Figure 5. Images of microvesicle samples obtained by atomic force microscopy: (**A**) MVs (naturally secreted from resting T cells); (**B**) AVs ChB (artificial vesicles generated with cytochalasin B from resting T cells); (**C**) AVs US (artificial vesicles generated with ultrasonication from resting T cells); (**D**) aMVs (MVs secreted by activated T cells); (**E**) AVs aChB (artificial vesicles generated with cytochalasin B from activated T cells); (**F**) AVs aUS (artificial vesicles generated with ultrasonication from activated T cells).

AFM was used to visualize the vesicles (Figure 5) as one of the recommended methods of single-particle study by MISEV2023 (Minimal Information for Studies of Extracellular Vesicles 2023). In general, the obtained images are consistent with the NTA results in terms of particle size and dispersion. The samples that were the most homogeneous and contained smaller particles were generated with cytochalasin B from resting T cells and with ultrasonication from activated T cells, while naturally secreted MVs from resting or activated T cells were more variable in size and larger in general. The mechanical properties of the vesicles, such as adhesion and deformation, were also evaluated by AFM (Figure 6). We found that vesicles from activated T cells had higher adhesion (Figure 6A) than vesicles from resting T cells, and this parameter also increased across the natural/ChB/US range. The AFM probe was made of silicon nitride and was negatively charged due to oxidation during the experiment, so this observed interaction may be electrostatic in nature [13]. The activation of T cells results in an increased presence of surface proteins such as T-cell receptor (TCR) or major histocompatibility complex (MHC) that, along with many other proteins, may contain positively charged motifs available for electrostatic interaction [14].

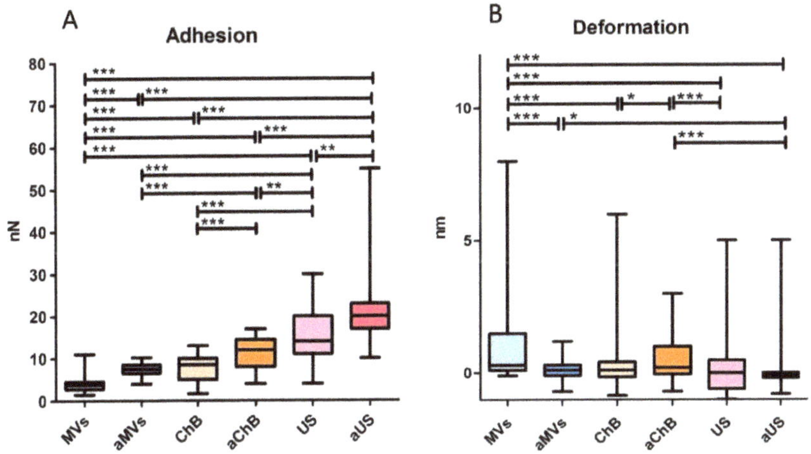

Figure 6. Adhesion and deformation properties of various microvesicles obtained by atomic force microscopy: (**A**) relative adhesion of microvesicles; (**B**) relative deformation of microvesicles, n = 85–220 depending on the sample. MVs (naturally secreted from resting T cells); AVs ChB (artificial vesicles generated with cytochalasin B from resting T cells); AVs US (artificial vesicles generated with ultrasonication from resting T cells); aMVs (MVs secreted by activated T cells); AVs aChB (artificial vesicles generated with cytochalasin B from activated T cells); AVs aUS (artificial vesicles generated with ultrasonication from activated T cells). p-value < 0.05 is marked *, p < 0.01 is marked **, and p < 0.001 is marked ***.

Despite significant differences in deformation properties observed in some of the samples (Figure 6B), there seems to be a minor tendency toward lower deformation in vesicles generated from activated T cells and across the natural/ChB/US range.

3.2. AVs from SupT1 Cells Contain Various Cellular Components of the Donor Cells

SupT1 cells were used to estimate the transfer of various cellular components into generated AVs using fluorometric assays and Western blot analysis. Several fluorescent probes were selected for the fluorometric assay, including Calcein AM cell-permeant dye used to determine cell viability, Katushka2S exogenous red fluorescent protein expressed in the cytoplasm, DiI lipophilic dye for membrane staining, and Hoechst 33342 for dsDNA staining. We also aimed to determine whether AVs were formed by the disruption of the cell membrane or by membrane budding. To achieve this, we collected AVs from an equal number of SupT1(Kat+) cells at different dilutions (10×10^6 cells/mL, 5×10^6 cells/mL, and 2.5×10^6 cells/mL) for samples stained with Calcein AM and DiI.

The total protein concentration measured in AVs by bicinchoninic acid assay confirmed that the yield was higher after US treatment compared to ChB, which is consistent with the NTA results. Furthermore, the yield was not affected by cell dilution for ChB-treated samples (Figures 7F and 8C,F). The differences between diluted US-treated samples can be explained by the variation in sample volume, which is critical due to the physical basis of the method.

Initially, SupT1 cells were simultaneously stained with DiI and Calcein AM, and then AVs were generated by ChB or US treatment. DiI fluorescence showed a much higher yield of the lipid component for AVs US at higher dilutions, whereas for Avs ChB, the maximum yield was in the middle of the concentration range (Figure 7A,D). By contrast, no significant difference in fluorescence was observed across samples stained with Calcein AM (Figure 7B). Interestingly, when the fluorescence of Calcein AM-stained cells was normalized to total protein or lipid (DiI fluorescence) levels, we observed a tendency for a decreased normalized Calcein AM signal for highly diluted samples (Figure 7C,E). This may indicate membrane disruption during AVs US formation. In addition, for Avs US the Calcein AM fluorescence normalized to total protein content was much lower than for AVs ChB, suggesting a greater loss of cytoplasmic content.

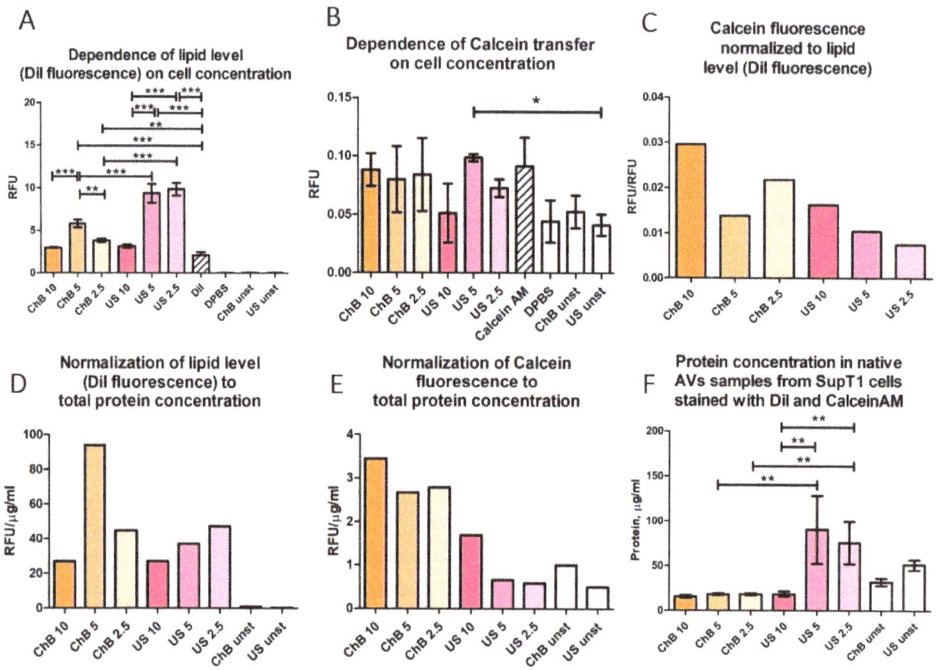

Figure 7. Transfer of SupT1 cytoplasmic compartments to AVs measured by fluorometric assay. ChB 10, ChB 5, and ChB 2.5 refer to AV samples obtained by cytochalasin B induction of cell suspensions diluted to 10×10^6 cells/mL, 5×10^6 cells/mL, or 2.5×10^6 cells/mL, respectively. US 10, US 5, US 2.5 refer to AV samples obtained by ultrasonication induction of cell suspensions diluted to 10×10^6 cells/mL, 5×10^6 cells/mL, or 2.5×10^6 cells/mL, respectively. All other samples were prepared from 5×10^6 cells/mL SupT1 suspension. Unst—vesicles obtained from unstained cells; DPBS—clear DPBS; DiI or Calcein—DPBS with dye at concentration used for staining: (**A**) fluorescence of DiI in samples obtained from different cell dilutions; (**B**) fluorescence of Calcein in samples obtained from different cell dilutions; (**C**) Calcein fluorescence normalized to lipid level; (**D**) lipid level normalized to total protein concentration; (**E**) Calcein fluorescence normalized to total protein concentration; (**F**) protein concentration in native samples obtained from different cell dilutions. All samples were analyzed in triplets. p-value < 0.05 is marked *, p < 0.01 is marked **, and p < 0.001 is marked ***.

From this point of view, the results for AVs obtained from SupT1(Kat+) cells may be somewhat ambiguous (Figure 8A–C). For both AVs ChB and AVs US an increase in Katushka2S fluorescence was observed, as the source cells were diluted. However, AVs US consistently showed lower Katushka2S fluorescence compared to AVs ChB, similar to that of Calcein AM staining.

Next, we determined whether the AVs contained residual parent cell DNA. To investigate this, AVs generated from SupT1 cells were stained with Hoechst 33258. The fluorometric assay showed that only AVs US, but not AVs ChB, contained dsDNA (Figure 8D–F). These results suggest that the method of AV induction can have a significant impact on the quality and cargo content of the resulting vesicles. Therefore, careful consideration of the method used for AV generation is critical for reliable experimental results.

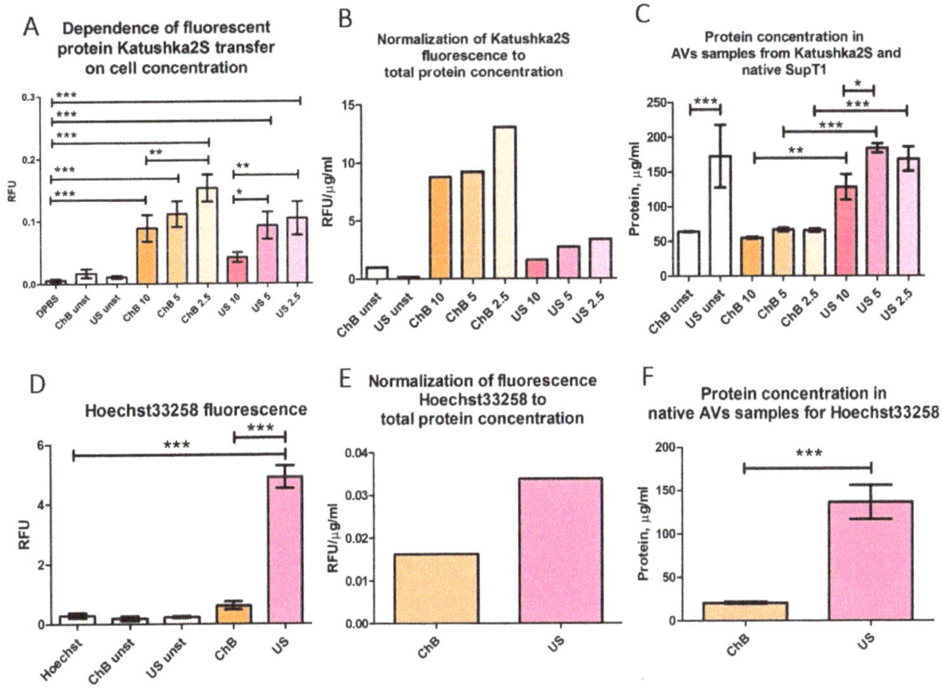

Figure 8. Transfer of SupT1 cytoplasmic fluorescent protein Katushka2S and nuclei to AVs measured by fluorometric assay: (**A–C**) Fluorometric data of Katushka2S transfer into AVs; ChB 10, ChB 5, and ChB 2.5 refer to AV samples induced with cytochalasin B from cell suspension diluted to 10×10^6 cells/mL, 5×10^6 cells/mL, or 2.5×10^6 cells/mL, respectively. US 10, US 5, and US 2.5 refer to AV samples induced with ultrasonication from cell suspension diluted to 10×10^6 cells/mL, 5×10^6 cells/mL, or 2.5×10^6 cells/mL, respectively. All other samples were obtained from SupT1 cells at 5×10^6 cells/mL. (**D–F**) Fluorometric data of AVs, stained by Hoechst33258 for detection of double-strand DNA. DPBS—clear DPBS; ChB unst, US unst—samples of vesicles, obtained from non-fluorescent or unstained cells; Hoechst—DPBS with dye at concentration used for staining. All samples were analyzed in triplets. p-value < 0.05 is marked *, $p < 0.01$ is marked **, and $p < 0.001$ is marked ***.

Western blot (WB) analysis also confirmed the transfer of various cellular components from the parental cells to AVs (Figure 9). All samples were normalized to total protein before loading; however, they had different β-actin contents, most likely due to the discrepancies in transfer efficiency during induction. Therefore, non-normalized data are also provided for diligent analysis.

Calnexin (90 kDa) is an important membrane-bound component of the endoplasmic reticulum (ER) [15] and is recommended by MISEV2023 (Minimal Information for Studies of Extracellular Vesicles 2023) guidelines as a marker of ER content in EVs. WB analysis showed that AVs ChB contained ER amounts comparable to that of the parental SupT1 cells when normalized to β-actin, whereas AVs US contained much higher ER amounts. However, in absolute amounts (not normalized to β-actin), AVs ChB and AVs US demonstrated comparable ER levels, which were higher than in SupT1 cells (Figure 9A).

Hsp70 (70 kDa) is a chaperone protein found in several cellular compartments, including the nucleus and mitochondria [16]. However, according to the MISEV2023 guidelines, Hsp70 should be considered a cytosolic protein found inside EVs. Our results showed that EVs ChB contained less Hsp70 than parental SupT1 cells after normalization to β-actin.

However, this may be due to the higher contents of β-actin in total protein rather than actual differences in Hsp70 levels. According to WB results, AVs US appeared to contain insignificant Hsp70 amounts, and it was difficult to distinguish this from the artifact signals of the non-specific binding (Figure 9B).

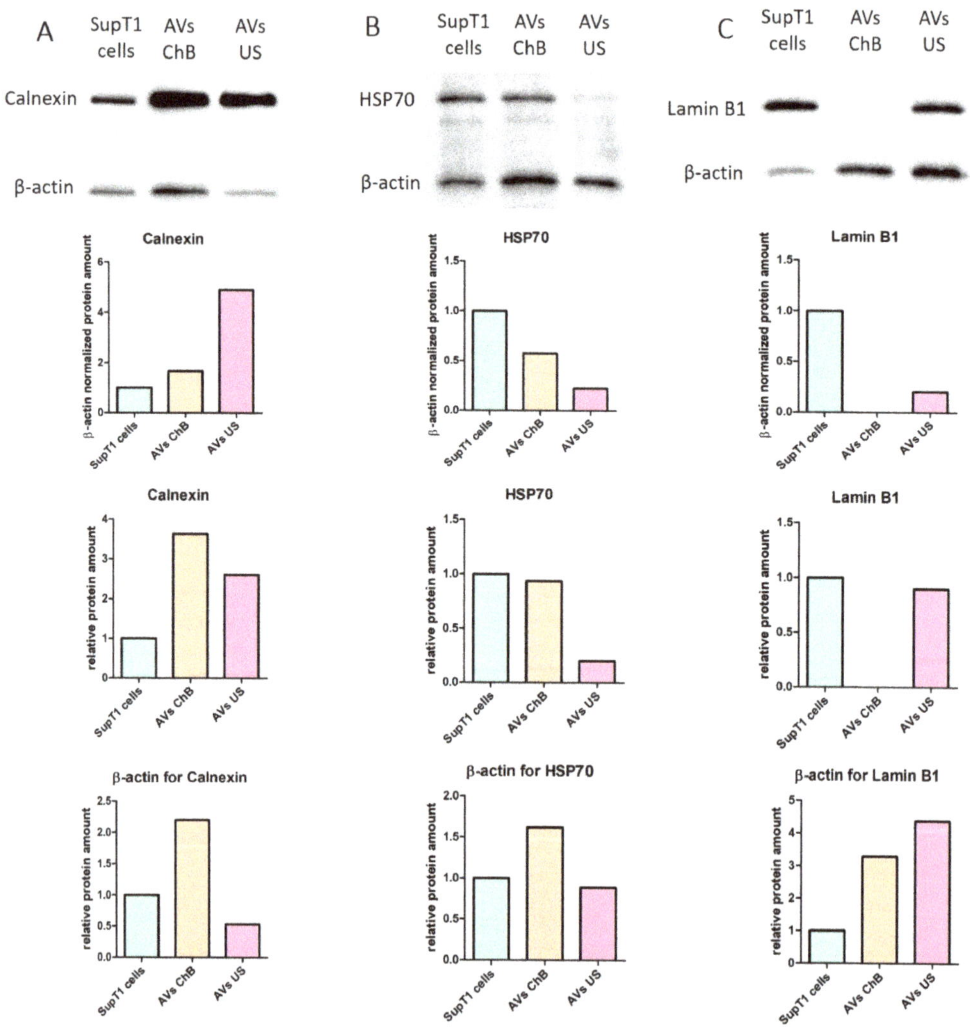

Figure 9. Transfer of SupT1 cell compartment into AVs measured by immunoblotting analysis: (**A**) immunoblotting analysis of calnexin (endoplasmic reticulum marker); (**B**) immunoblotting analysis of Hsp70 (cytosolic marker); (**C**) immunoblotting analysis of lamin B1 (nuclear marker). Data include immunoblotting images, calculated levels of the normalized target protein, and β-actin.

Lamin B1 is a key component of the nuclear lamina, which comprises the inner nuclear membrane and nucleoplasm [17]. The lack of Lamin B1 in AVs ChB suggests the absence of the nuclear fraction, consistent with the presumed induction mechanism (Figure 9C). Meanwhile, AVs US contained nuclear components from the parental cells, albeit at lower levels than in the cells themselves. Further investigation is required to determine the exact mechanism underlying the transfer of nuclear components in AVs US and whether this is due to the cell isolation process or a natural feature associated with their formation.

In summary, AVs ChB appear to be strikingly similar to their parental cells in terms of content, except for nuclear components. In contrast, AVs US were found to consist mainly of membranes and membrane-bound components of the parental cells. Further research is needed to fully understand the formation mechanism, composition, and functions of these types of AVs.

3.3. AVs from Primary T Cells Generated with Cytochalasin B or Ultrasonication Carry Key Functional Proteins

We also investigated whether T cell-derived extracellular vesicles contained functionally important proteins. The expression of CD3 on the surface of T cells is well known to become enhanced upon activation [18]. We aimed to determine whether CD3 is detectable on T cell-derived EVs. For that, we performed WB analysis and normalized the data to β-actin. Our results showed a relative increase in CD3 levels in all types of vesicles tested, especially in the case of AVs aUS obtained from activated T cells. Notably, natural MVs showed the highest absolute levels of CD3 (Figure 10A).

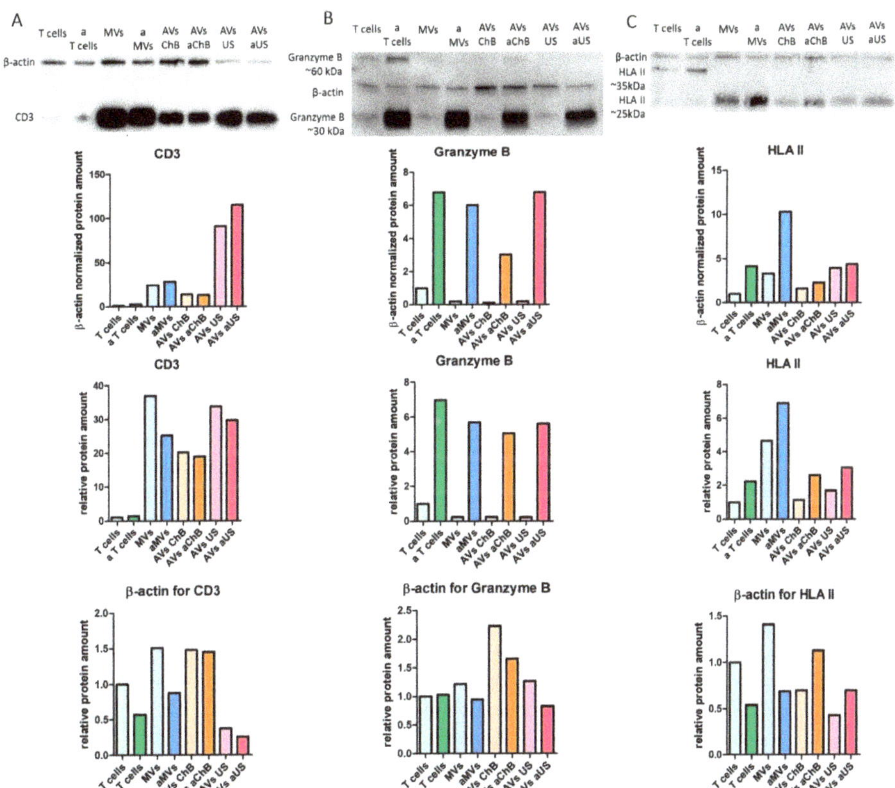

Figure 10. Functionally important proteins (CD3, granzyme B, and HLA II) presented in different types of AVs, obtained from resting T cells (MVs, AVs ChB, and AVs US) or activated T cells (aMVs, AVs aChB, and AVs aUS): (**A**) immunoblotting analysis of CD3; (**B**) immunoblotting analysis of granzyme B; (**C**) immunoblotting analysis of HLA II. Data include immunoblotting images, calculated levels of the normalized target protein, and β-actin.

Granzyme B (30 kDa) is one of the major effectors of cytotoxic T lymphocyte (CTL)-mediated cell death that is released into the extracellular space upon T-cell activation, where it penetrates target tumor cells via perforin-mediated entry [19]. Our results showed that all vesicles obtained from activated T cells had similar levels of granzyme B (Figure 10B). The 60 kDa bands observed in the T-cell samples most likely represent dimers [20] that did not dissociate under SDS-PAGE conditions. However, no such dimers were found in the vesicle samples, except for AVs aChB.

HLA II expression reflects the antigen-presenting function of T lymphocytes and is predominantly known as a characteristic of $CD4^+$ Th cells, which increases after activation [21]. HLA II is a heterodimer consisting of α-chain (approximately 35 kDa) and β-chain (approximately 25 kDa) that normally dissociates after boiling under SDS-PAGE conditions [22]. Interestingly, we found that the 35 kDa subunit was predominantly present in T-cell samples, whereas the 25 kDa subunit was much more abundant in microvesicle samples (Figure 10C). Nevertheless, the overall HLA II content in microvesicles appeared to be high, especially in the case of microvesicles generated from pre-activated T cells.

4. Discussion

The relatively well-established field of natural EVs is now being complemented by industry-oriented approaches to generate artificial vesicles with uniform properties and high yields. In this study, we aimed to evaluate the induction of T-cell microvesicles using cytochalasin B and ultrasonication and to compare the resulting products with natural EVs and parental cells.

We have shown that both cytochalasin B and ultrasonication can induce the formation of artificial vesicles (AVs) (Figure 11). Considering the number of particles and the total protein content, ultrasonication appears to be more efficient in producing higher quantities of AVs. However, in terms of the quality of the resulting AVs, these two induction methods yielded different results. In contrast, AVs induced by ultrasonication showed higher self-inclusion of membrane-bound proteins and parental cell DNA and had lower content of cytosolic and cytoplasmic proteins. Importantly, membrane disruption during ultrasonication could potentially be exploited to enhance AVs with therapeutic or otherwise functional payload, e.g., small-molecule drugs, genetic vectors, proteins, fluorescent compounds, etc.

In the biopharmaceutical industry, the manufacturing of AVs requires high efficiency, scalability, simplicity of technology, and a minimal chemical footprint. These features are necessary to make upstream and downstream processes cost-effective while ensuring that the final product is functional and safe. From this perspective, ultrasonication as an induction method appears to be one of the most attractive techniques for producing AVs for therapeutic purposes.

Cell-free therapy modality in the context of T cells is a highly promising technology. Nowadays, T cells are used and studied for the treatment of various diseases such as oncology, autoimmune disorders, and many others. In all these fields, artificial vesicles could contribute to significant progress, for example, by facilitating access through dense solid tumor microenvironment, overcoming immunosuppressive tumor resistance to CAR-T therapy, providing increased safety, and presenting the possibility of allogeneic production.

However, significant research gaps remain to be addressed by the scientific community. These include the need to investigate the content of AVs as a time- and cell-type dependent process and its impact on the properties of the resulting AVs, especially for activated immune cells as a source. In addition, the functional capacity of AVs is an open question that requires further investigation. The wide range of technology implementation gives rise to a number of promising research directions. Different cell sources, genetic modification of parent cells (e.g., to achieve allogeneicity or to increase specificity or efficacy), and additional loading with small molecules are promising but not limited avenues for further development.

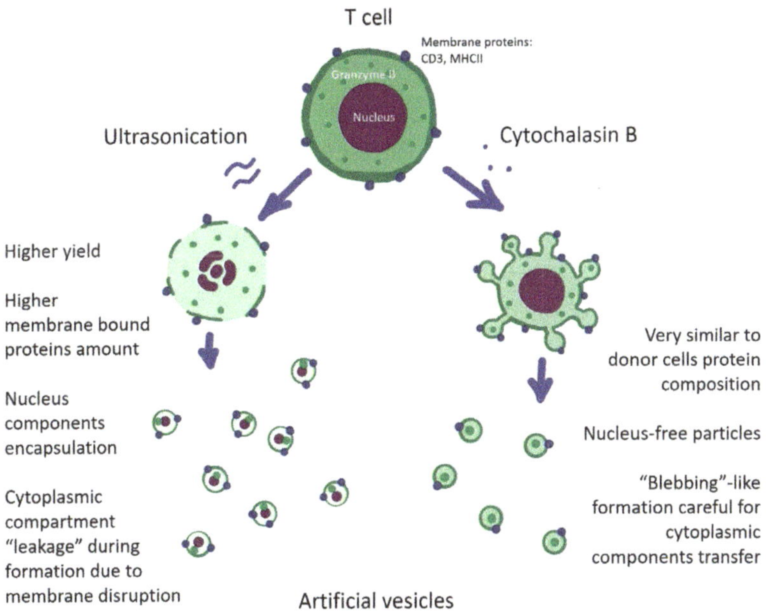

Figure 11. Formation of artificial vesicles from T cells using physical induction by ultrasonication and chemical induction by cytochalasin B. Ultrasonication causes disruption of the cell membrane with partial leakage of cell contents, while membrane proteins are transferred to vesicles. Cytochalasin B induces vesiculation from the cell surface with effective intracellular transfer of cytoplasmic contents. In both cases, functional components such as granzyme B are transferred to the resulting vesicles.

Supplementary Materials: The following supporting information can be downloaded at: https://www.mdpi.com/article/10.3390/biomedicines12040919/s1, Figure S1: Flow cytometry phenotyping of T cells used for AV generation, A—CD3$^+$ stained T-cells, B—CD4$^+$ and CD8$^+$ subpopulations of CD3$^+$ T-cells. Figure S2: Percentage of Katushka2S-positive cells in SupT1 cells used for AV generation.

Author Contributions: Conceptualization, E.A.Z. and E.R.B.; data curation, E.A.Z., S.A.M., I.A.G., E.M.G., E.T.S. and A.A.K.; formal analysis, E.A.Z., E.T.S., A.A.K. and M.P.K.; funding acquisition, investigation, E.A.Z.; methodology, E.A.Z., E.T.S., A.A.K., Y.Y. and E.R.B.; project administration, E.A.Z. and E.R.B.; resources, E.R.B.; supervision, E.R.B.; validation, E.A.Z.; visualization, E.A.Z.; writing—original draft preparation, E.A.Z.; writing—review and editing, E.A.Z. and E.R.B. All authors have read and agreed to the published version of the manuscript.

Funding: This research was funded by Russian Science Foundation grant #23-24-00224 and the APC was funded by the Russian Science Foundation grant #23-24-00224.

Institutional Review Board Statement: This study was conducted in accordance with the Declaration of Helsinki and approved by the Local Ethics Committee of Kazan Federal University (protocol N27; 28 December 2020).

Informed Consent Statement: Informed consent was obtained from all subjects involved in the study.

Data Availability Statement: The data that support the findings of this study are not openly available and are available from the corresponding author upon reasonable request.

Conflicts of Interest: The authors have no conflicts of interest to declare that are relevant to the content of this article.

References

1. Bahmani, L.; Ullah, M. Different Sourced Extracellular Vesicles and Their Potential Applications in Clinical Treatments. *Cells* **2022**, *11*, 1989. [CrossRef] [PubMed]
2. Vergani, E.; Daveri, E.; Vallacchi, V.; Bergamaschi, L.; Lalli, L.; Castelli, C.; Rodolfo, M.; Rivoltini, L.; Huber, V. Extracellular vesicles in anti-tumor immunity. *Semin. Cancer Biol.* **2022**, *86 Pt 1*, 64–79. [CrossRef] [PubMed]
3. Zhang, F.; Guo, J.; Zhang, Z.; Duan, M.; Wang, G.; Qian, Y.; Zhao, H.; Yang, Z.; Jiang, X. Application of engineered extracellular vesicles for targeted tumor therapy. *J. Biomed. Sci.* **2022**, *29*, 14. [CrossRef] [PubMed]
4. Ramos-Zaldívar, H.M.; Polakovicova, I.; Salas-Huenuleo, E.; Corvalán, A.H.; Kogan, M.J.; Yefi, C.P.; Andia, M.E. Extracellular vesicles through the blood-brain barrier: A review. *Fluids Barriers CNS* **2022**, *19*, 60. [CrossRef] [PubMed]
5. Chen, J.; Tan, Q.; Yang, Z.; Jin, Y. Engineered extracellular vesicles: Potentials in cancer combination therapy. *J. Nanobiotechnol.* **2022**, *20*, 132. [CrossRef] [PubMed]
6. Estes, S.; Konstantinov, K.; Young, J.D. Manufactured extracellular vesicles as human therapeutics: Challenges, advances, and opportunities. *Curr. Opin. Biotechnol.* **2022**, *77*, 102776. [CrossRef] [PubMed]
7. Syromiatnikova, V.; Prokopeva, A.; Gomzikova, M. Methods of the Large-Scale Production of Extracellular Vesicles. *Int. J. Mol. Sci.* **2022**, *23*, 10522. [CrossRef] [PubMed]
8. Khannanov, A.; Burmatova, A.; Ignatyeva, K.; Vagizov, F.; Kiiamov, A.; Tayurskii, D.; Cherosov, M.; Gerasimov, A.; Vladimir, E.; Kutyreva, M. Effect of the Synthetic Approach on the Formation and Magnetic Properties of Iron-Based Nanophase in Branched Polyester Polyol Matrix. *Int. J. Mol. Sci.* **2022**, *23*, 14764. [CrossRef] [PubMed]
9. Malloy, A.; Hole, P.; Carr, B. NanoParticle Tracking Analysis. *Halo System MRS Online Proc. Libr.* **2006**, *952*, 204. [CrossRef]
10. Dragovic, R.A.; Gardiner, C.; Brooks, A.S.; Tannetta, D.S.; Ferguson, D.J.; Hole, P.; Carr, B.; Redman, C.W.; Harris, A.L.; Dobson, P.J.; et al. Sizing and phenotyping of cellular vesicles using Nanoparticle Tracking Analysis. *Nanomedicine* **2011**, *7*, 780–788. [CrossRef]
11. Wang, L.; Abhange, K.K.; Wen, Y.; Chen, Y.; Xue, F.; Wang, G.; Tong, J.; Zhu, C.; He, X.; Wan, Y. Preparation of Engineered Extracellular Vesicles Derived from Human Umbilical Cord Mesenchymal Stem Cells with Ultrasonication for Skin Rejuvenation. *ACS Omega* **2019**, *4*, 22638–22645. [CrossRef] [PubMed]
12. Nair, A.; Bu, J.; Rawding, P.A.; Do, S.C.; Li, H.; Hong, S. Cytochalasin B Treatment and Osmotic Pressure Enhance the Production of Extracellular Vesicles (EVs) with Improved Drug Loading Capacity. *Nanomaterials* **2022**, *12*, 3. [CrossRef] [PubMed]
13. Mueller, H.; Butt, H.-J.; Bamberg, E. Force Measurements on Myelin Basic Protein Adsorbed to Mica and Lipid Bilayer Surfaces Done with the Atomic Force Microscope. *Biophys. J.* **1999**, *76*, 1072–1079. [CrossRef] [PubMed]
14. Ma, Y.; Poole, K.; Goyette, J.; Gaus, K. Introducing Membrane Charge and Membrane Potential to T Cell Signaling. *Front. Immunol.* **2017**, *8*, 1513. [CrossRef] [PubMed]
15. Kozlov, G.; Gehring, K. Calnexin cycle—Structural features of the ER chaperone system. *FEBS J.* **2020**, *287*, 4322–4340. [CrossRef] [PubMed]
16. Longshaw, V.M.; Chapple, J.P.; Balda, M.S.; Cheetham, M.E.; Blatch, G.L. Nuclear translocation of the Hsp70/Hsp90 organizing protein mSTI1 is regulated by cell cycle kinases. *J. Cell Sci.* **2004**, *117 Pt 5*, 701–710. [CrossRef] [PubMed]
17. Evangelisti, C.; Rusciano, I.; Mongiorgi, S.; Ramazzotti, G.; Lattanzi, G.; Manzoli, L.; Cocco, L.; Ratti, S. The wide and growing range of lamin B-related diseases: From laminopathies to cancer. *Cell Mol. Life Sci.* **2022**, *79*, 126. [CrossRef] [PubMed]
18. Blanchard, N.; Lankar, D.; Faure, F.; Regnault, A.; Dumont, C.; Raposo, G.; Hivroz, C. TCR Activation of Human T Cells Induces the Production of Exosomes Bearing the TCR/CD3/ζ Complex. *J. Immunol.* **2002**, *168*, 3235–3241. [CrossRef] [PubMed]
19. Afonina, I.S.; Cullen, S.P.; Martin, S.J. Cytotoxic and non-cytotoxic roles of the CTL/NK protease granzyme B. *Immunol. Rev.* **2010**, *235*, 105–116. [CrossRef]
20. Estébanez-Perpiña, E.; Fuentes-Prior, P.; Belorgey, D.; Braun, M.; Kiefersauer, R.; Maskos, K.; Huber, R.; Rubin, H.; Bode, W. Crystal structure of the caspase activator human granzyme B, a proteinase highly specific for an Asp-P1 residue. *Biol. Chem.* **2000**, *381*, 1203–1214. [CrossRef]
21. Holling, T.M.; van der Stoep, N.; Quinten, E.; van den Elsen, P.J. Activated Human T Cells Accomplish MHC Class II Expression Through T Cell-Specific Occupation of Class II Transactivator Promoter III. *J. Immunol.* **2002**, *168*, 763–770. [CrossRef] [PubMed]
22. Serra, P.; Garabatos, N.; Singha, S.; Fandos, C.; Garnica, J.; Solé, P.; Parras, D.; Yamanouchi, J.; Blanco, J.; Tort, M.; et al. Increased yields and biological potency of knob-into-hole-based soluble MHC class II molecules. *Nat. Commun.* **2019**, *10*, 4917. [CrossRef] [PubMed]

biomedicines

MDPI

Article

Extracellular Vesicles Derived from Osteogenic-Differentiated Human Bone Marrow-Derived Mesenchymal Cells Rescue Osteogenic Ability of Bone Marrow-Derived Mesenchymal Cells Impaired by Hypoxia

Chenglong Wang [1], Sabine Stöckl [1], Girish Pattappa [2], Daniela Schulz [3], Korbinian Hofmann [1], Jovana Ilic [4], Yvonne Reinders [5], Richard J. Bauer [3], Albert Sickmann [5,6,7] and Susanne Grässel [1,*]

1 Department of Orthopedic Surgery, Experimental Orthopedics, Center for Medical Biotechnology (ZMB), Biopark 1, University of Regensburg, 93053 Regensburg, Germany; chenglong.wang@ukr.de (C.W.); sabine.stoeckl@ukr.de (S.S.); korbinian.hofmann@stud.uni-regensburg.de (K.H.)
2 Department of Trauma Surgery, Center for Medical Biotechnology (ZMB), Biopark 1, University of Regensburg, 93053 Regensburg, Germany; girish.pattappa@ukr.de
3 Department of Oral and Maxillofacial Surgery, Center for Medical Biotechnology (ZMB), Biopark 1, University Hospital Regensburg, 93053 Regensburg, Germany; daniela.schulz@ukr.de (D.S.); richard.bauer@ukr.de (R.J.B.)
4 IZKF Group Tissue Regeneration in Musculoskeletal Diseases, University Hospital & Bernhard-Heine-Centrum for Locomotion Research, University of Würzburg, 97070 Würzburg, Germany; j-ilic.klh@uni-wuerzburg.de
5 Leibniz-Institut für Analytische Wissenschaften—ISAS—e.V., Bunsen-Kirchhoff-Straße 11, 44139 Dortmund, Germany; yvonne.reinders@isas.de (Y.R.); albert.sickmann@isas.de (A.S.)
6 Medizinisches Proteom-Center, Ruhr-Universität Bochum, 44801 Bochum, Germany
7 Department of Chemistry, College of Physical Sciences, University of Aberdeen, Aberdeen AB24 3FX, UK
* Correspondence: susanne.graessel@ukr.de

Abstract: In orthopedics, musculoskeletal disorders, i.e., non-union of bone fractures or osteoporosis, can have common histories and symptoms related to pathological hypoxic conditions induced by aging, trauma or metabolic disorders. Here, we observed that hypoxic conditions (2% O_2) suppressed the osteogenic differentiation of human bone marrow-derived mesenchymal cells (hBMSC) in vitro and simultaneously increased reactive oxygen species (ROS) production. We assumed that cellular origin and cargo of extracellular vesicles (EVs) affect the osteogenic differentiation capacity of hBMSCs cultured under different oxygen pressures. Proteomic analysis revealed that EVs isolated from osteogenic differentiated hBMSC cultured under hypoxia (hypo-osteo EVs) or under normoxia (norm-osteo EVs) contained distinct protein profiles. Extracellular matrix (ECM) components, antioxidants and pro-osteogenic proteins were decreased in hypo-osteo EVs. The proteomic analysis in our previous study revealed that under normoxic culture conditions, pro-osteogenic proteins and ECM components have higher concentrations in norm-osteo EVs than in EVs derived from naïve hBMSCs (norm-naïve EVs). When selected for further analysis, five anti-hypoxic proteins were significantly upregulated (response to hypoxia) in norm-osteo EVs. Three of them are characterized as antioxidant proteins. We performed qRT-PCR to verify the corresponding gene expression levels in the norm-osteo EVs' and norm-naïve EVs' parent cells cultured under normoxia. Moreover, we observed that norm-osteo EVs rescued the osteogenic ability of naïve hBMSCs cultured under hypoxia and reduced hypoxia-induced elevation of ROS production in osteogenic differentiated hBMSCs, presumably by inducing expression of anti-hypoxic/ antioxidant and pro-osteogenic genes.

Keywords: extracellular vesicles; BMSC; osteogenic differentiation; hypoxia; normoxia; ROS; antioxidants

1. Introduction

Poor blood circulation affects tissue oxygen saturation levels in the human body, creating hypoxic pathological conditions that are the underlying cause of many human diseases, such as brain ischemia, heart attack and acute lung and kidney injury [1,2]. In orthopedics, many diseases have common pathological conditions related to hypoxia. For example, femoral head osteonecrosis can develop due to blood supply disruption, which results in hypoxic injury to the femoral head. The bone mineral loss, which arises from arteriosclerosis of the lower limbs, together with hypoxic ischemia, can induce osteoporosis [3]. In addition, basic reports [4,5] support the theory that these orthopedic diseases' pathological conditions are related to hypoxia. Hypoxia is able to impair bone regeneration by reducing the differentiation capacity of bone marrow-derived mesenchymal cells (BMSC) toward osteoblasts [6]. However, there are also other reports showing conflicting and inconsistent results regarding the influence of hypoxia on the osteogenic differentiation of precursor cells. Wagegg et al. [7] showed that osteogenic differentiation of naïve human (h)BMSCs is enhanced under hypoxic conditions compared to normoxic conditions. They concluded that hypoxia promotes osteogenesis of hBMSCs in a hypoxia-inducible factor (HIF)-1-dependent manner. HIFs are proteins that respond to changes in oxygen concentration and are subjected to proteosomal degradation under normoxia while they are stabilized under hypoxia [8].

'Reactive oxygen species' (ROS) is an umbrella term for an array of derivatives of molecular oxygen, including hydrogen peroxide (H_2O_2) and the superoxide anion radical (O_2^-). Changes in ROS production were shown to modulate diverse physiological processes [9,10], as excessive production of ROS is suggested to inhibit bone formation [11,12]. In general, hypoxic conditions affect ROS levels [13,14], suggesting that the ROS level is increased under hypoxia. Contrary, reports from other studies [15,16] showed that hypoxia caused a ROS level decrease compared to normoxic conditions in a pre-osteoblastic cell line and in macrophages. Thus, our **first aim** was to determine how hypoxia would affect the osteogenic differentiation ability of naïve hBMSCs and if it increases ROS production.

Extracellular vesicles (EVs) are enclosed by a lipid bilayer and released by a wide range of cell types (under physiological and pathological conditions), with diameters ranging from 50 to 200 nm [17,18]. EVs carry a wide range of bioactive molecules, including proteins, lipids, mRNAs, microRNAs (miRNAs), and long noncoding RNAs (lncRNAs), with EVs' cargo being directly dependent on the metabolic condition or the differentiation status of their parental cells [19–21]. Moreover, EVs, which function as cell-to-cell communicators, have emerged as an important route for interchanging proteins, lipids and genetic material between cells and tissues, similar to neurotransmitters acting as chemical messengers transmitting information between neurons [1,21]. In previous years, many therapeutic approaches for musculoskeletal disorders have been focused on MSC-based cell therapies due to their differentiation and immunomodulatory properties. MSC-EVs may account for a large part of these functions and are, therefore, under investigation as an alternative therapeutic approach to cell therapies. Immigrating MSCs into the bone defect secrete large amounts of EVs, and it was shown that MSC-EV-based approaches have the potential to promote bone regeneration [19].

EVs may play a pivotal role in cancer cell growth, progression, and metastasis in solid tumors [22]. It is well established that cell proliferation is rapid in tumors, but the vasculature formed is insufficient to maintain a sufficient oxygen level, leading to the development of a hypoxic tumor microenvironment [23,24]. The alteration in the composition and function of tumor-derived EVs mediated by hypoxia allows the tumor cells to respond to hypoxia and to modify their surrounding microenvironment [22,24]. Furthermore, several in vitro studies [25,26] suggested that EVs derived from tumor cells under hypoxia contain a unique protein signature that significantly enhances invasion compared to EVs from tumor cells grown under normoxia. However, according to our current knowledge, none of those studies addressed the analysis of EVs from osteogenic differentiated BMSCs under hypoxia. Therefore, the **second aim** of this study was to analyze the proteomes of EVs derived from osteogenic differentiated hBMSCs under normoxic or hypoxic conditions and to investigate whether osteogenic EVs generated under hypoxia are loaded with unique proteomic signatures, which would allow the cells to respond to hypoxia.

EVs are envisioned as promising bioactive effectors to promote the osteogenic differentiation capacity of MSCs, which induce the efficient repair of bone injuries [27,28]. Further, MSC-EVs can promote new bone formation with supporting vascularization and displaying improved morphological, biomechanical, and histological outcomes, coupled with positive effects on cell survival, proliferation, migration, osteogenesis, and angiogenesis [19].

Our previous study [29] showed that under normoxic conditions, EVs, isolated from hBMSCs at a late-stage of osteogenic differentiation, promote the osteogenic differentiation capacity of hBMSCs and, at the same time, have negative effects on the adipogenic differentiation capacity of hBMSCs. Current knowledge of the underlying molecular mechanisms of these pro-osteogenic and anti-adipogenic effects of EVs under hypoxia is very limited. Thus, in this study, the **third aim** was to further investigate why and how EVs derived from hBMSCs at late-stage osteogenic differentiation under normoxia enhance the osteogenic capacity of naïve hBMSCs cultured under hypoxia. The three aims of this study are summarized in Figure 1.

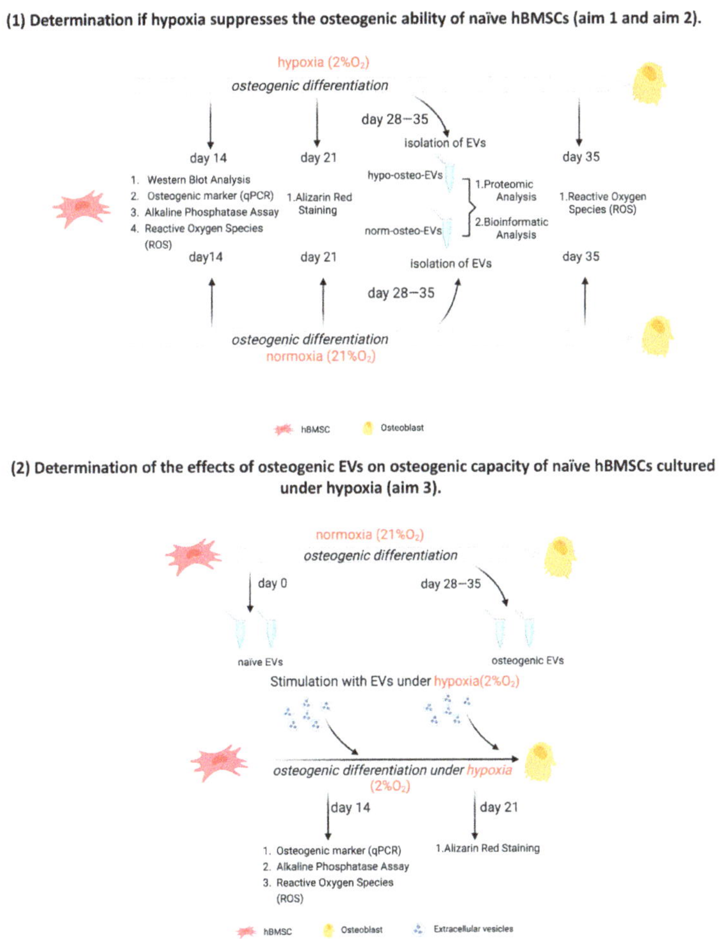

Figure 1. Overview of experimental set-up; EVs = extracellular vesicles.

2. Materials and Methods

A graphical illustration of the experimental set-up is shown in Figure 1.

2.1. Ethical Statement

This study has been approved by the local ethics committee (MSCs: Ethikkommission, No. 14-101-0189, University of Regensburg), and all patients' written informed consent was obtained before undergoing surgery (email: ethikkommission@klinik.uni-regensburg.de).

2.2. Isolation, Culture and Characterization of Immunophenotype of Human BMSCs

hBMSCs were prepared from frozen stocks obtained from the femoral bone marrow aspirate of twelve patients undergoing hip replacement surgery (mean age: 60.4 ± 8.7 years, range: 46–73 years, male: 50%). Density gradient centrifugation was used to isolate the hBMSCs according to established protocols [30–32]. hBMSCs were expanded until 80% confluency (passage 1–4) in StemMACS^{TM} MSC expansion medium (Miltenyi Biotec, Bergisch Gladbach, Germany) with the following composition: L-glutamine, fetal calf serum (FCS) (Sigma-Aldrich GmbH, Bergisch Gladbach, Germany), phenol red and supplemented with 0.2% MycoZap (Lonza, Basel, Switzerland). Flow cytometric analysis of hBMSC with specific antibodies against MSC positive marker (CD44, CD73) and negative marker (CD19, CD34) is shown in Supplementary Figure S1.

2.3. Generation of EVs-Depleted FCS

EVs-depleted FCS (FCS$^{depl\text{-}uc}$) was prepared according to established protocols [33,34]. In short, FCS was diluted in α-MEM medium to a final concentration of 20% and subsequently ultra-centrifuged at 120,000× *g* (Beckman Coulter, Brea, CA, USA) overnight (18 h) at 4 °C to generate EV-depleted FCS. FCS$^{depl\text{-}uc}$ was stored in aliquots at −20 °C. Medium used for EV collection and hBMSC stimulation was supplemented with 10% FCS$^{depl\text{-}uc}$.

2.4. Osteogenic Differentiation of Human BMSCs

For harvesting the conditioned medium (CM) for EV isolation, 3×10^6 hBMSCs (passage 4) were cultured in growth medium in triple T175 flasks (ThermoFisher, Dreieich, Germany) until 80% confluency before onset of osteogenic differentiation. To induce osteogenic differentiation of hBMSCs according to established protocols [32,34], the expansion medium was changed to osteogenic differentiation medium (α-MEM (Sigma-Aldrich, Steinheim, Germany), 10% FCS$^{depl\text{-}uc}$ or 10% regular FCS, 4 mM GlutaMAXTM-I (Gibco, Paisley, UK), 1% penicillin–streptomycin (P/S), 10 µM ascorbic acid-2-phosphate, 10 mM ß-glycerophosphate and 100 nM dexamethasone (all from Sigma-Aldrich, Steinheim, Germany). Osteogenic differentiation was terminated after a maximum of 35 days (medium was replaced every 3 days).

2.5. Induction of Hypoxia

A total of 2% oxygen is defined as a hypoxic condition according to published protocols [35,36]. For osteogenic differentiation under hypoxia, hBMSCs were cultured in a hypoxia incubator (ThermoFisher Scientific, Langenselbold, Germany) set at 2% O_2 and 5% CO_2 levels, balanced with 93% N_2. Normoxic control BMSCs were incubated in a standard cell culture incubator set at 20% oxygen, 5% CO_2 and 75% N_2.

2.6. Collection of Conditioned Medium for EV Isolation

Worth noting, 3×10^6 hBMSCs (passage 4) were expanded in triple T175 flasks in growth medium until 80% confluency under normoxia.

For harvesting the norm-naïve EVs, conditioned medium (CM) for EV isolation from undifferentiated naïve hBMSCs (i.e., norm-naïve EVs = naïve hBMSCs derived EVs) under normoxia, growth medium was replaced by α-MEM medium with 1% P/S, 10% FCS$^{depl\text{-}uc}$ and 4 mM GlutaMAXTM-I. After 48 h incubation under normoxic conditions, CM was stored immediately at −80 °C for subsequent EV isolation.

Osteogenic differentiation of hBMSCs was induced under normoxic or hypoxic conditions, respectively. For harvesting osteogenic CM under normoxia and hypoxia, regular FCS was replaced by 10% FCS$^{depl\text{-}uc}$ in the osteogenic medium on days 26, 28, 30 and 33 of culture. After 48 h incubation, CM was collected on days 28, 30, 32 and 35 under normoxic and hypoxic conditions, respectively. (i.e., hypo-osteo EVs containing CM = harvesting and pooling of CM from hBMSCs undergoing osteogenic differentiation from 28–35 days under hypoxia; norm-osteo EVs containing CM = harvesting and pooling CM after 28–35 days under normoxia) and stored at −80 °C for further processing.

2.7. EV Isolation

To isolate hypo-osteo EVs, norm-naïve EVs and norm-osteo EVs from the respective CM, ultracentrifugation was performed according to our previously published protocol [34,37]. In brief, the respective CM was centrifuged at 300× *g* (Sigma, Osterodea, Harz, Germany) for 10 min at 4 °C to remove intact cells. The supernatant was transferred to a new falcon tube and centrifuged again at 2000× *g* to remove dead cells. Afterward, the supernatant was transferred to a new tube and centrifuged for 30 min at 10,000× *g* to remove cell debris, and the subsequent supernatant was filtered (Filtropur S plus 0.2 µm; Sarstedt, Nümbrecht, Germany) into an ultracentrifugation tube (Polypropylene Centrifuge Tubes; Beckman Coulter, Brea, CA, USA) and was subjected to ultracentrifugation once at 120,000× *g* for 70 min at 4 °C. Following careful aspiration of the supernatant, the pellet was washed with PBS and centrifuged again (120,000× *g* for 70 min at 4 °C). The resulting EV pellets were resuspended in the presence of 25 mM trehalose (Carl Roth, Karlsruhe, Germany) in PBS. Protein concentration was measured using BCA Protein Assay Kit Pierce (Thermo Scientific, Rockford, IL, USA).

2.8. Conditioned Medium pH under Hypoxia and Normoxia

CM for isolation of hypo-osteo EVs and norm-osteo EVs was obtained as described above. Osteogenic medium with 10% FCS$^{depl\text{-}uc}$, kept in T75 flasks for two days either under hypoxia or normoxia (without cells), was set as control groups. Subsequently, all CM groups were collected, and pH of each CM was determined using a pH meter (Hanna Instruments, Nusfalau, Romania).

2.9. Subcellular Protein Extraction

Nuclear protein extracts were obtained using the NE-PER™ Nuclear and Cytoplasmic Extraction Kit and Halt™ Protease Inhibitor Cocktail according to the manufacturer's instructions. The nuclear protein isolates were determined using a BCA Protein Assay Kit (all reagents are from Thermo Scientific, Rockford, IL, USA).

2.10. Western Blotting Analysis

2.10.1. Detection of EV Markers

From each sample, 10 µg purified EVs were loaded onto and separated by 15% SDS-PAGE. After electrophoretic separation, proteins were blotted onto 0.22 µm PVDF membranes (Carl Roche, Karlsruhe, Germany). The PVDF membranes were stained with Ponceau S staining solution (Sigma-Aldrich, Steinheim, Germany) and documented by photography for blotting efficiency and total protein expression analysis. Subsequently, the membranes were washed and blocked with 5% BSA (Carl Roth, Karlsruhe, Germany) in 0.1% Tween Tris Buffered Saline (T-TBS) for 1 h at RT and consecutively incubated with the following primary antibodies in 5% BSA/T-TBS overnight at 4 °C: anti-CD9 (1:1000), anti-CD63 (1:500) and anti-CD81 (1:1000) antibodies (all Thermo Fisher Scientific, Rockford, IL, USA) overnight at 4 °C. After three washing steps, 10 min each, membranes were incubated with horseradish peroxidase coupled secondary antibody (1:10,000) (Jackson Immuno Research, West Grove, PA, USA) for 1 h at RT. Protein bands were visualized with ECL detection reagents and SuperSignal™ West Femto Maximum Sensitivity Substrate (both Thermo Fisher Scientific, Rockford, IL, USA). Semi-quantitative analysis was performed with ImageJ 1.54 software (Bio-Rad, Hercules, CA, USA).

2.10.2. Detection of HIF-1α and RUNX2

Then, 3 × 10^5 hBMSCs were cultured in growth medium (T75) until 80% confluency. Growth medium was exchanged with osteogenic differentiation medium containing 10% FCS under either normoxia or hypoxia, and cells were cultured for 14 days. Nuclear proteins were isolated using the NE-PER™ Nuclear and Cytoplasmic Extraction Kit. From each sample, 30 µg of nuclear protein was loaded onto and separated by 4–15% Mini-PROTEAN® TGX™ Precast Protein Gels (Bio-Rad, Hercules, CA, USA). Western blot was performed as described above using anti-HIF-1α (1:1000), anti-RUNX2 (1:1000) and anti-Histone H3 (1:1000) antibodies (all Cell Signaling Technology, Danvers, MA, USA).

2.11. *EV Uptake Test*

Similar volumes of hypo-osteo EVs (15 µg) and norm-osteo EVs (15 µg) were labeled with PKH26 Red Fluorescent Cell Linker Mini Kit for general cell membrane labeling (Sigma-Aldrich, Saint Louis, MO, USA) according to our previous publication [29]. Subsequently, 2 × 10^4 naïve hBMSCs were cultured in growth medium in eight-well chamber slides (Falcon, Big Flats, NY, USA) for 48 h. Cells were washed with PBS, and the pre-stained EVs (15 µg) were added for 24 h. Nuclei of cells were counterstained with DAPI (Molecular Probes, Eugene, OR, USA) and the cytoskeleton with Phalloidin (Abcam, Malvern, UK), then staining was analyzed using a fluorescence microscope (Eclipse TE2000-U; Nikon, Tokyo, Japan).

2.12. *Nanoparticle Tracking Analysis (NTA)*

The concentration and particle size distribution of the purified EV fractions were analyzed using The NanoSight NS300 (Malvern Instruments, Malvern, UK) following the manufacturer's instructions. Briefly, the accuracy of NTA was confirmed with 100 nm polystyrene beads (Sigma-Aldrich, Saint Louis, MO, USA), then EV samples were diluted 1:100 in PBS at RT and a total of five 30 s videos were recorded.

2.13. *Alkaline Phosphatase Assay*

Intracellular alkaline phosphatase (ALP) enzyme activity was determined with QuantiChrom™ Alkaline Phosphatase Assay Kit (BioAssay Systems, Hayward, CA, USA). Moreover, 1 × 10^4 hBMSCs were cultured in 24-well plates in growth medium under normoxia until 80% confluency.

Then, growth medium was replaced by osteogenic differentiation medium with 10% FCS under either normoxia or hypoxia (2% O_2), and cell culture was continued for two weeks. For EV treatment, hBMSCs were cultured under hypoxia for two weeks in osteogenic differentiation medium containing 10% $FCS^{depl\text{-}uc}$ and were treated with the different EV groups (10 µg/mL) or PBS (no EVs) from days 8 to 14 (fresh EVs were added every two days). hBMSCs kept in osteogenic differentiation medium containing 10% $FCS^{depl\text{-}uc}$ under normoxia for two weeks were set as positive control group (no EVs). Afterward, intracellular ALP enzyme activity was quantified in all groups. Data were calculated either as percentage of the 'no EVs' group under hypoxia (negative control group) or as percentage of normoxia group (no EV treatment = positive control).

2.14. *Alizarin Red Staining*

For analyzing calcification levels, 3 × 10^4 hBMSCs were cultured in 12-well plates in growth medium until 80% confluency. For comparison of hypoxic and normoxic conditions, growth medium was replaced by osteogenic differentiation medium containing 10% FCS under either normoxia or hypoxia for three weeks.

For EV treatment, cells were cultured under hypoxia with osteogenic differentiation medium containing 10% $FCS^{depl\text{-}uc}$ for 3 weeks and stimulated with the different EV groups (10 μg/mL) or PBS (no EVs) from days 5 to 21 (fresh EVs and PBS were added every two days). Cells, which were kept in osteogenic differentiation medium containing 10% FCS$^{depl\text{-}uc}$ under normoxia for three weeks, were set as positive control group (no EVs). Subsequently, cells were washed and fixed with glutaraldehyde for 15 min at RT. After a washing step with PBS (pH = 4.2), cells were incubated for 20 min with Alizarin Red-S staining solution (1%, Carl Roth, Karlsruhe, Germany) at RT. Afterward, quantitative analysis was performed as described previously [34]. Results were further calculated as percentage of the 'no EVs group' under hypoxia (negative control group).

2.15. RNA Isolation and Real-Time -qPCR

For analyzing gene expression, 6 × 10^4 hBMSCs were cultured in growth medium (6-well plates) until 80% confluency. For comparison of hypoxic and normoxic conditions, growth medium was exchanged for osteogenic differentiation medium containing 10% FCS under either normoxia or hypoxia for two weeks. For EV treatment, growth medium was exchanged to osteogenic differentiation medium with 10% FCS$^{depl\text{-}uc}$, and cells were cultured for 2 weeks under hypoxia and treated with the different EV groups (10 μg/mL) or PBS (no EVs) from day 12 on. Cells kept in osteogenic differentiation medium containing 10% FCS$^{depl\text{-}uc}$ under normoxia for two weeks were set as positive control group (no EVs). Afterward, RNA was isolated using Absolutely RNA™ Microprep Kit (Agilent Technologies, Cedar Creek, TX, USA), and cDNA was prepared using AffinityScript QPCR cDNA Synthesis Kit (Agilent Technologies, Cedar Creek, TX, USA) as recommended by manufacturer's protocol. RT-qPCR was performed in duplicates using the Brilliant III Ultra-Fast SYBR Green QPCR Master Mix with an Agilent PCR-System (Agilent Technologies, Cedar Creek, TX, USA). All genes were analyzed relatively in relation to GAPDH and TATA-binding protein (TBP) expression (normalizer). All genes were set to the expression of the calibrator ('no EVs' group under hypoxia).

For validation of proteomics data, norm-naïve EVs parent cells (undifferentiated, naïve hBMSCs) were harvested for RNA isolation under normoxia. For harvesting RNA of the norm-osteo EVs' parent cells, the growth medium was replaced by osteogenic medium with 10% FCS$^{depl\text{-}uc}$ and cells were cultured for either 14 or 35 days under normoxia. All genes were analyzed and calibrated to the expression in naïve hBMSCs under normoxia (calibrator). Primers are listed in Supplementary Table S2.

2.16. Measurement of Reactive Oxygen Species (ROS) Level

Extracellular ROS level was measured with the OxiSelect™ in vitro ROS/RNS Assay Kit (Cell Biolabs Inc., San Diego, CA, USA). 1 × 10^4 hBMSCs were cultured in 24-well plates in growth medium under normoxia until 80% confluency. Growth medium was replaced by osteogenic differentiation medium, which was changed every third day.

For comparison of hypoxic and normoxic conditions, hBMSCs were cultured in osteogenic differentiation medium containing 10% FCS for either 14 or 35 days under either normoxia or hypoxia. Osteogenic differentiation medium was changed every third day. After 48 h incubation at day 12 and day 33, the osteogenic supernatants were collected subsequently on days 14 and 35.

For EV treatment, hBMSCs were cultured under hypoxia for two weeks in osteogenic differentiation medium containing 10% FCS$^{depl\text{-}uc}$. The different EV groups (10 μg/mL) or PBS (no EVs) were added from days 12 to 14. hBMSCs, which were kept in osteogenic differentiation medium containing 10% FCS$^{depl\text{-}uc}$ under normoxia for two weeks, were set as positive control group (no EVs). Results were further calculated as percentage of the 'no EVs group' under hypoxia (negative control group).

Extracellular ROS was quantified according to manufacturer's instructions. Briefly, 50 μL of cell supernatants were added into a 96-well black-bottom fluorescence plate (NunclonTM, Thermo Fisher Scientific, Roskilde, Denmark), and 50 μL of catalyst were added to each well and incubated for 5 min at RT. Afterward, 100 μL of DCFH was added at RT for 15 min in the dark. Fluorescence was measured using a SpectraMax® iD3 plate reader (Molecular Devices, San Jose, CA, USA) at 480 nm excitation/530 nm emission. Fluorescence intensity is proportional to the total ROS levels within the sample.

2.17. Proteomic Analysis

2.17.1. Sample Preparation of EVs for Proteomics Analysis

EV samples were purified from the culture supernatant of the corresponding three cell donors, and total protein concentration was measured using the BCA assay. Briefly, 5 μg EV protein was reduced in 10 mM dithiothreitol (DTT) at 56 °C for 30 min and consecutively alkylated in 30 mM of iodoacetamide (IAA) at RT for 30 min in the dark. The remaining IAA was quenched with 30 mM DTT at RT for 15 min. Afterward, EV proteins were digested using the S-Trap™ (ProtiFi, Fairport, NY, USA) mini procedure according to the manufacturer's protocol.

2.17.2. Quantitative Proteomic Analysis by LC-MS/MS

From each EV sample, 500 ng per protein was analyzed by nano LC-MS/MS. EV samples were loaded on an Ultimate 3000 Rapid Separation Liquid chromatography (RSLC) nano system with a ProFlow flow control device coupled to a Lumos Fusion orbitrap mass spectrometer (both from Thermo Scientific). Peptides dissolved in 0.1% TFA were placed onto a trapping column (Acclaim PepMap100 C18, 100 μm × 2 cm, Thermo Scientific, Bremen, Germany) at a flow rate of 10 μL/min. Afterward, peptides were separated on a phase column (Acclaim PepMap100 C18, 75 μm × 50 cm, Thermo Scientific, Bremen, Germany) using a binary gradient.

2.17.3. Database Search and Bioinformatics Analysis

All MS raw data were identified using the Proteome Discoverer software 2.3.0.523 (Thermo Scientific, Bremen, Germany), and it is MASCOT algorithm against a human UniprotKB database (http://www.uniprot.org; downloaded 21 November 2019). The search parameters were 0.5 Da for MS and MS/MS and precursor and fragment ion tolerances of 10 ppm, respectively. Carbamidomethylation of cysteine was set as fixed modification, and oxidation of methionine was set as dynamic modification. Trypsin was set as enzyme with a maximum of two missed cleavages, using Percolator false discovery rate (strict) set to 0.01 for both peptide and protein identification. Label-free quantification (LFQ) analysis was performed, including replicates for each condition. Proteins with more than 2-fold change were considered as distinct proteins. All distinct upregulated and downregulated proteins in hypo-osteo EVs compared with those in norm-osteo EVs were then subjected to Kyoto Encyclopedia of Genes and Genomes (KEGG) and Gene Ontology (GO) analyses. The following bioinformatic analyses include Venn diagram, heatmap, KEGG and GO databases. Among them, Venn diagram was conducted with the bioinformatics platform jvenn [38] (http://jvenn.toulouse.inra.fr/app/index.html, accessed on 21 November 2019), and the heatmap was constructed with the software TBtools 1.0 [39]. GO and KEGG analysis of annotated proteins were conducted with the bioinformatics platform STRING database (http://string-db.org, accessed on 21 November 2019) and visualized using following bioinformatics platform (https://www.bioinformatics.com.cn, accessed on 21 November 2019). In order to obtain a better idea of the potential relationships between the proteins, protein–protein interaction networks of the identified proteins were constructed with the STRING database with default parameters and visualized using Cytoscape software 3.9.1.

2.18. Statistical Analysis

Prism 8.21 software (GraphPad, San Jose, CA, USA) was used for statistical analysis. Differences between groups were assessed by One sample t-test and Wilcoxon test or by one-way ANOVA with Dunn's multiple comparisons test when appropriate. $p < 0.05$ was considered statistically significant.

3. Results

3.1. Generating Conditioned Medium for Preparation of Osteogenic EVs from a Hypoxic (Hypo-Osteo EVs) Environment and Osteogenic EVs from a Normoxic (Norm-Osteo EVs) Environment

Representative images in Supplementary Figure S2 show that the color of conditioned medium (CM) from osteogenic differentiated hBMSCs under hypoxic conditions is distinct from CM under normoxic conditions and also distinct from osteogenic medium (OM) (no cells) subjected to both hypoxic and normoxic conditions (Supplementary Figure S2A). In order to explain the different medium colors under normoxic and hypoxic conditions, the pH-values of CM and OM were determined. As shown in Supplementary Figure S2B, the pH of CM from osteogenic differentiated hBMSCs under hypoxia decreased significantly compared to CM recovered from osteogenic differentiated hBMSCs under normoxia and from both OM subjected to both hypoxia and normoxia.

3.2. Characterization of EVs

3.2.1. NTA Evaluation of EVs

We determined the particle concentration, distribution and size of hypo-osteo EVs and norm-osteo EVs via nanoparticle tracking analysis (NTA). The average particle size of hypo-osteo EVs (n = 3) was smaller by trend than their norm-osteo-EV counterparts, although both representatively shown EV groups correspond to the standard size of EVs (Figure 2A,B,D). However, there is no statistically significant difference in counts and size between hypo-osteo EVs and norm-osteo EVs (Figure 2C,D).

3.2.2. Uptake of EVs by Naïve hBMSCs

In order to evaluate the cellular internalization of EVs, naïve hBMSCs were incubated with PKH-26 stained hypo-osteo EVs and norm-osteo EVs for 24 h. Intracellular fluorescence labeling (red) revealed that the internalized hypo-osteo EVs and norm-osteo EVs accumulated in the cytoplasm (Figure 2E,F "merge") of the target hBMSCs with no obvious differences between both groups.

3.2.3. Surface Markers of EVs

The presence of the most common canonical EV membrane markers CD9, CD63 and CD81 was analyzed via Western blotting. Positive bands for CD9, CD63 and CD81 were detected in both hypo-osteo-EV and norm-osteo-EV groups (Figure 2G). Supplementary Figure S2A,B show the respective uncropped Western blot membranes after development and the respective blot membranes stained with Ponceau S as loading control. The quantification of each marker band intensity showed that CD9, CD63 and CD81 protein expression levels were significantly decreased in hypo-osteo EVs compared to norm-osteo EVs (Figure 2H–J). Quantitative proteomic analyses confirmed the presence of CD9, CD63 and CD81 in the EV samples (Figure 2K). Uncropped Western blot membranes and Ponceau S stained loading control images are shown in Supplementary Figure S3.

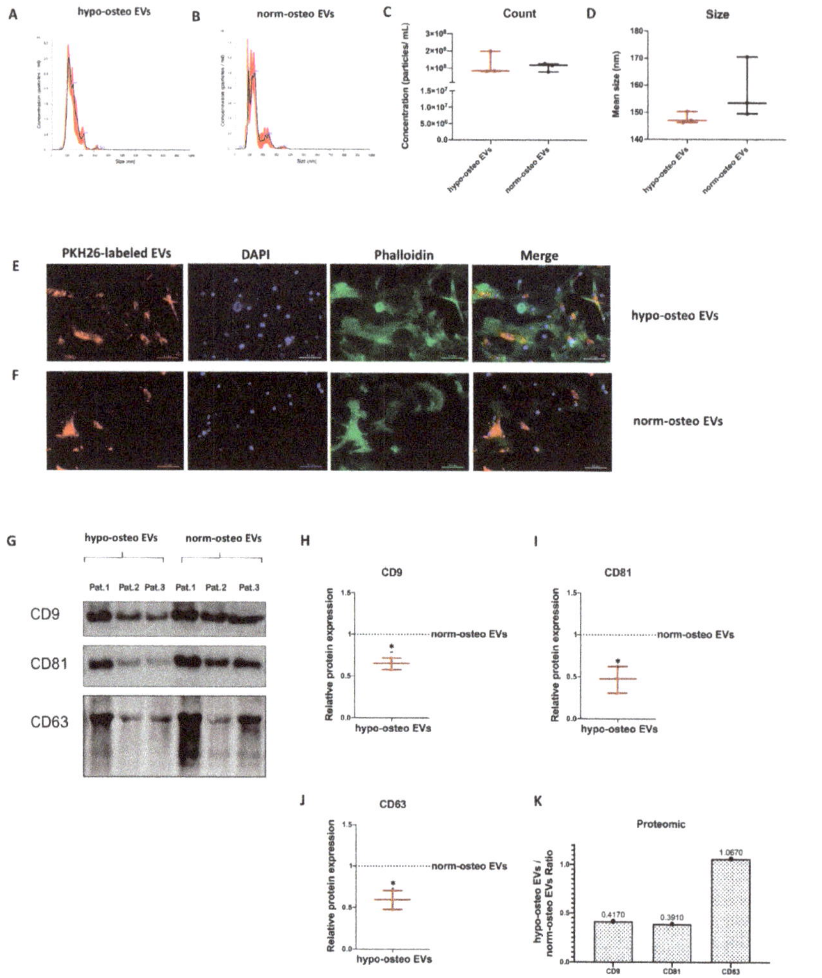

Figure 2. Characterization of the EV groups. (**A**,**B**) Representative particle size distribution of hypo-osteo EVs and norm-osteo EVs was measured by NTA; n = 3. (**C**,**D**) Quantitative comparison between hypo-osteo EVs and norm-osteo EVs in count and size measured; n = 3. (**E**,**F**) Uptake of EVs by naïve hBMSCs. PKH26-labeled hypo-osteo EVs (**E**) and norm-osteo EVs (**F**) were internalized by naïve hBMSCs and visualized with fluorescence microscopy. Cell nuclei were stained with DAPI, and structure of the cytoskeleton was visualized with Phalloidin staining. 20 × 10 magnification; Scale bar 100 μm; n = 3. (**G**) Western blot image showing bands of standard surface markers (CD9, CD81 and CD63) of hypo-osteo EVs and norm-osteo EVs; n = 3; Pat. = patient. (**H**–**J**) Relative quantitation of western blot image band intensities; n = 3. (**K**) The expression/level ratio of CD9, CD81 and CD63 proteins in hypo-osteo EVs was compared with that in norm-osteo EVs (proteomics data); n = 3. Results were calculated as percentage of the unstimulated control group (norm-osteo EVs, shown by the dotted line); * = $p < 0.05$.

3.3. Osteogenic Differentiation of hBMSCs under Hypoxia

To assess the influence of hypoxia on the matrix calcification ability of osteogenic differentiated hBMSCs, analysis of calcified matrix nodules after 21 days of osteogenic differentiation under normoxia and hypoxia was conducted via Alizarin Red staining. Figure 3A demonstrates that calcium deposits in the hypoxia sample groups decreased in intensity and area compared to the normoxia samples, even though the staining intensity showed inter-sample differences. In general, the quantification of the Alizarin Red staining intensity and amount confirmed that the BMSCs of all five donors cultured under hypoxia have significantly decreased calcium deposits compared to those cultured under normoxia after 21 days of osteogenic differentiation. Results from different donors were combined for quantification (Figure 3B). Alkaline phosphatase (ALP) enzyme activity level serves as an indicator of bone formation and correlates with osteoblast activity [40]. Here, the ALP activity assay revealed that compared to the normoxia group, hypoxia significantly suppresses ALP activity in hBMSCs after 14 days of osteogenic differentiation (Figure 3C). To assess whether hypoxia influences the ROS level of osteogenic differentiated hBMSCs, we performed a ROS assay after 14 and 35 days of osteogenic differentiation under hypoxic and normoxic conditions. Supplementary Figure S4A shows that the extracellular ROS level was already significantly increased after 14 days of osteogenic differentiation of hBMSCs under hypoxic conditions compared to normoxic conditions. Moreover, excessive production of ROS was maintained up to 35 days of osteogenic differentiation under hypoxia (Supplementary Figure S4B).

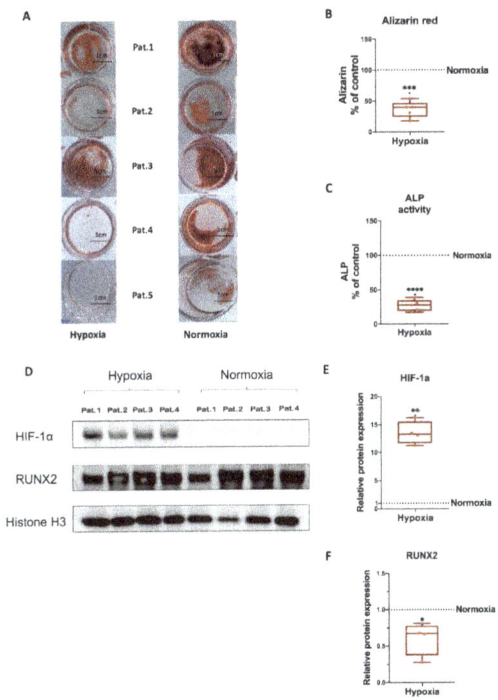

Figure 3. Evaluation of osteogenic differentiation ability of naïve hBMSCs under hypoxia and normoxia. (**A**) Alizarin Red staining of hBMSCs after 3 weeks of osteogenic differentiation under hypoxia or normoxia. Shown are the individual results from five different donors. Macroscopic view (scale bar 1 cm); n = 5; Pat. = patient. (**B**) Quantification of Alizarin Red staining; n = 5. (**C**) Quantification of Alkaline Phosphatase (ALP) activity of hBMSCs after 2 weeks of osteogenic differentiation under hypoxia or normoxia; n = 5. (**D**) Representative Western blot images of HIF-1α and RUNX2 after 2 weeks of osteogenic differentiation of hBMSCs under hypoxia and normoxia; n = 4. (**E**,**F**) Relative quantitation of Western blot image band intensities relative to Histone H3; n = 4. Results were calculated as percentage of the unstimulated control group (osteogenic differentiation of hBMSCs under normoxia, shown by the dotted line); * = $p < 0.05$; ** = $p < 0.01$; *** = $p < 0.001$; **** = $p < 0.0001$.

We further analyzed gene expression levels of the osteogenic markers BGLAP (Osteocalcin), RUNX2 (Runt-related transcription factor 2), ALP, COL1A1 (Collagen alpha-1(I) chain) and OPN (Osteopontin). Besides OPN, the expression of all analyzed genes revealed a significant decrease under hypoxia compared to normoxia (Supplementary Figure S4C–G).

3.4. HIF-1α and RUNX2 Protein Expression in hBMSCs Undergoing Osteogenic Differentiation under Hypoxia

In order to evaluate if a 2% O_2 condition is effective for induction of hypoxia in cells, we analyzed hypoxia-inducible factor-1α (HIF-1α) protein expression, and if hypoxia influences osteogenic differentiation of hBMSCs, we analyzed RUNX2 protein expression. Western blotting analysis showed that hypoxia induces HIF-1α protein expression and downregulates RUNX2 protein expression in hBMSCs undergoing osteogenic differentiation. Nuclear protein Histone H3 served as loading control. Results from four different donors were combined for quantification (Figure 3D–F). Uncropped Western blot membranes and Ponceau S-stained loading control images are shown in Supplementary Figure S5.

3.5. Proteomic Analysis of Osteogenic EVs Produced under Hypoxia and Normoxia

3.5.1. Summary of the Proteomic Profiles

To investigate whether osteogenic EVs from a hypoxic environment are loaded with unique proteomic signatures, we performed quantitative proteomic analysis to identify the protein profiles of hypo-osteo EVs (n = 3) and norm-osteo EVs (n = 3). The Venn diagram in Figure 4A shows that 52 unique proteins were identified in the norm-osteo EV group, and 11 unique proteins were identified in the hypo-osteo EV group. Moreover, the norm-osteo EV group has 913 proteins in common with the hypo-osteo EV group. Analysis of distinct proteins with at least a 2-fold change between the hypo-osteo EV group and the norm-osteo EV group revealed that the protein levels of 67 proteins were increased and the levels of 377 proteins were decreased in the hypo-osteo EVs compared to the norm-osteo EVs (Supplementary Table S1). As shown in Figure 4B, the detailed list of the distinct proteins (more than a 2-fold change) and their abundance is presented in the heatmap. We identified 21 pro-osteogenic proteins, 21 proteins involved in ECM remodeling and five antioxidant proteins, which were decreased in hypo-osteo EVs compared to that in norm-osteo EVs (Tables 1–3). The hypo-osteo EVs/norm-osteo EVs ratios measured for these proteins ranged from a 100-fold to a 2008-fold reduction. The five decreased antioxidant proteins are: 5′-AMP-activated protein kinase catalytic subunit alpha-1 (PRKAA1), NAD(P)H dehydrogenase 1 (NQO1), Annexin A1 (ANXA1), 40S ribosomal protein S3 and Peroxiredoxin-1 (RPS3) and Peroxiredoxin-1 (PRDX1).

Table 1. The expression/level ratio of selected downregulated pro-osteogenic proteins in hypo-osteo EVs compared with those in norm-osteo EVs.

UniProt	Protein Names	Gene Names	Hypo-Osteo EVs/Norm-Osteo EVs Ratio (Fold Change)
Q92896	Golgi apparatus protein 1	GLG1	0.01
Q4V9L6	Transmembrane protein 119	TMEM119	0.106
P05186	Alkaline phosphatase	ALPL	0.154
P17813	Endoglin	ENG	0.245
Q04771	Activin receptor type-1	ACVR1	0.265
Q9ULC3	Ras-related protein Rab-23	RAB23	0.287
P26373	60S ribosomal protein L13	RPL13	0.292
P20020	Plasma membrane calcium-transporting ATPase 1	ATP2B1	0.303

Table 1. *Cont.*

UniProt	Protein Names	Gene Names	Hypo-Osteo EVs/Norm-Osteo EVs Ratio (Fold Change)
P35222	**Catenin beta-1**	**CTNNB1**	0.304
P00533	**Epidermal growth factor receptor**	**EGFR**	0.305
Q16610	Extracellular matrix protein 1	ECM1	0.326
P50281	Matrix metalloproteinase-14	MMP14	0.331
P08133	Annexin A6	ANXA6	0.356
P07355	Annexin A2	ANXA2	0.362
P13797	Plastin-3	PLS3	0.387
Q16832	Discoidin domain-containing receptor 2	DDR2	0.401
P22413	Ectonucleotide pyrophos-phatase/phosphodiesterase family member 1	ENPP1	0.438
Q5JWF2	Guanine nucleotide-binding protein G(s) subunit alpha isoforms XLas	GNAS	0.448
O00299	Chloride intracellular channel protein 1	CLIC1	0.458
Q13491	Neuronal membrane glycoprotein M6-b	GPM6B	0.494
P61586	Transforming protein RhoA	RHOA	0.498

Table 2. The expression/level ratio of selected downregulated ECM proteins in hypo-osteo EVs compared with that in norm-osteo EVs.

UniProt	Protein Names	Gene Names	Hypo-Osteo EVs /Norm-Osteo EVs Ratio (Fold Change)
Q12965	Unconventional myosin-Ie	MYO1E	0.01
P02458	Collagen alpha-1(II) chain	COL2A1	0.01
Q01955	Collagen alpha-3(IV) chain	COL4A3	0.01
Q12965	Unconventional myosin-Ie	MYO1E	0.01
Q16610	Extracellular matrix protein 1	ECM1	0.326
O75578	Integrin alpha-10	ITGA10	0.189
P17813	Endoglin	ENG	0.245
P26006	Integrin alpha-3	ITGA3	0.256
P06756	Integrin alpha-V	ITGAV	0.323
Q13683	Integrin alpha-7	ITGA7	0.326
P50281	Matrix metalloproteinase-14	MMP14	0.331
P18084	Integrin beta-5	ITGB5	0.347
P98095	Fibulin-2	FBLN2	0.347

Table 2. *Cont.*

UniProt	Protein Names	Gene Names	Hypo-Osteo EVs /Norm-Osteo EVs Ratio (Fold Change)
Q08722	Leukocyte surface antigen CD47	CD47	0.352
P07355	Annexin A2	ANXA2	0.362
Q14112	Nidogen-2	NID2	0.379
P24821	Tenascin	TNC	0.396
Q16832	Discoidin domain-containing receptor 2	DDR2	0.401
P16070	CD44 antigen	CD44	0.412
O14672	Disintegrin and metalloproteinase domain-containing protein 10	ADAM10	0.428
P08648	Integrin alpha-5	ITGA5	0.498

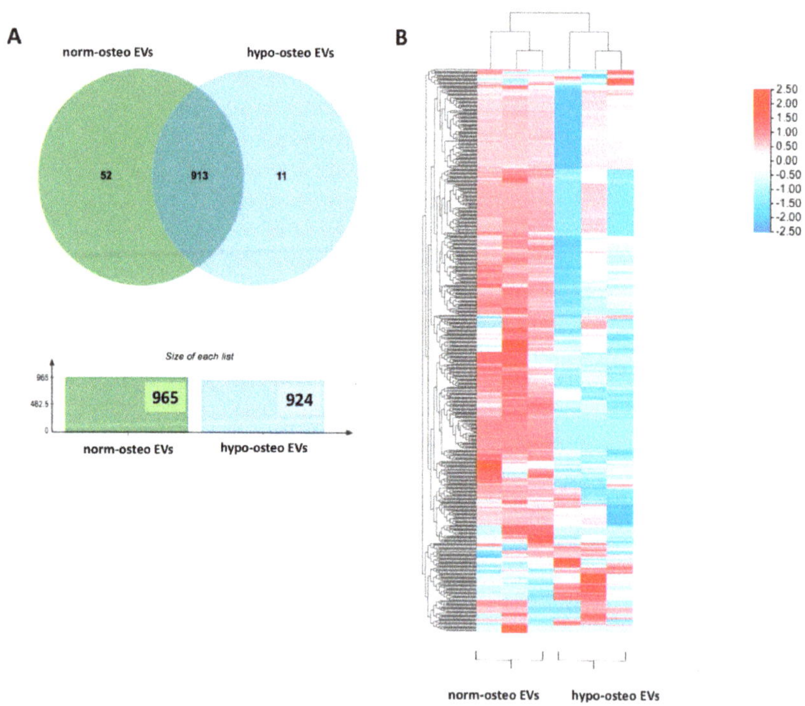

Figure 4. Venn diagram of total proteins and heatmap of distinct proteins identified in hypo-osteo EVs and norm-osteo EVs. (**A**) The distinct profiles (Venn diagram) of total proteins in hypo-osteo EVs and norm-osteo EVs; n = 3. (**B**) The distinct protein (more than 2-fold change) profiles of norm-osteo EVs and hypo-osteo EVs (heatmap); n = 3. The color code indicates the log2 (FC) difference of the proteins for those two EV groups: red means enriched in EVs, and blue means depleted in EVs.

Table 3. The expression/level ratio of selected downregulated antioxidant proteins in hypo-osteo EVs compared with that in norm-osteo EVs.

UniProt	Protein Names	Gene Names	Hypo-Osteo EVs /Norm-Osteo EVs Ratio (Fold Change)
Q13131	5′-AMP-activated protein kinase catalytic subunit alpha-1	PRKAA1	0.143
P15559	NAD(P)H dehydrogenase [quinone] 1	NQO1	0.298
P04083	Annexin A1	ANXA1	0.343
P23396	40S ribosomal protein S3	RPS3	0.438
Q06830	Peroxiredoxin-1	PRDX1	0.485

3.5.2. GO and KEGG Enrichment Analyses

GO (Gene Ontology) terms were performed for annotation of the differentially expressed proteins (more than 2-fold change) in norm-osteo EVs and hypo-osteo EVs, which are divided into three categories (biological processes, molecular functions and cell components). GO biological processes analysis of upregulated and downregulated proteins in hypo-osteo EVs were compared with that in norm-osteo EVs. Among them, upregulated proteins matched 42 significant GO terms (no GO terms related to bone regeneration). The top 19 upregulated Go terms are shown in Figure 5A. Downregulated proteins matched 650 significant GO terms, and the significant downregulated GO terms related to bone regeneration (ECM, osteogenesis, ROS, adhesion and angiogenesis) are also shown in Figure 5A. GO analysis revealed information about all upregulated and downregulated molecular functions, specifically concerning the downregulated cell-to-cell and cell-to-matrix binding processes (Figure 5B) and cellular components (Figure 5C) in hypo-osteo EVs compared to norm-osteo EVs. KEGG pathway analysis identified significantly downregulated and upregulated enriched pathways in hypo-osteo EVs compared to that in norm-osteo EVs (Figure 5D). The pathways, shown in Figure 5D, revealed that especially the 'PI3K-Akt signaling', 'ECM-receptor interaction' 'cGMP-PKG signaling pathway' and 'growth hormone synthesis, secretion and action', were significantly downregulated in hypo-osteo EVs compared with norm-osteo EVs.

3.5.3. Hub Proteins

Protein–protein interaction (PPI) networks of all the differently expressed proteins (more than a 2-fold change) were created using the STRING database and visualized using Cytoscape with unconnected nodes excluded. Altogether, 520 nodes (62 upregulated and 358 downregulated proteins in hypo-osteo EVs compared to that in norm-osteo EVs) and 2680 interaction pairs were identified in the PPI network of the distinct proteins (Figure 6A). Hub nodes contain the key genes of the PPI network. The top 20 hub proteins of the whole PPI network were identified using the Degree and CytoHubba plug-ins in Cytoscape (Figure 6B). Among them, the two most highly correlated hub proteins are epidermal growth factor receptor (EGFR) and catenin beta-1 (CTNNB1), which are downregulated in hypo-osteo EVs compared to norm-osteo EVs. Notably, EGFR was identified in the context of GO terms 'cellular response to reactive oxygen species', pro-osteogenic and pro-angiogenic proteins'. Moreover, CTNNB1 was identified in the context of pro-osteogenic and pro-angiogenic proteins (Table 1). As shown in Figure 6B, the two hub proteins are marked with a yellow box.

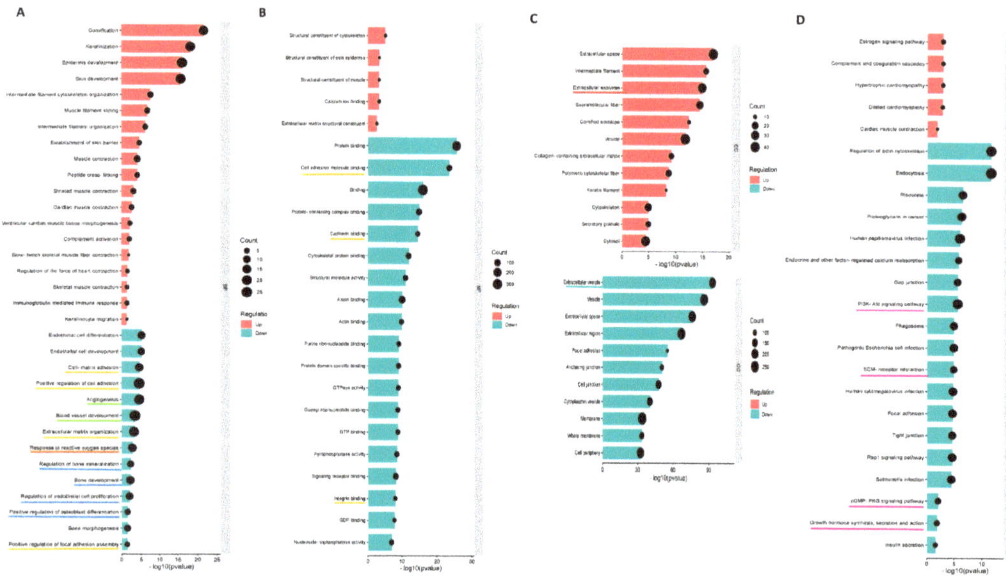

Figure 5. Functional enrichment analysis of distinct regulated and downregulated proteins in hypo-osteo EVs compared with that in norm-osteo EVs. Gene ontology (GO) analysis of the upregulated and downregulated biological processes (**A**), molecular functions (**B**), hypo-osteo EVs compared with that in norm-osteo EVs for upregulated and downregulated proteins were clustered; n = 3. (**C**) Cellular components in hypo-osteo EVs compared with that in norm-osteo EVs with the KEGG (**D**) enrichment analyses data for upregulated and downregulated proteins were clustered; n = 3. KEGG = Kyoto Encyclopedia of Genes and Genomes. Pathways related to bone regeneration are marked with pink lines. BP = biological processes; MF = molecular functions; CC = cellular components. GO terms related to bone regeneration (ECM, osteogenesis, angiogenesis, ROS and adhesion) and EV are marked with different colored lines.

3.6. Effects of EVs Derived from Late Stage Osteogenic-Differentiated hBMSCs under Normoxia on Osteogenic Ability of hBMSCs Cultured under Hypoxia

To investigate the capability of norm-osteo EVs to influence matrix calcification of osteogenic differentiated hBMSCs impaired by hypoxia, Alizarin Red staining of calcified matrix was evaluated after 21 days of osteogenic differentiation under hypoxia and simultaneous EV stimulation (EVs from osteogenic differentiated and naïve hBMSCs cultured under normoxia) for the last 16 culture days. Representative images showing calcium deposits revealed that norm-osteo EVs induced increased intensity and area of calcification compared to the negative control group (no EVs under hypoxia) and compared to EVs isolated from undifferentiated naïve hBMSCs (norm-naïve EVs) when added to hBMSCs (Figure 7A). The quantification of the Alizarin Red staining intensity was consistent with these results. The norm-osteo EV group significantly increased calcium deposits compared to the negative control group (no EVs under hypoxia) and the norm-naïve EV group when added to hBMSCs; however, the area of calcium deposits was still smaller compared to the positive culture group (no EVs under normoxia) (Figure 7B). 14 days of osteogenic differentiation of hBMSCs in the presence of norm-naïve EVs and norm-osteo EVs (applied for the last six culture days), resulted in increased ALP activity compared to the negative control group (Figure 7C). In addition, the 'no EV' treatment group cultured under normoxia still displayed a higher ALP activity level in comparison to stimulation with norm-naïve EVs and norm-osteo EVs under hypoxia.

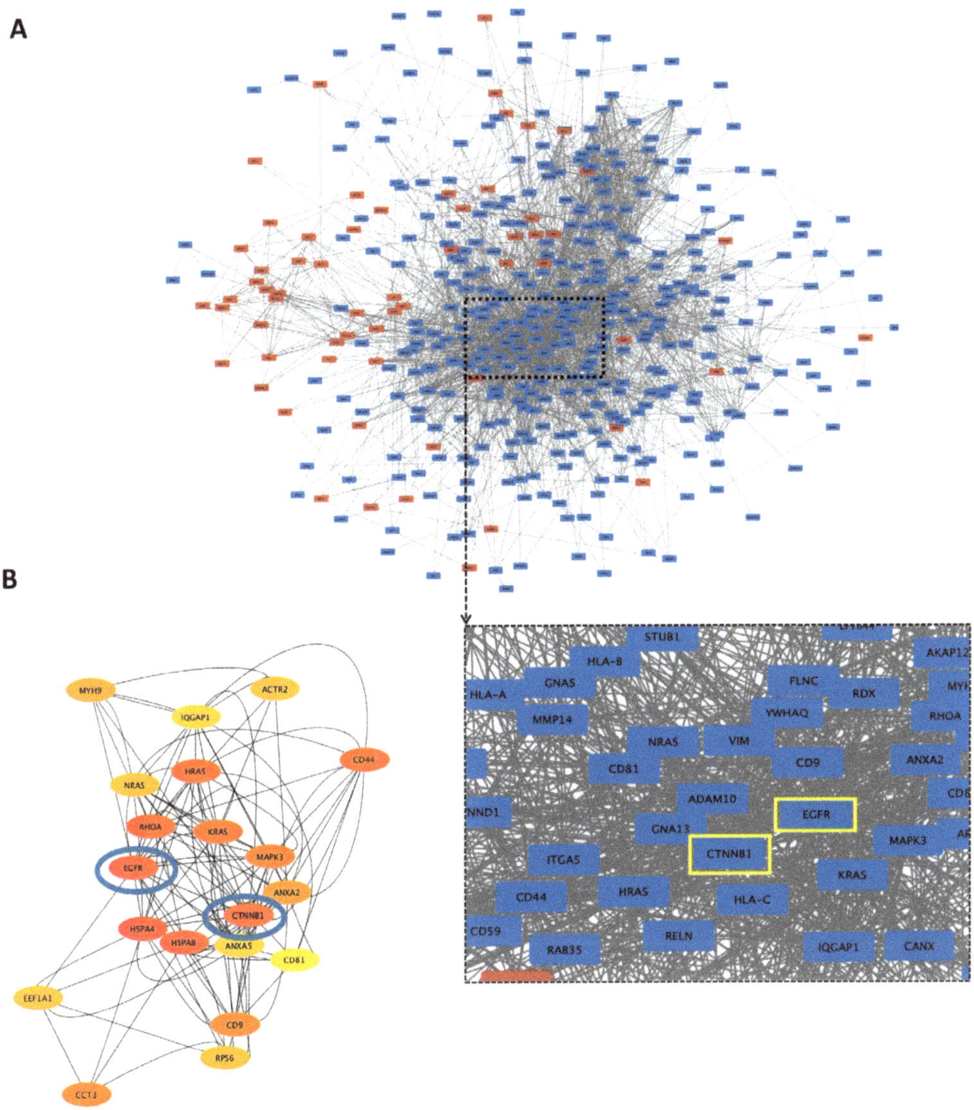

Figure 6. Protein–protein interaction (PPI) network of the identified proteins and hub proteins in hypo-osteo EVs compared with that in norm-osteo EVs. (**A**) Interactions between upregulated and downregulated proteins in hypo-osteo EVs compared with that in norm-osteo EVs; n = 3; Red nodes indicate upregulated proteins and blue nodes indicate downregulated proteins. (**B**) The 20 most highly correlated hub proteins in PPI network. The colors indicate the strength of correlated hub proteins of top 20 hub proteins; red is the highest correlated hub. The top two hub proteins (EGFR and CTNNB1) are marked with blue circles and yellow boxes.

To investigate the capability of norm-osteo EVs to reduce elevated ROS levels in osteogenic differentiated hBMSCs under hypoxia, ROS concentration was determined after 14 days of osteogenic differentiation under hypoxia and simultaneous EV stimulation. Figure 8D showed that the norm-osteo EV group and norm-naïve EV group significantly reduced ROS levels compared to the negative control group (no EVs under hypoxia).

Furthermore, there was no significant difference in ROS production among the two EV groups and the positive control group.

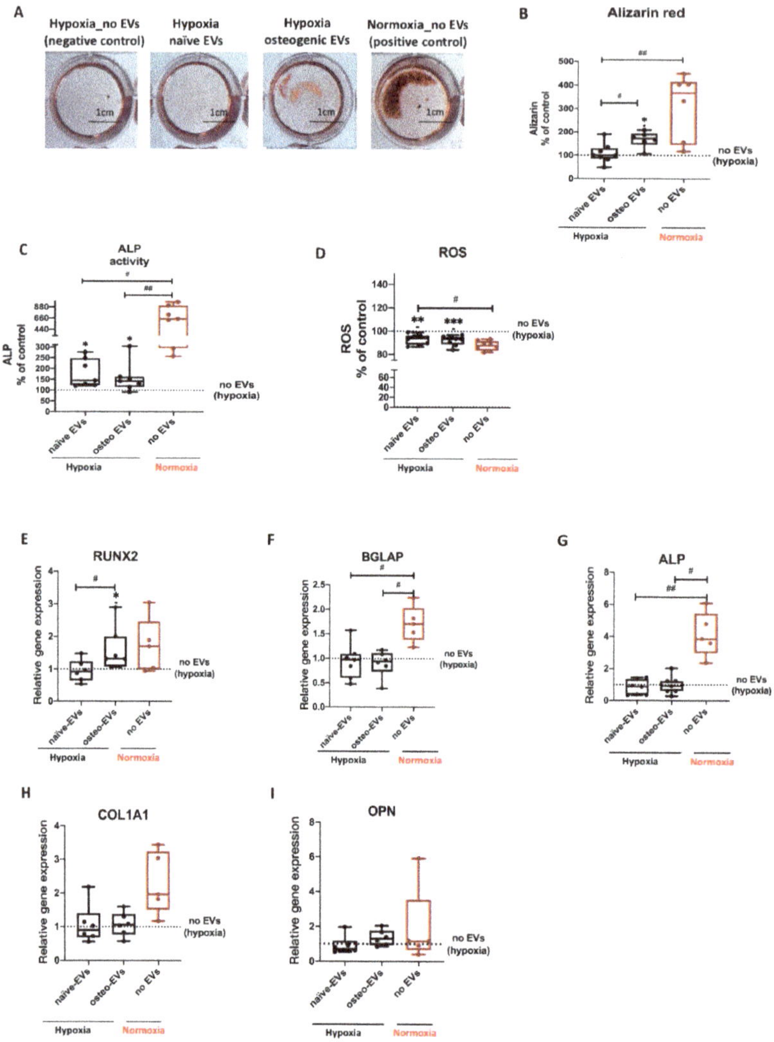

Figure 7. Evaluation of osteogenic differentiation ability of hBMSCs after EV treatment under hypoxia. (A) Alizarin Red staining of hBMSCs after 3 weeks of osteogenic differentiation and simultaneous stimulation with the different EV groups (scale bar 1 cm); n = 6–7. (B) Quantification of Alizarin Red staining; n = 6–7. (C) Quantification of ALP activity of hBMSC after 2 weeks of osteogenic differentiation and simultaneous stimulation with the different EV groups under hypoxia; n = 7. (D) ROS production of hBMSCs after 2 weeks of osteogenic differentiation and simultaneous stimulation with the different EV groups under hypoxia; n = 8. (E–I) Gene expression of the osteogenic marker genes (RUNX2, BGLAP, ALP, COL1A1 and OPN) were analyzed after 2 weeks of osteogenic differentiation of hBMSCs and simultaneous treatment with the different EV groups under hypoxia; n = 5–6. Results were calculated as percentage of the negative control group (no EVs under hypoxia, shown by the dotted line). Difference to the negative control: * = $p < 0.05$; ** = $p < 0.01$; *** = $p < 0.001$; difference between groups: # = $p < 0.05$; ## = $p < 0.01$.

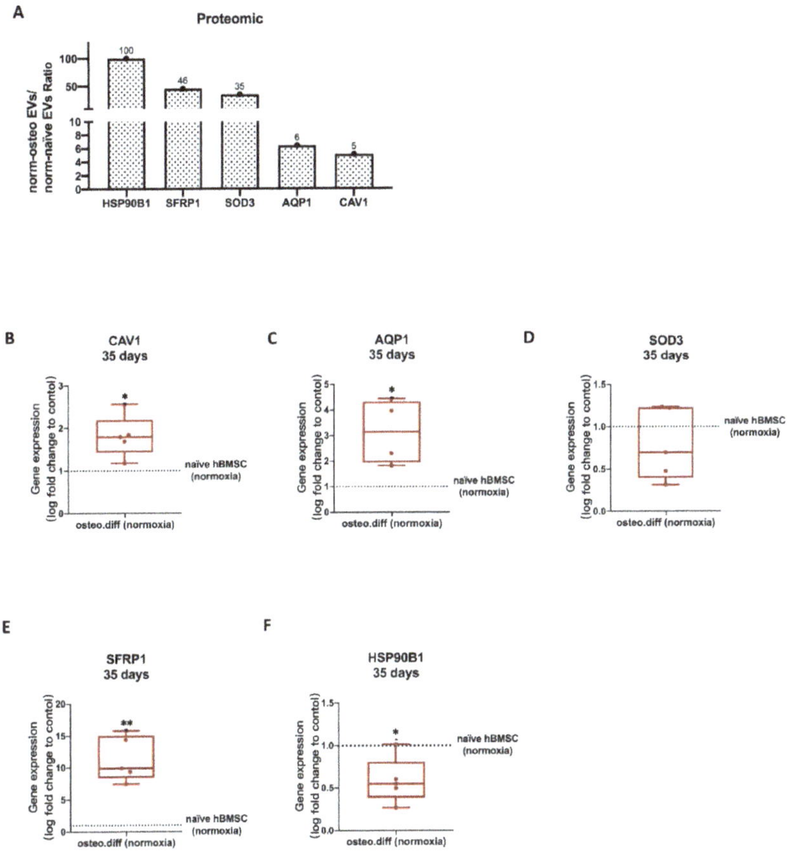

Figure 8. Validation of selected proteomic data obtained from norm-naïve EVs and norm-osteo EVs by gene expression analysis of hBMSCs. (**A**) The expression/level ratio of the five identified anti-hypoxic proteins (CAV1, SFRP1, SOD3, HSP90B1 and AQP1) in norm-osteo EVs compared with that in norm-naïve EVs (proteomics data); n = 3. (**B–F**) Gene expression of the five anti-hypoxic genes (CAV1, SFRP1, SOD3, HSP90B1 and AQP1) were analyzed in hBMSCs after 35 days of osteogenic differentiation and in naïve hBMSCs both cultured under normoxia; n = 4–5. Results were calculated as percentage of the control group (naïve hBMSCs under normoxia, shown by the dotted line); * = $p < 0.05$; ** = $p < 0.01$.

Analysis of osteogenic markers revealed that treatment with the norm-osteo EVs significantly increased RUNX2 expression in hBMSCs compared to the norm-naïve EVs and no EVs control groups under hypoxia (Figure 7E). No significant difference was found in ALP, OPN, BGLAP and COL1A1 gene expression between hBMSCs stimulated with hypo-naïve and hypo-osteo EVs (Figure 7F–I), whereas ALP and BGLAP gene expression in the positive control group (no EVs under normoxia) was significantly higher.

3.6.1. GO Enrichment Analyses and Protein–Protein Interaction (PPI) Network Analyses of Norm-Naïve EVs and norm-Osteo EVs

Our previous study [29] revealed that norm-osteo EVs and norm-naïve EVs contained distinct protein profiles, with pro-osteogenic proteins and ECM components highly enriched in norm-osteo EVs. In order to determine the potential molecules that mediate the effects of osteogenic EVs in rescuing the osteogenic ability of hBMSCs impaired by hypoxia, GO biological processes analysis of upregulated proteins in norm-osteo EVs compared to that in norm-naïve EVs were further analyzed, and the five significant GO terms related to hypoxia and osteogenesis are shown in Supplementary Figure S6A. To further investigate the potential molecular factors contained in norm-osteo EVs that suppress hypoxia and promote osteogenesis, we performed Venn diagram (Supplementary Figure S6B) and PPI network analyses on upregulated proteins in norm-osteo EVs associated with 'response to hypoxia', 'ossification', 'skeletal system development', 'osteoblast differentiation' and 'extracellular matrix (ECM) organization' (Supplementary Figure S6C–G). Four protein interaction networks at significant levels (PPI enrichment p value < 0.05) and one protein interaction network (response to hypoxia) at no significant level (PPI enrichment p value = 0.102) were constructed. As shown in Supplementary Figure S6G, 'response to hypoxia' has three proteins (Caveolin-1 (CAV1)/Secreted frizzled-related protein 1 (SFRP1) and/or matrix metalloproteinase-2 (MMP-2) in common with the 'ossification', 'skeletal system development', 'osteoblast differentiation' or 'ECM organization'. The analysis indicates a significant relationship between the CAV1/SFRP1/MMP-2 and the other proteins in the four GO terms related to osteogenesis and ECM (PPI enrichment p value < 0.05).

3.6.2. Hub Proteins

The Cytoscape platform confirmed 148 nodes (96 upregulated and 52 downregulated proteins in norm-osteo EVs compared to those in norm-naïve EVs), and 653 interaction pairs were identified in the PPI network of the distinct proteins (Supplementary Figure S7A). The top 20 hub proteins of the whole PPI network were identified using the Degree and CytoHubba plug-ins in Cytoscape (Supplementary Figure S7B). Among them, 11 hub proteins (Caveolin-1, Fibulin-1, Collagen alpha-1(VI) chain, Nidogen-2, Collagen alpha-3(VI) chain, 72 kDa type IV collagenase, Elastin, Decorin, Fibronectin, Basement membrane-specific heparan sulfate proteoglycan core protein, MAGUK p55 subfamily member 2) related to hypoxia or osteogenesis, were increased in the norm-osteo EVs group compared to the norm-naïve EVs group.

3.6.3. Anti-Hypoxic Proteins

As shown in Supplementary Figure S6G, a total of nine proteins were identified in the GO terms related to 'response to hypoxia', which are highly enriched in norm-osteo EVs compared with that in norm-naïve EVs, and they were selected for further analysis. Among them, five anti-hypoxic proteins were experimentally determined in the previous studies [41–45], which are Caveolin-1, Secreted frizzled-related protein 1, Extracellular superoxide dismutase (SOD), Endoplasmin (i.e., 94 kDa glucose-regulated protein or HSP90B) and Aquaporin-1 (AQP1). Three of these five proteins (Caveolin-1, Extracellular superoxide dismutase-3 and Endoplasmin) are also classified as antioxidant proteins [46–48]. In this line, the norm-osteo EVs/norm-naïve EVs ratios measured for these five proteins ranged from a 5.09-fold to a 100-fold increase (Figure 8A).

3.7. *Validation of Proteomics Data*

3.7.1. Anti-Hypoxic Gene Expression Levels in the EVs' Parent Cells

To assess the reliability of the proteomic data from norm-osteo EVs and norm-naïve EVs, we selected the five anti-hypoxic genes (CAV1, SFRP1, SOD3, HSP90B1 and AQP1) and further performed qRT-PCR to verify their relative expression levels in the norm-osteo EVs' and norm-naïve EVs' parent cells cultured under normoxia. We observed that CAV1, SFRP1, and AQP1 gene expression was significantly increased after 14 days (Supplementary Figure S8A–E) and after 35 days (Figure 8B–F) of osteogenic differentiation of hBMSC compared to naïve hBMSC both cultured under normoxia.

3.7.2. Anti-Hypoxic Gene Expression Levels in hBMSCs Undergoing Osteogenic Differentiation under Hypoxia after EV Treatment

Under hypoxia, gene expression analysis of these five anti-hypoxic genes (CAV1, SFRP1, SOD3, HSP90B1 and AQP1) revealed that stimulation with both the norm-naïve

EV and norm-osteo EV groups significantly increased CAV1 and HSP90B1 expression in hBMSCs compared to the negative control group (no EVs under hypoxia). Moreover, the SFRP1 gene expression level after norm-osteo EV stimulation was significantly increased compared to the negative control group. SOD3 gene expression level in hBMSCs after norm-naïve EVs stimulation was significantly increased compared to the negative control group (Figure 9A–E).

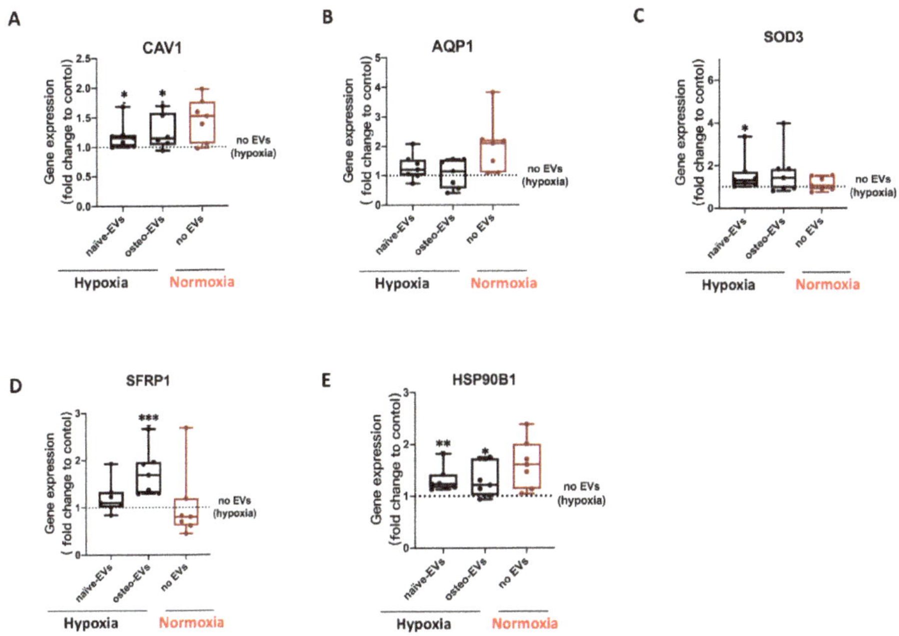

Figure 9. Evaluation of gene expression of the five anti-hypoxic proteins during osteogenic differentiation of hBMSCs under hypoxia after EVs stimulation. (**A–E**) Expression levels of the five anti-hypoxic genes were analyzed after 2 weeks of osteogenic differentiation in hBMSCs and simultaneous treatment with the different EV groups under hypoxia; n = 6–7. Results were calculated as percentage of the negative control group (no EVs under hypoxia, shown by the dotted line); Difference to the negative control: * = $p < 0.05$; ** = $p < 0.01$, ***= $p < 0.001$.

4. Discussion

We characterized EVs isolated from naïve or osteogenic differentiated hBMSCs cultured under normoxia and hypoxia and confirmed their purity and identity in line with our previous studies [42,43,46]. Hypoxia can suppress the osteogenic differentiation capacity of naïve hBMSCs, correlated to decreased calcium deposits, reduced ALP activity and downregulation of gene/protein expression of the osteogenic markers BGLAP, RUNX2, ALP, and COL1A1. This confirms an earlier study by Pattappa et al. [49], who showed that hypoxia may enhance long-term MSC expansion and reduce cell senescence but results in a population with impaired osteogenic differentiation potential. Our proteomic data supported these findings, revealing that hypoxia affected EVs' protein cargo. Moreover, 21 pro-osteogenic proteins were reduced in hypo-osteo EVs compared to norm-osteo EVs (Table 1). In particular, Golgi apparatus protein 1 (GLG1), Transmembrane protein 119 (TMEM119) and alkaline phosphatase, tissue-nonspecific isozyme (ALPL) concentration were reduced about 6.5-fold to 100-fold in hypo-osteo EVs compared to norm-osteo EVs. GLG1 (alternative name: E-selectin ligand 1 = ESL-1) was recently described as an important regulator of bone remodeling, and loss of GLG1 in osteoblasts is leading to delayed differentiation and mineralization [50]. TMEM119 (alternative name: Osteoblast induction factor = OBIF) is an osteoblast differentiation factor that plays a vital role in bone formation and osteoblast differentiation [51], and ALPL (i.e., ALP) as an indicator of bone formation can reflect the activity of the osteoblasts [30]. Here, we clearly demonstrated that a hypoxic culture environment reduced the osteogenic activity of hBMSCs-derived EVs as it significantly suppressed ALP enzyme activity, expression of osteogenic genes, and ALP protein amount in hypo-osteo EVs' cargo. Furthermore, the top two hub proteins, EGFR and CTNNB1, which were less concentrated in hypo-osteo EVs, are pro-osteogenic proteins. EGFR is critically important for osteogenesis, as EGFR deficiency leads to irregular mineralization of bone in mice [52]. CTNNB1 can upregulate osteogenic differentiation and mineralization via FOXQ1, which also promotes the nuclear translocation of CTNNB1 in murine (m)BMSCs, enhancing Wnt/β-catenin signaling, which was also shown to be essential for the osteogenic differentiation-promoting effect of FOXQ1 in mBMSCs [53]. In bone, the ECM is an intricate dynamic structure that plays an important role by instructing the osteogenic differentiation process of BMSCs [54]. The proteomic profiling of EVs showed that the concentration of 21 ECM proteins was decreased in hypo-osteo EVs compared to norm-osteo EVs (Table 2), and subsequent KEGG pathways analysis confirmed that ECM-receptor interaction pathways were significantly reduced in hypo-osteo EVs compared with norm-osteo EVs. ECM macromolecules promote the osteogenic differentiation process of BMSCs through ECM–receptor interaction, e.g., via integrin receptors. Integrins are heterodimeric cell surface receptors that mediate cell–ECM contact and subsequent adhesion and are critical in signal transduction from the ECM into the cells and vice versa [55,56]. CD9, CD81 and CD63 members of the tetraspan superfamily are associated with integrins and form different complexes with different members of the integrin family [57–60]. CD81 and CD9 identified as hub proteins in the PPI network, were decreased in hypo-osteo EVs compared to norm-osteo EVs, as validated with proteomic profiling and Western blot analysis. We assume that CD81 and CD9 are associated with osteogenesis, which is consistent with the study of Singh et al. [61], showing that osteo-chondro-progenitor cells expressing CD9 were readily differentiated to osteoblasts compared to cells without CD9, both in vitro and in vivo.

Cellular oxidative stress may be defined as an imbalance between free radicals (i.e., ROS) and antioxidant proteins in favor of free radicals, potentially leading to oxidative damage of cell membranes and intracellular organelles [62,63]. In our study, hypoxia increased ROS production and secretion. Supported by our proteomic data, we demonstrated that hypoxia reduced the amount of several antioxidant proteins in the EVs' cargo. Five antioxidants (5′-AMP-activated protein kinase catalytic subunit alpha-1 = PRKAA1, NAD(P)H quinone dehydrogenase 1 = NQO1, Annexin A1 = ANXA1, 40S ribosomal protein S3 = RPS3, Peroxiredoxin-1 = PRDX1) were clearly reduced in hypo-osteo EVs compared to norm-osteo EVs (Table 3). Zhu et al. [64] reported that PRKAA1 inactivation led to enhanced mitochondrial ROS production. NQO1, a superoxide scavenger, assists cells in handling ROS [65] and ANXA1, as an anti-inflammatory agent, can interfere with the generation of ROS [66]. RPS3 exerts antioxidative functions and protects cells against oxidative stress [67]. PRDX1 is described as a scavenger of ROS, and loss of PRDX1 in mice leads to an elevation of ROS. Thus, the proteomic analysis of hypo-osteo EVs provided novel insights into the putative mechanisms by which hypoxia can increase ROS production because antioxidant proteins were less abundant in hypo-osteo EVs, disturbing the subtle balance between extracellular ROS level and the intercellular transported antioxidants inside the EVs.

EVs derived from distinct cell types preferring a hypoxic environment, such as cancer cells, MSCs and cardiac cells, significantly increased angiogenesis compared to their normoxic EV controls [1,68]. Notably, our proteomic data revealed that the GO terms related to angiogenesis were significantly downregulated in hypo-osteo EVs derived from osteogenic differentiated BMSCs under hypoxia compared to the norm-osteo EV counterparts. Moreover, the top hub protein in our proteomic analysis is EGFR, a pro-angiogenic protein, which was less abundant in hypo-osteo EVs compared to norm-osteo EVs. It is known that osteonecrosis and osteoporosis pathogenesis are promoted by blood supply disruption, which results in hypoxic injury in bone. Thus, we speculate that under hypoxic pathological conditions in bone tissue, the alteration in the composition/cargo and function of osteogenic EVs, mediated by hypoxia, affects bone homeostasis, which in turn affects osteogenesis and angiogenesis negatively. Moreover, in our study, pro-angiogenic proteins were enriched in norm-osteo EVs, consistent with the study of Narayanan et al. [69], showing that norm-osteo EVs have a strong capacity for promoting vascularization in vivo.

We clearly demonstrated that norm-osteo EVs, harvested at a late stage of osteogenic differentiation of hBMSCs under normoxia, can rescue the osteogenic ability of hBMSCs impaired by hypoxia. This was demonstrated by increased calcium deposits, enhanced ALP activity and the induction of gene expression of the osteogenic transcription factor RUNX2. Our previous study [29] revealed that under normoxic culture conditions, pro-osteogenic proteins were enriched in norm-osteo EVs in comparison to norm-naïve EVs from undifferentiated hBMSCs. Here, we further suggest that the five anti-hypoxic proteins (Caveolin-1 = CAV1, Secreted frizzled-related protein 1 = SFRP1, Extracellular superoxide dismutase-3 = SOD3, Endoplasmin = HSP90B1 and Aquaporin-1 = AQP1), which were highly enriched in norm-osteo EVs, might prevent cell damage or mitigated altered response to external stimuli inflicted by hypoxia. Caveolin-1 can reduce HIF1-α transcriptional activity under hypoxia by reducing HIF-1α S-nitrosylation in vitro and in vivo [35]. For secreted frizzled-related protein 1, it was recently reported that it can directly protect cells from apoptosis during hypoxia and reoxygenation [32]. Overexpression of SOD3 (i.e., EcSOD) suppressed the hypoxia-induced accumulation of HIF-1α in cells. When neurons were exposed to hypoxia/reoxygenation, cells with overexpression of HSP90B1 (i.e., GRP94) were resistant to apoptosis induced by hypoxia/reoxygenation [31]. Aquaporin 1 is a water and oxygen channel that can suppress hyperglycemia-induced cellular hypoxia [34]. The gene expression levels of CAV1, SFRP1 and AQP1 analyzed in the EVs' parent cells (naïve and osteogenic differentiated hBMSCs kept under normoxia) followed the same trend as those indicated by the proteomic data of norm-osteo EVs and norm-naïve EVs supporting our proteomic data. In addition, after stimulation of hBMSCs kept under hypoxic conditions with EVs, we observed that norm-osteo EVs induced CAV1, SFRP1 and HSP90B gene expression in the osteogenic differentiated hBMSCs. Hence, we speculate that norm-osteo EVs are able to transfer CAV1, SFRP1 and HSP90B1 cargo to target cells in a hypoxic environment, and we hypothesize that the cargo of osteogenic EVs enable them to rescue the osteogenic ability of hBMSCs by transferring these and other proteins to the target cells. Moreover, our data suggest that norm-naïve EVs can also promote the anti-hypoxic capacity of a cell by the induction of the expression of CAV1, SOD3 and HSP90B1 in the target cells. That is a likely reason why norm-naïve EVs were able to promote ALP activity in hBMSCs cultured under hypoxia.

Interestingly, three (CAV1, SOD3 and HSP90B1) of the five identified anti-hypoxic proteins are also known to act as antioxidants [36–38,70]. In our study, norm-osteo EVs could inhibit hypoxia-induced elevation of ROS produced by osteogenic differentiated hBMSCs, presumably by an increased antioxidant gene expression (CAV1 and HSP90B1). Moreover, norm-naïve EVs suppressed hypoxia-induced elevation of ROS levels in cultures of osteogenic differentiated hBMSCs, presumably by the increased antioxidant gene expression of SOD3, CAV1 and HSP90B1. Our results are consistent with the study of Khanh et al. [71], showing that EVs from infant MSCs rescued elderly MSCs from oxidative cell damage due to the elevation of ROS via upregulation of SOD1 and SOD3 protein expression. Furthermore, Ma et al. [14] reported that Icariin, a major bioactive pharmaceutical constituent isolated from Chinese medicine Horny Goat Weed, rescued the osteogenic ability of osteoblasts impaired by hypoxia via reducing the production of ROS, increasing SOD and ALP activity and forming a mineralized matrix. Thus, we speculate that norm-osteo EVs and norm-naïve EVs rescued the ALP activity of hBMSCs impaired by hypoxia by reducing the production of ROS. However, norm-naïve EVs were not able to rescue the mineralization ability of osteogenic differentiated hBMSCs impaired by hypoxia.

According to our previous study [29], together with the current data presented here, a possible reason for that might be the fact that ECM components, pro-osteogenic proteins and anti-hypoxic proteins were less abundant in norm-naïve EVs compared to norm-osteo EVs.

5. Conclusions

In conclusion, the proteomic analysis of hypo-osteo EVs provides novel insights into how hypoxia can suppress the osteogenic ability of hBMSCs and simultaneously promote ROS production and secretion. The present study provides evidence that ECM macromolecules and -receptors, antioxidant- and pro-osteogenic proteins are decreased in hypo-osteo EVs, which otherwise would allow the osteogenic differentiated hBMSCs to respond to hypoxia and to accommodate to their surrounding microenvironment. These novel findings add to the understanding that the production of particular hypo-osteo EVs under hypoxic conditions contributes to impaired osteogenesis of mesenchymal precursor cells. Furthermore, norm-osteo EVs rescued the osteogenic ability of hBMSCs, impaired by hypoxia, by inducing expression of anti-hypoxic genes (CAV1, SFRP1, HSP90B1) and reversed hypoxia-induced elevation of ROS production in osteogenic differentiated hBMSCs.

Supplementary Materials: The following supporting information can be downloaded at: https://www.mdpi.com/article/10.3390/biomedicines11102804/s1, Figure S1: Flow cytometric analysis of hBMSC with specific antibodies against positive MSC markers (CD44, CD73) and negative MSC markers (CD19, CD34); Figure S2: Conditioned medium from hypo-osteo EVs and norm-osteo EVs; Figure S3: The uncropped Western blot membranes of Figure 3G and respective Ponceau S stained loading control images below; Figure S4: Evaluation of secreted reactive oxygen species (ROS), and osteogenic marker gene expression in osteogenic differentiated hBMSCs under hypoxia and normoxia; Figure S5: The uncropped Western blot membrane of Figure 3D and respective Ponceau S stained loading control images below; Figure S6: Enrichment analyses and protein–protein interaction (PPI) network analyses of norm-naïve EVs and norm-osteo EVs; Figure S7: PPI network of the distinct proteins and hub proteins identified in norm-osteo EVs compared with that in norm-naïve EVs; Figure S8: Validation of the proteomic data obtained from norm-naïve EVs and norm-osteo EVs by gene expression analysis in hBMSC. Table S1: Distinct proteins identified in hypo-osteo EVs and norm-osteo EVs (attached excel file); Table S2; Primer sequences for qPCR.

Author Contributions: C.W.: methodology, validation, formal analysis, investigation, data curation, writing—original draft and editing; S.S.: conceptualization, writing—review and editing; G.P.: methodology and resources; D.S.: methodology and resources; K.H.: resources; J.I.: methodology, NTA analysis; Y.R.: proteomic analysis and data evaluation; R.J.B.: resources. A.S.: proteomic analysis and data evaluation; S.G.: conceptualization, writing—review and editing, project administration, funding acquisition. All authors have read and agreed to the published version of the manuscript.

Funding: This research was funded by a grant from the German Society of Orthopedics and Orthopedic Surgery (Deutsche Gesellschaft für Orthopädie und Orthopädische Chirurgie; DGOOC) to S.G. Y.R. and A.S. acknowledge the support from the "Ministerium für Kultur undWissenschaft des Landes Nordrhein-Westfalen" and "Der Regierende Bürgermeister von Berlin, Senatskanzlei Wissenschaft und Forschung".

Institutional Review Board Statement: The studies involving human participants were reviewed and approved by the Ethikkommission, University Hospital Regensburg, email: ethikkommission@klinik.uni.regensburg.de.

Informed Consent Statement: Informed consent was obtained from all subjects involved in the study.

Data Availability Statement: Not applicable.

Acknowledgments: We thank Mandy Vogel and Claudia Göttl for their excellent technical assistance.

Conflicts of Interest: The authors declare no conflict of interest.

References

1. Bister, N.; Pistono, C.; Huremagic, B.; Jolkkonen, J.; Giugno, R.; Malm, T. Hypoxia and extracellular vesicles: A review on methods, vesicular cargo and functions. *J. Extracell. Vesicles* **2020**, *10*, e12002. [CrossRef] [PubMed]
2. Lee, J.W.; Ko, J.; Ju, C.; Eltzschig, H.K. Hypoxia signaling in human diseases and therapeutic targets. *Exp. Mol. Med.* **2019**, *51*, 1–13. [CrossRef] [PubMed]
3. Laroche, M.; Moulinier, L.; Leger, P.; Lefebvre, D.; Mazieres, B.; Boccalon, H. Bone mineral decrease in the leg with unilateral chronic occlusive arterial disease. *Clin. Exp. Rheumatol.* **2003**, *21*, 103–106.
4. Salim, A.; Nacamuli, R.P.; Morgan, E.F.; Giaccia, A.J.; Longaker, M.T. Transient changes in oxygen tension inhibit osteogenic differentiation and Runx2 expression in osteoblasts. *J. Biol. Chem.* **2004**, *279*, 40007–40016. [CrossRef] [PubMed]
5. Li, L.J.; Jiang, D.M. Hypoxia-responsive miRNA-21-5p inhibits Runx2 suppression by targeting SMAD7 in MC3T3-E1 cells. *J. Cell. Biochem.* **2019**, *120*, 16867–16875. [CrossRef]
6. Qin, Q.Y.; Liu, Y.P.; Yang, Z.; Aimaijiang, M.; Ma, R.; Yang, Y.X.; Zhang, Y.D.; Zhou, Y.M. Hypoxia-Inducible Factors Signaling in Osteogenesis and Skeletal Repair. *Int. J. Mol. Sci.* **2022**, *23*, 11201. [CrossRef]
7. Wagegg, M.; Gaber, T.; Lohanatha, F.L.; Hahne, M.; Strehl, C.; Fangradt, M.; Tran, C.L.; Schonbeck, K.; Hoff, P.; Ode, A.; et al. Hypoxia Promotes Osteogenesis but Suppresses Adipogenesis of Human Mesenchymal Stromal Cells in a Hypoxia-Inducible Factor-1 Dependent Manner. *PLoS ONE* **2012**, *7*, e46483. [CrossRef]
8. Ivan, M.; Kondo, K.; Yang, H.F.; Kim, W.; Valiando, J.; Ohh, M.; Salic, A.; Asara, J.M.; Lane, W.S.; Kaelin, W.G. HIF alpha targeted for VHL-mediated destruction by proline hydroxylation: Implications for O-2 sensing. *Science* **2001**, *292*, 464–468. [CrossRef]
9. Sies, H.; Jones, D.P. Reactive oxygen species (ROS) as pleiotropic physiological signalling agents. *Nat. Rev. Mol. Cell Biol.* **2020**, *21*, 363–383. [CrossRef]
10. Gorlach, A.; Dimova, E.Y.; Petry, A.; Martinez-Ruiz, A.; Hernansanz-Agustin, P.; Rolo, A.P.; Palmeira, C.M.; Kietzmann, T. Reactive oxygen species, nutrition, hypoxia and diseases: Problems solved? *Redox Biol.* **2015**, *6*, 372–385. [CrossRef]
11. Hannah, S.S.; McFadden, S.; McNeilly, A.; McClean, C. "Take My Bone Away?" Hypoxia and bone: A narrative review. *J. Cell. Physiol.* **2021**, *236*, 721–740. [CrossRef] [PubMed]
12. Badila, A.E.; Radulescu, D.M.; Ilie, A.; Niculescu, A.G.; Grumezescu, A.M.; Radulescu, A.R. Bone Regeneration and Oxidative Stress: An Updated Overview. *Antioxidants* **2022**, *11*, 318. [CrossRef] [PubMed]
13. Balogh, E.; Toth, A.; Mehes, G.; Trencsenyi, G.; Paragh, G.; Jeney, V. Hypoxia Triggers Osteochondrogenic Differentiation of Vascular Smooth Muscle Cells in an HIF-1 (Hypoxia-Inducible Factor 1)-Dependent and Reactive Oxygen Species-Dependent Manner. *Arterioscler. Thromb. Vasc. Biol.* **2019**, *39*, 1088–1099. [CrossRef] [PubMed]
14. Ma, H.P.; Ma, X.N.; Ge, B.F.; Zhen, P.; Zhou, J.; Gao, Y.H.; Xian, C.J.; Chen, K.M. Icariin attenuates hypoxia-induced oxidative stress and apoptosis in osteoblasts and preserves their osteogenic differentiation potential in vitro. *Cell Prolif.* **2014**, *47*, 527–539. [CrossRef]
15. Matic, S.; Dia, V.P. Bovine milk exosomes affected proliferation of macrophages under hypoxia. *Curr. Res. Food Sci.* **2022**, *5*, 2108–2113. [CrossRef]
16. Nicolaije, C.; Koedam, M.; van Leeuwen, J. Decreased oxygen tension lowers reactive oxygen species and apoptosis and inhibits osteoblast matrix mineralization through changes in early osteoblast differentiation. *J. Cell. Physiol.* **2012**, *227*, 1309–1318. [CrossRef]
17. Colombo, M.; Raposo, G.; Thery, C. Biogenesis, Secretion, and Intercellular Interactions of Exosomes and Other Extracellular Vesicles. *Annu. Rev. Cell Dev. Biol.* **2014**, *30*, 255–289. [CrossRef]
18. Edgar, J.R. Q&A: What are exosomes, exactly? *BMC Biol.* **2016**, *14*, 46. [CrossRef]
19. Herrmann, M.; Diederichs, S.; Melnik, S.; Riegger, J.; Trivanovic, D.; Li, S.; Jenei-Lanzl, Z.; Brenner, R.E.; Huber-Lang, M.; Zaucke, F.; et al. Extracellular Vesicles in Musculoskeletal Pathologies and Regeneration. *Front. Bioeng. Biotechnol.* **2021**, *8*, 624096. [CrossRef]
20. Wang, X.Q.; Omar, O.; Vazirisani, F.; Thomsen, P.; Ekstrom, K. Mesenchymal stem cell-derived exosomes have altered microRNA profiles and induce osteogenic differentiation depending on the stage of differentiation. *PLoS ONE* **2018**, *13*, e0193059. [CrossRef]
21. Van Niel, G.; D'Angelo, G.; Raposo, G. Shedding light on the cell biology of extracellular vesicles. *Nat. Rev. Mol. Cell Biol.* **2018**, *19*, 213–228. [CrossRef] [PubMed]
22. An, T.; Qin, S.; Xu, Y.; Tang, Y.; Huang, Y.; Situ, B.; Inal, J.M.; Zheng, L. Exosomes serve as tumour markers for personalized diagnostics owing to their important role in cancer metastasis. *J. Extracell. Vesicles* **2015**, *4*, 27522. [CrossRef] [PubMed]
23. McKeown, S.R. Defining normoxia, physoxia and hypoxia in tumours-implications for treatment response. *Br. J. Radiol.* **2014**, *87*, 20130676. [CrossRef] [PubMed]
24. Yaghoubi, S.; Najminejad, H.; Dabaghian, M.; Karimi, M.H.; Abdollahpour-Alitappeh, M.; Rad, F.; Mahi-Birjand, M.; Mohammadi, S.; Mohseni, F.; Lari, M.S.; et al. How hypoxia regulate exosomes in ischemic diseases and cancer microenvironment? *IUBMB Life* **2020**, *72*, 1286–1305. [CrossRef]
25. Dorayappan, K.D.P.; Wanner, R.; Wallbillich, J.J.; Saini, U.; Zingarelli, R.; Suarez, A.A.; Cohn, D.E.; Selvendiran, K. Hypoxia-induced exosomes contribute to a more aggressive and chemoresistant ovarian cancer phenotype: A novel mechanism linking STAT3/Rab proteins. *Oncogene* **2018**, *37*, 3806–3821. [CrossRef]

26. Ramteke, A.; Ting, H.; Agarwal, C.; Mateen, S.; Somasagara, R.; Hussain, A.; Graner, M.; Frederick, B.; Agarwal, R.; Deep, G. Exosomes secreted under hypoxia enhance invasiveness and stemness of prostate cancer cells by targeting adherens junction molecules. *Mol. Carcinog.* **2015**, *54*, 554–565. [CrossRef]
27. Li, Q.; Yu, H.L.; Sun, M.Y.; Yang, P.; Hu, X.Q.; Ao, Y.F.; Cheng, J. The tissue origin effect of extracellular vesicles on cartilage and bone regeneration. *Acta Biomater.* **2021**, *125*, 253–266. [CrossRef]
28. Zhang, L.; Jiao, G.; Ren, S.; Zhang, X.; Li, C.; Wu, W.; Wang, H.; Liu, H.; Zhou, H.; Chen, Y. Exosomes from bone marrow mesenchymal stem cells enhance fracture healing through the promotion of osteogenesis and angiogenesis in a rat model of nonunion. *Stem Cell Res. Ther.* **2020**, *11*, 38. [CrossRef]
29. Wang, C.L.; Stockl, S.; Li, S.S.; Herrmann, M.; Lukas, C.; Reinders, Y.; Sickmann, A.; Grässel, S. Effects of Extracellular Vesicles from Osteogenic Differentiated Human BMSCs on Osteogenic and Adipogenic Differentiation Capacity of Naive Human BMSCs. *Cells* **2022**, *11*, 2491. [CrossRef]
30. Leyh, M.; Seitz, A.; Durselen, L.; Springorum, H.R.; Angele, P.; Ignatius, A.; Grifka, J.; Grässel, S. Osteoarthritic cartilage explants affect extracellular matrix production and composition in cocultured bone marrow-derived mesenchymal stem cells and articular chondrocytes. *Stem Cell Res. Ther.* **2014**, *5*, 77. [CrossRef]
31. Leyh, M.; Seitz, A.; Duerselen, L.; Schaumburger, J.; Ignatius, A.; Grifka, J.; Grässel, S. Subchondral bone influences chondrogenic differentiation and collagen production of human bone marrow-derived mesenchymal stem cells and articular chondrocytes. *Arthritis Res. Ther.* **2014**, *16*, 453. [CrossRef] [PubMed]
32. Grässel, S.; Stockl, S.; Jenei-Lanzl, Z. Isolation, culture, and osteogenic/chondrogenic differentiation of bone marrow-derived mesenchymal stem cells. *Methods Mol. Biol.* **2012**, *879*, 203–267. [CrossRef] [PubMed]
33. Li, S.; Stöckl, S.; Lukas, C.; Goetz, J.; Herrmann, M.; Federlin, M.; Grässel, S. hBMSC-Derived Extracellular Vesicles Attenuate IL-1 beta-Induced Catabolic Effects on OA-Chondrocytes by Regulating Pro-inflammatory Signaling Pathways. *Front. Bioeng. Biotechnol.* **2020**, *8*, 603598. [CrossRef] [PubMed]
34. Niedermair, T.; Lukas, C.; Li, S.; Stoeckl, S.; Craiovan, B.; Brochhausen, C.; Federlin, M.; Herrmann, M.; Grässel, S. Influence of Extracellular Vesicles Isolated from Osteoblasts of Patients with Cox-Arthrosis and/or Osteoporosis on Metabolism and Osteogenic Differentiation of BMSCs. *Front. Bioeng. Biotechnol.* **2020**, *8*, 615520. [CrossRef] [PubMed]
35. Pattappa, G.; Schewior, R.; Hofmeister, I.; Seja, J.; Zellner, J.; Johnstone, B.; Docheva, D.; Angele, P. Physioxia Has a Beneficial Effect on Cartilage Matrix Production in Interleukin-1 Beta-Inhibited Mesenchymal Stem Cell Chondrogenesis. *Cells* **2019**, *8*, 936. [CrossRef]
36. Pattappa, G.; Reischl, F.; Jahns, J.; Schewior, R.; Lang, S.G.; Zellner, J.; Johnstone, B.; Docheva, D.; Angele, P. Fibronectin Adherent Cell Populations Derived from Avascular and Vascular Regions of the Meniscus Have Enhanced Clonogenicity and Differentiation Potential Under Physioxia. *Front. Bioeng. Biotechnol.* **2022**, *9*, 789621. [CrossRef]
37. Li, S.S.; Stockl, S.; Lukas, C.; Herrmann, M.; Brochhausen, C.; Konig, M.A.; Johnstone, B.; Grässel, S. Curcumin-primed human BMSC-derived extracellular vesicles reverse IL-1 beta-induced catabolic responses of OA chondrocytes by upregulating miR-126-3p. *Stem Cell Res. Ther.* **2021**, *12*, 252. [CrossRef]
38. Bardou, P.; Mariette, J.; Escudie, F.; Djemiel, C.; Klopp, C. jvenn: An interactive Venn diagram viewer. *BMC Bioinform.* **2014**, *15*, 293. [CrossRef]
39. Chen, C.J.; Chen, H.; Zhang, Y.; Thomas, H.R.; Frank, M.H.; He, Y.H.; Xia, R. TBtools: An Integrative Toolkit Developed for Interactive Analyses of Big Biological Data. *Mol. Plant* **2020**, *13*, 1194–1202. [CrossRef]
40. Vanstraalen, J.P.; Sanders, E.; Prummel, M.F.; Sanders, G.T.B. Bone-alkaline phosphatase as indicator of bone-formation. *Clin. Chim. Acta* **1991**, *201*, 27–34. [CrossRef]
41. Bando, Y.; Katayama, T.; Kasai, K.; Taniguchi, M.; Tamatani, M.; Tohyama, M. GRP94 (94 kDa glucose-regulated protein) suppresses ischemic neuronal cell death against ischemia/reperfusion injury. *Eur. J. Neurosci.* **2003**, *18*, 829–840. [CrossRef] [PubMed]
42. Tao, J.; Abudoukelimu, M.; Ma, Y.T.; Yang, Y.N.; Li, X.M.; Chen, B.D.; Liu, F.; He, C.H.; Li, H.Y. Secreted frizzled related protein 1 protects H9C2 cells from hypoxia/re-oxygenation injury by blocking the Wnt signaling pathway. *Lipids Health Dis.* **2016**, *15*, 72. [CrossRef] [PubMed]
43. Sibenaller, Z.A.; Welsh, J.L.; Du, C.B.; Witmer, J.R.; Schrock, H.E.; Du, J.; Buettner, G.R.; Goswami, P.C.; Cieslak, J.A.; Cullen, J.J. Extracellular superoxide dismutase suppresses hypoxia-inducible factor-1 alpha in pancreatic cancer. *Free. Radic. Biol. Med.* **2014**, *69*, 357–366. [CrossRef]
44. Sada, K.; Nishikawa, T.; Kukidome, D.; Yoshinaga, T.; Kajihara, N.; Sonoda, K.; Senokuchi, T.; Motoshima, H.; Matsumura, T.; Araki, E. Hyperglycemia Induces Cellular Hypoxia through Production of Mitochondrial ROS Followed by Suppression of Aquaporin-1. *PLoS ONE* **2016**, *11*, e0158619. [CrossRef]
45. Sanhueza, C.; Bennett, J.C.; Valenzuela-Valderrama, M.; Contreras, P.; Lobos-Gonzalez, L.; Campos, A.; Wehinger, S.; Lladser, A.; Kiessling, R.; Leyton, L.; et al. Caveolin-1-Mediated Tumor Suppression Is Linked to Reduced HIF1 alpha S-Nitrosylation and Transcriptional Activity in Hypoxia. *Cancers* **2020**, *12*, 2349. [CrossRef] [PubMed]
46. Martinez-Outschoorn, U.E.; Balliet, R.M.; Rivadeneira, D.B.; Chiavarina, B.; Pavlides, S.; Wang, C.G.; Whitaker-Menezes, D.; Daumer, K.M.; Lin, Z.; Witkiewicz, A.K.; et al. Oxidative stress in cancer associated fibroblasts drives tumor-stroma co-evolution A new paradigm for understanding tumor metabolism, the field effect and genomic instability in cancer cells. *Cell Cycle* **2010**, *9*, 3256–3276. [CrossRef]

47. Fukai, T.; Ushio-Fukai, M. Superoxide Dismutases: Role in Redox Signaling, Vascular Function, and Diseases. *Antioxid. Redox Signal.* **2011**, *15*, 1583–1606. [CrossRef]
48. Pizzo, P.; Scapin, C.; Vitadello, M.; Florean, C.; Gorza, L. Grp94 acts as a mediator of curcumin-induced antioxidant defence in myogenic cells. *J. Cell. Mol. Med.* **2010**, *14*, 970–981. [CrossRef]
49. Pattappa, G.; Thorpe, S.D.; Jegard, N.C.; Heywood, H.K.; de Bruijn, J.D.; Lee, D.A. Continuous and uninterrupted oxygen tension influences the colony formation and oxidative metabolism of human mesenchymal stem cells. *Tissue Eng. Methods* **2013**, *19*, 68–79. [CrossRef]
50. Yang, T.; Grafe, I.; Bae, Y.J.; Chen, S.; Chen, Y.Q.; Bertin, T.K.; Jiang, M.M.; Ambrose, C.G.; Lee, B. E-selectin ligand 1 regulates bone remodeling by limiting bioactive TGF-beta in the bone microenvironment. *Proc. Natl. Acad. Sci. USA* **2013**, *110*, 7336–7341. [CrossRef]
51. Mizuhashi, K.; Kanamoto, T.; Ito, M.; Moriishi, T.; Muranishi, Y.; Omori, Y.; Terada, K.; Komori, T.; Furukawa, T. OBIF, an osteoblast induction factor, plays an essential role in bone formation in association with osteoblastogenesis. *Dev. Growth Differ.* **2012**, *54*, 474–480. [CrossRef] [PubMed]
52. Linder, M.; Hecking, M.; Glitzner, E.; Zwerina, K.; Holcmann, M.; Bakiri, L.; Ruocco, M.G.; Tuckermann, J.; Schett, G.; Wagner, E.F.; et al. EGFR controls bone development by negatively regulating mTOR-signaling during osteoblast differentiation. *Cell Death Differ.* **2018**, *25*, 1094–1106. [CrossRef] [PubMed]
53. Xiang, L.S.; Zheng, J.M.; Zhang, M.D.; Ai, T.T.; Cai, B. FOXQ1 promotes the osteogenic differentiation of bone mesenchymal stem cells via Wnt/beta-catenin signaling by binding with ANXA2. *Stem Cell Res. Ther.* **2020**, *11*, 403. [CrossRef]
54. Lin, X.; Patil, S.; Gao, Y.G.; Qian, A.R. The Bone Extracellular Matrix in Bone Formation and Regeneration. *Front. Pharmacol.* **2020**, *11*, 757. [CrossRef]
55. Volloch, V.; Olsen, B.R. Why cellular stress suppresses adipogenesis in skeletal tissue, but is ineffective in adipose tissue: Control of mesenchymal cell differentiation via integrin binding sites in extracellular matrices. *Matrix Biol.* **2013**, *32*, 365–371. [CrossRef] [PubMed]
56. Docheva, D.; Popov, C.; Alberton, P.; Aszodi, A. Integrin signaling in skeletal development and function. *Birth Defects Res.-Embryo Today-Rev.* **2014**, *102*, 13–36. [CrossRef]
57. Hirano, T.; Higuchi, T.; Ueda, M.; Inoue, T.; Kataoka, N.; Maeda, M.; Fujiwara, H.; Fujii, S. CD9 is expressed in extravillous trophoblasts in association with integrin alpha(3) and integrin alpha(5). *Mol. Hum. Reprod.* **1999**, *5*, 162–167. [CrossRef]
58. Justo, B.L.; Jasiulionis, M.G. Characteristics of TIMP1, CD63, and beta 1-Integrin and the Functional Impact of Their Interaction in Cancer. *Int. J. Mol. Sci.* **2021**, *22*, 9319. [CrossRef]
59. Stipp, C.S.; Hemler, M.E. Transmembrane-4-superfamily proteins CD151 and CD81 associate with alpha 3 beta 1 integrin, and selectively contribute to alpha 3 beta 1-dependent neurite outgrowth. *J. Cell Sci.* **2000**, *113*, 1871–1882. [CrossRef]
60. Horvath, G.; Serru, V.; Clay, D.; Billard, M.; Boucheix, C.; Rubinstein, E. CD19 is linked to the integrin-associated tetraspans CD9, CD81, and CD82. *J. Biol. Chem.* **1998**, *273*, 30537–30543. [CrossRef]
61. Singh, A.; Lester, C.; Drapp, R.; Hu, D.Z.; Glimcher, L.H.; Jones, D. Tetraspanin CD9 and ectonucleotidase CD73 identify an osteochondroprogenitor population with elevated osteogenic properties. *Development* **2015**, *142*, 438–443. [CrossRef] [PubMed]
62. Forman, H.J.; Torres, M. Reactive oxygen species and cell signaling—Respiratory burst in macrophage signaling. *Am. J. Respir. Crit. Care Med.* **2002**, *166*, S4–S8. [CrossRef] [PubMed]
63. Sies, H. Oxidative stress: Oxidants and antioxidants. *Exp. Physiol.* **1997**, *82*, 291–295. [CrossRef] [PubMed]
64. Zhu, H.P.; Foretz, M.; Xie, Z.L.; Zhang, M.; Zhu, Z.R.; Xing, J.J.; Leclerc, J.; Gaudry, M.; Viollet, B.; Zou, M.H. PRKAA1/AMPK alpha 1 is required for autophagy-dependent mitochondrial clearance during erythrocyte maturation. *Autophagy* **2014**, *10*, 1522–1534. [CrossRef]
65. Siegel, D.; Gustafson, D.L.; Dehn, D.L.; Han, J.Y.; Boonchoong, P.; Berliner, L.J.; Ross, D. NAD(P)H: Quinone oxidoreductase 1: Role as a superoxide scavenger. *Mol. Pharmacol.* **2004**, *65*, 1238–1247. [CrossRef]
66. Kiani-Esfahani, A.; Sheykhshabani, S.K.; Peymani, M.; Hashemi, M.S.; Ghaedi, K.; Nasr-Esfahani, M.H. Overexpression of Annexin A1 Suppresses Pro-Inflammatory Factors in PC12 Cells Induced by 1-Methyl-4-Phenylpyridinium. *Cell J.* **2016**, *18*, 197.
67. Ahn, E.H.; Kim, D.W.; Shin, M.J.; Kim, Y.N.; Kim, H.R.; Woo, S.J.; Kim, S.M.; Kim, D.S.; Kim, J.; Park, J.; et al. PEP-1-ribosomal protein S3 protects dopaminergic neurons in an MPTP-induced Parkinson's disease mouse model. *Free. Radic. Biol. Med.* **2013**, *55*, 36–45. [CrossRef]
68. Svensson, K.J.; Kucharzewska, P.; Christianson, H.C.; Skold, S.; Lofstedt, T.; Johansson, M.C.; Morgelin, M.; Bengzon, J.; Ruf, W.; Belting, M. Hypoxia triggers a proangiogenic pathway involving cancer cell microvesicles and PAR-2-mediated heparin-binding EGF signaling in endothelial cells. *Proc. Natl. Acad. Sci. USA* **2011**, *108*, 13147–13152. [CrossRef]
69. Narayanan, R.; Huang, C.-C.; Ravindran, S. Hijacking the Cellular Mail: Exosome Mediated Differentiation of Mesenchymal Stem Cells. *Stem Cells Int.* **2016**, *2016*, 3808674. [CrossRef]

70. Varadaraj, K.; Kumari, S.S. Lens aquaporins function as peroxiporins to facilitate membrane transport of hydrogen peroxide. *Biochem. Biophys. Res. Commun.* **2020**, *524*, 1025–1029. [CrossRef]
71. Khanh, V.C.; Yamashita, T.; Ohneda, K.; Tokunaga, C.; Kato, H.; Osaka, M.; Hiramatsu, Y.; Ohneda, O. Rejuvenation of mesenchymal stem cells by extracellular vesicles inhibits the elevation of reactive oxygen species. *Sci. Rep.* **2020**, *10*, 17315. [CrossRef] [PubMed]

biomedicines

MDPI

Article

The Influence of Exercise-Associated Small Extracellular Vesicles on Trophoblasts *In Vitro*

Shuhiba Mohammad [1], Jayonta Bhattacharjee [1], Velislava Tzaneva [1], Kelly Ann Hutchinson [1], Madeeha Shaikh [1], Danilo Fernandes da Silva [1], Dylan Burger [2] and Kristi B. Adamo [1,*]

1 School of Human Kinetics, Faculty of Health Sciences, University of Ottawa, Ottawa, ON K1N 6N5, Canada
2 Kidney Research Centre, Department of Cellular and Molecular Medicine, The Ottawa Hospital Research Institute, University of Ottawa, Ottawa, ON K1H 8L6, Canada
* Correspondence: kadamo@uottawa.ca

Abstract: Exercise induces the release of small extracellular vesicles (sEVs) into circulation that are postulated to mediate tissue cross-talk during exercise. We previously reported that pregnant individuals released greater levels of sEVs into circulation after exercise compared to matched non-pregnant controls, but their biological functions remain unknown. In this study, sEVs isolated from the plasma of healthy pregnant and non-pregnant participants after a single bout of moderate-intensity exercise were evaluated for their impact on trophoblasts *in vitro*. Exercise-associated sEVs were found localized within the cytoplasm of BeWo choriocarcinoma cells, used to model trophoblasts in vitro. Exposure to exercise-associated sEVs did not significantly alter BeWo cell proliferation, gene expression of angiogenic growth factors *VEGF* and *PLGF*, or the release of the hormone human chorionic gonadotropin. The results from this pilot study support that exercise-associated sEVs could interact with trophoblasts in vitro, and warrant further investigation to reveal their potential role in communicating the effects of exercise to the maternal–fetal interface.

Keywords: exercise; physical activity; small extracellular vesicles; placenta; trophoblast; pregnancy

1. Introduction

Exercise during pregnancy is well known to bestow benefits on both mother and fetus, potentially improving health across two generations. To promote maternal health and as a front-line therapy for mitigating the risk of pregnancy disorders, the 2019 Canadian Guideline for Physical Activity throughout Pregnancy recommends that those without contraindications should engage in at least 150 min of moderate-intensity physical activity per week [1]. Maternal physical activity is associated with decreased risk of pregnancy complications, including preeclampsia, gestational diabetes mellitus, and gestational hypertension [2], and improvement of prenatal depressive symptoms [3] while reducing blood glucose levels [4]. Prenatal physical activity is also associated with beneficial neonatal outcomes such as reduced odds of macrosomia [5] and fat mass at birth [6]. While the advantages are numerous and well established, the biological mechanisms by which these benefits are communicated to the mother and fetus are not well understood.

Exercise has been posited to alter the structure and physiology of the placenta [7], the critical interface between mother and fetus chiefly responsible for maternal–fetal communication. The placenta supports fetal growth and survival by mediating the exchange of gases, nutrients, and waste, while providing endocrine and immune support. As a transient discoid organ anchored to the maternal uterus, the placenta is composed of a heterogeneous population of cells organized in a manner to ensure sufficient maternal–fetal exchange between the juxtaposed maternal and fetal circulatory systems. In the placenta, maternal exercise has been shown to impact oxidative stress [8], nutrient transporters [9,10], and angiogenic growth factors [11,12]. Data from exercise interventions also show beneficial effects on placental growth [13] and volume available for maternal–fetal exchange [14,15]. While it is evident that exercise impacts placental function, the biological mechanisms contributing to these changes are less clear.

The benefits of exercise are hypothesized to be mediated in part by the release of bioactive molecules into circulation after exercise, including myokines (cytokines produced and released by skeletal muscle) [16,17] and small extracellular vesicles (sEVs) [18,19]. sEVs (historically referred to as "exosomes" [20]) are lipid membrane-enclosed particles (~20–120 nm in diameter) secreted by cells into extracellular space and contain bioactive compounds such as nucleic acids (i.e., mRNAs and miRNAs), lipids, and proteins [21,22]. sEVs are theorized to facilitate long-distance intercellular communication by interaction or transfer of their biological cargo from donor to target cells [23,24]. Data from both human and animal studies demonstrate that sEVs are released into circulation after exercise (reviewed by [19]) and contain biological molecules potentially involved in tissue cross-talk in response to exercise [18]. We previously reported that pregnant individuals release greater levels of sEVs into circulation compared to non-pregnant individuals after a single bout of moderate-intensity exercise [25]. The potential biological function and cellular targets of circulating sEVs released in response to maternal exercise are unknown. Since the placenta can release and take up sEVs as a part of maternal–fetal communication [26,27], exercise-associated sEVs could possibly act on the placenta. Therefore, circulating sEVs may represent a potential mechanism involved in improving placental function in the context of maternal exercise.

In this study, we examined in pilot experiments whether exposure to circulating sEVs obtained after acute exercise affected trophoblasts *in vitro*. Trophoblast cells are specialized epithelial cells that constitute the maternal–fetal interface and are responsible for hormone production and the exchange of gases, nutrients, and waste between mother and fetus. First, we determined whether circulating exercise-associated sEVs from healthy pregnant and non-pregnant individuals could interact with trophoblasts *in vitro*. Further, we evaluated whether exposure to exercise-associated plasma sEVs could influence metrics of trophoblast biology, including proliferation, expression of angiogenic growth factors known to be altered in the placenta of physically active vs. inactive mothers [11], and secretion of the major pregnancy hormone, human chorionic gonadotropin (b-hCG). Treatment with sEVs from healthy non-pregnant controls was used to determine whether the potential effects on trophoblast biology were associated with pregnancy status or exercise stimulus. In this set of pilot experiments, we hypothesized that exercise-associated sEVs from pregnant individuals would elicit greater effects on trophoblast biology compared to exercise-associated sEVs from non-pregnant controls.

2. Materials and Methods

2.1. Ethical Approval and Study Participants

Experimental procedures were approved by the University of Ottawa Research Ethics Board (file number: H-06-18-634). All protocols were performed in fulfillment of the guidelines described in the Declaration of Helsinki. Informed written consent was secured from participants after an explanation of the study procedures. Pregnant and non-pregnant individuals were recruited from the Ottawa area (ON, Canada) for participation in the study. Healthy individuals without contraindication to exercise between the ages of 18 and 40 were eligible for inclusion, with a self-reported pre- or non-pregnant body mass index (BMI) of 18.5–29.9 kg/m^2. Participants were required to be weight-stable ($\pm$5 kg) for approximately six months before the study. Pregnant participants needed to be between 13 and 28 weeks gestation carrying a singleton fetus to participate in the study. Those with chronic health conditions including hypertension, diabetes (pre/non-pregnant or gestational diabetes), and untreated thyroid disease and frequent users of tobacco, drugs, or alcohol were excluded from participation.

2.2. Acute Exercise Procedure

The acute exercise stimulus followed procedures outlined by Hutchinson et al. (2019) [28] and Mohammad et al. (2021) [25]. Briefly, participants were requested to refrain from exercise and food for 8 h before the acute exercise session. Participants were provided with a standardized snack, after which resting heart rate was determined as previously described [25,28]. A target range of 40–59% of heart rate (HR) reserve was used to specify moderate-intensity exercise [29,30], where HR reserve was calculated using the Karvonen equation [31] as described previously [25,28]. The moderate-intensity acute exercise session consisted of a brisk 30 min treadmill walk with continuous HR monitoring using a Polar V800 HR monitor (Polar Electro, Lachine, QC, Canada). A short warm-up (3 min at 2% incline at a speed of 2 miles per hour (mph)) was followed by an incremental phase (6% incline), where treadmill speed was increased by 0.2 mph every minute until the upper range of moderate-intensity HR reserve (59%) was met. Once this range was met, the participants continued to exercise for 30 min. Blood was collected (10 mL) immediately before (at rest) and after the exercise session from the median cubital vein using potassium EDTA blood collection tubes (#367863; BD Biosciences, Mississauga, ON, Canada). Plasma was promptly processed by centrifugation at 1700× *g* for 15 min at 4 °C, and samples were stored at −80 °C until further analyses.

2.3. sEV Isolation and Labeling

Isolation of sEVs from plasma was performed using differential ultracentrifugation as described previously [25,32,33]. Plasma samples (1.0 mL) were thawed rapidly at 37 °C, then kept on ice for all remaining procedures. Samples were first centrifuged at 20,000× *g* for 20 min at 4 °C to remove large EVs and apoptotic bodies. The remaining supernatant was centrifuged at a speed of 100,000× *g* using a Beckman Coulter Optima MAX ultracentrifuge (Beckman Coulter Inc., Brea, CA, USA) equipped with a TLA-55 rotor (Beckman Coulter) for 90 min at 4 °C. The resulting pellet of sEVs was washed with 1.0 mL of 0.1 μm filtered phosphate-buffered saline (PBS) and then centrifuged at 100,000× *g* as described above. The final residual pellet of sEVs was resuspended in 100 μL of 0.1 μm filtered PBS. Aliquots of 10 μL of this suspension were separated and frozen at −80 °C for further analysis. One 10 μL aliquot was used for protein extraction and quantification to standardize sEV treatment concentrations for subsequent functional assays. To extract protein, 1 μL of 10× radioimmunoprecipitation assay (RIPA) buffer with protease inhibitor cocktail (MilliporeSigma Canada Co., #P8340, Oakville, ON, Canada) was added to a 10 μL sEV aliquot. Samples were sonicated using a bath sonicator for 1 min to achieve EV and protein lysis and subsequently were incubated on ice for 30 min before protein quantification using a DC protein assay (Bio-Rad Laboratories, #5000112, Mississauga, ON, Canada). sEVs from this cohort were previously validated to be the expected size (~100–120 nm) and displayed characteristics confirming the presence of these particles (i.e., expression of classical sEV protein markers TSG-101 and flotillin-1, absence of non-sEV marker calnexin, and intact membrane integrity and characteristic size as determined by transmission electron microscopy [25]. Where indicated, sEVs were fluorescently labeled with PKH26, a lipophilic membrane dye, using the PKH26 Red Fluorescent Cell Linker Kit according to the manufacturer's instructions (Phanos Technologies, MilliporeSigma Canada Co., #MINI26-1KT). Following the incorporation of the dye, the labeled sEVs were centrifuged at 100,000× *g* for 90 min at 4 °C, and the resulting sEV pellets were resuspended in 100 μL of 0.1 μm filtered PBS and stored at −80 °C for subsequent sEV internalization and interaction fluorescence assays.

2.4. Cell Culture

BeWo choriocarcinoma cells were obtained from the American Type Culture Collection (ATCC CCL-98, Manassas, VA, USA) and grown in Ham's F-12K (Kaighn's) medium (Gibco, Thermo Fisher Scientific, #21127022, Waltham, MA, USA) supplemented with 10% fetal bovine serum (FBS) and incubated at 37 °C and 5% CO_2 in a humidified environment.

For all sEV treatment experiments, cells from passages 7–12 were used in the presence of F-12K medium supplemented with 10% EV-depleted FBS. EV-depletion of undiluted FBS was achieved by ultracentrifugation at 100,000× *g* for 90 min at 4 °C [34] and retention of the resulting supernatant, confirmed by nanoparticle tracking analysis. Cells were experimentally manipulated 48 h post-seeding.

2.5. sEV Localization by Fluorescence Confocal Microscopy

BeWo cells (2.5×10^4) were plated in 8-well chamber slides (ibidi USA, #80826, Fitchburg, WI, USA) and incubated with 2.5 µg/mL of PKH26-labeled sEVs (or PBS control) overnight (16 h) at 37 °C and 5% CO_2. The cell culture supernatant was removed, and wells were vigorously washed five times with PBST and then fixed with 10% buffered formalin for 10 min at room temperature. All subsequent steps were conducted at room temperature with three PBST washes between each step unless noted otherwise. Fixative was removed, and then cells were permeabilized using 0.1% Triton X-100 in PBS for 5 min. Next, slides were incubated with phalloidin-iFluor 488 Reagent (1:1000; Abcam Inc., #ab176753, Cambridge, MA, USA) in 1% BSA in PBS for 25 min. Finally, 1 drop of NucBlue Fixed Cell ReadyProbes Reagent (DAPI) (Invitrogen, Thermo Fisher Scientific, #R37606) was added to each well for 5 min. Mounting media (ibidi USA, #500001) were added to each well before imaging using an inverted Zeiss LSM 880 AxioObserver Z1 laser-scanning confocal microscope with Airyscan FAST detector equipped with Zen Black software (version 2.3, Carl Zeiss Microscopy GmbH, Jena, Germany). Images were taken using a 63× oil-immersion objective lens (Carl Zeiss Microscopy GmbH, Plan Apochromat 63/1.4 NA oil) with optical slices (z-stacks) at a thickness of 0.20 µm. The confocal was equipped with lasers emitting at 405, 488, and 561 nm which were used for the excitation of each fluorophore: DAPI (Ex/Em 405/450 nm), phalloidin (Ex/Em 488/516 nm), and PKH26 (Ex/Em 561/579 nm). Each confocal microscopy image was acquired using the same imaging parameters. Images were subjected to linear unmixing of the measured spectral profiles for each fluorophore (DAPI, phalloidin, and PKH26) using Zen Black software (version 2.3) to account for signal crossover between spectral channels. Representative maximum intensity projections were acquired from a subset of z-stacks corresponding to the middle of the cells. For each condition, a minimum of three random fields of view were selected and examined for sEV localization. To increase the quality of the images for display purposes, lookup tables for the phalloidin channel image were set to "Magenta" and for the PKH26 channel image were set to "Green" using Fiji software (version 2.3.0/1.53f, U.S. National Institutes of Health, Bethesda, Maryland, USA).

For the localization experiments, a range of PKH26-labeled sEV concentrations was initially tested (1, 2.5, 5, and 10 µg/mL) for visualization by confocal microscopy. The concentration of 2.5 µg/mL of sEVs incubated overnight (16 h) was found to be the exposure with the best signal-to-noise ratio.

2.6. Proliferation Assessment by Ki67 Immunostaining

To assess the influence of exercise-associated plasma sEVs on BeWo cell proliferation in vitro, Ki67 immunostaining was used. BeWo cells (2.5×10^4) were seeded onto 8-well chamber slides (ibidi USA, #80826) and incubated with 10 µg/mL sEVs (or PBS control) for 24 h at 37 °C and 5% CO_2 in duplicate. Then, the cell culture supernatant was removed and wells were washed three times with PBST. All of the following steps were carried out at room temperature unless stated otherwise. Cells were fixed with 10% formalin for 10 min and then washed three times with PBST. Cells were then permeabilized using 0.1% Triton X-100 in PBS for 5 min followed by three washes with PBST. Cells were blocked for 30 min with BlockAid Blocking Solution (Invitrogen, Thermo Fisher Scientific, #B10710) and then incubated with recombinant anti-Ki67 rabbit monoclonal antibody (SP6) (1:250; Abcam Inc, #ab16667) at 4 °C in PBST overnight. Negative controls omitted the primary antibody. The following day, wells were washed three times with PBST and then incubated with goat AlexaFluor 488 anti-rabbit IgG (H+L) Superclonal recombinant secondary antibody (1:1000; Invitrogen, Thermo Fisher Scientific, #A27034) in PBST for 60 min. Wells were washed three times with PBST and then incubated with 1 drop of NucBlue Fixed Cell ReadyProbes Reagent (DAPI) (Invitrogen, Thermo Fisher Scientific, #R37606) per well for 5 min. Mounting media (ibidi USA, #500001) were added to each well before imaging using a ThermoFisher FL Auto 2 inverted automated epifluorescent microscope equipped with version Auto2 software (Invitrogen, Thermo Fisher Scientific). Each well was divided into four quadrants, with one image taken at 20× magnification per quadrant for a total of four images per well. All experiments were performed in triplicate. A ratio of Ki67 immunostaining intensity to nuclear area was measured using Fiji software (version 2.3.0/1.53f, U.S. National Institutes of Health).

2.7. RNA Isolation and Quantitative Real-Time Polymerase Chain Reaction (qPCR)

BeWo cells were seeded at a density of 1.0×10^5 in 12-well dishes; 48 h later, they were treated with 10 μg/mL plasma sEVs (or PBS control) for 24 h at 37 °C and 5% CO_2. Cell culture supernatant was collected and stored at −80 °C for downstream b-hCG analysis described below. Cells were washed twice with cold sterile PBS and then lysed for total RNA isolation using an Illustra RNAspin Mini isolation kit (Cytiva Life Sciences, Fisher Scientific Company, #25050071, Ottawa, ON, Canada) as per the manufacturer's instructions. Isolated total RNA was eluted in RNase-free water and was analyzed for concentration and purity using spectrophotometry (Take3, Gen5 software version 1.11.5, BioTek Instruments Inc., Winooski, VT, USA). RNA integrity was verified using a 2% agarose gel stained with SYBR Safe DNA gel stain (Invitrogen, Thermo Fisher Scientific, #S33102) and electrophoresis of bromophenol blue-labeled RNA aliquots at 100 V for 30 min in TAE (Tris-acetate-EDTA) buffer. RNA bands were visualized by ultraviolet transillumination using a ChemiDoc XRS+ system (Bio-Rad Laboratories, Mississauga, ON, Canada). Then, 0.5 μg of RNA was reverse transcribed into cDNA using an iScript cDNA synthesis kit (Bio-Rad Laboratories, #1708891) and a Biometra TPersonal Combi Thermocycler (Analytik Jena, Jena, Germany) according to the manufacturer's protocol, and then stored at −20 °C until further analysis. A total of 25 ng of cDNA was used for quantitative polymerase chain reaction (qPCR) using TaqMan Advanced Master Mix (Applied Biosystems, Thermo Fisher Scientific, #444557). Samples were loaded into a Rotor-Gene 3000 real-time DNA detection system with Rotor-Gene software (version 6.1.93, Corbett Research, Sydney, Australia). The expression of angiogenic growth factors *VEGF* and *PLGF* was measured relative to an endogenous control, *GAPDH*. Taqman gene expression assay probes labeled with 6-FAM (6-carboxyfluorescein) fluorescent dye were used for the detection of *VEGF* (Hs00900055_m1), *PLGF* (Hs00182176_m1), and *GAPDH* (Hs02786624_g1). The qPCR reaction was as follows: hold at 50 °C for 2 min, then hold at 95 °C for 2 min, followed by 40 cycles consisting of denaturing at 95 °C for 3 s and hold at 60 °C for 30 s. All qPCR reactions were performed in duplicate with appropriate controls (no cDNA reverse transcriptase cDNA control and no template qPCR control), and all experiments were conducted in triplicate. Corresponding threshold cycle (CT) values were recorded, and relative gene expression was calculated using the $2^{-\Delta\Delta CT}$ method [35]. Data from the target genes (*VEGF* and *PLGF*) were expressed as a ratio to *GAPDH* gene expression for normalization. Gene expression values from PBS control treatment conditions were considered as control.

2.8. b-hCG Assay

Cell culture supernatant collected from the gene expression analyses described above were used to determine the effect of sEV treatment on b-hCG production in BeWo cells after 24 h of exposure using a DRG b-hCG ELISA kit (DRG International, #EIA-1911, Springfield, NJ, USA) as per the manufacturer's instructions. b-hCG concentration was normalized to mg of total RNA isolated from the corresponding gene expression experiments and is presented in mIU/mL.

2.9. Statistical Analysis

All data are presented as mean ± standard deviation (SD) from three independent experiments. All statistical analyses and graphs were generated using GraphPad Prism version 9.3 (GraphPad Software, La Jolla, CA, USA). A one-way ANOVA with Tukey's post-test (if applicable) was used to compare whether no treatment (PBS control) was different from exposure to exercise-associated sEVs from pregnant and non-pregnant individuals. The homogeneity assumption was confirmed by Levene's test. Statistical significance was considered when $p < 0.05$.

3. Results

3.1. Exercise-Associated sEVs Interact with BeWo Cells

We first examined whether circulating sEVs obtained from pregnant and non-pregnant individuals after a bout of acute moderate-intensity exercise could be found within trophoblast-like cells *in vitro*. Representative images obtained by confocal microscopy show that PKH26-labeled sEVs from both pregnant and non-pregnant individuals obtained post-exercise localized within the cytoplasm of BeWo cells after overnight incubation (Figure 1).

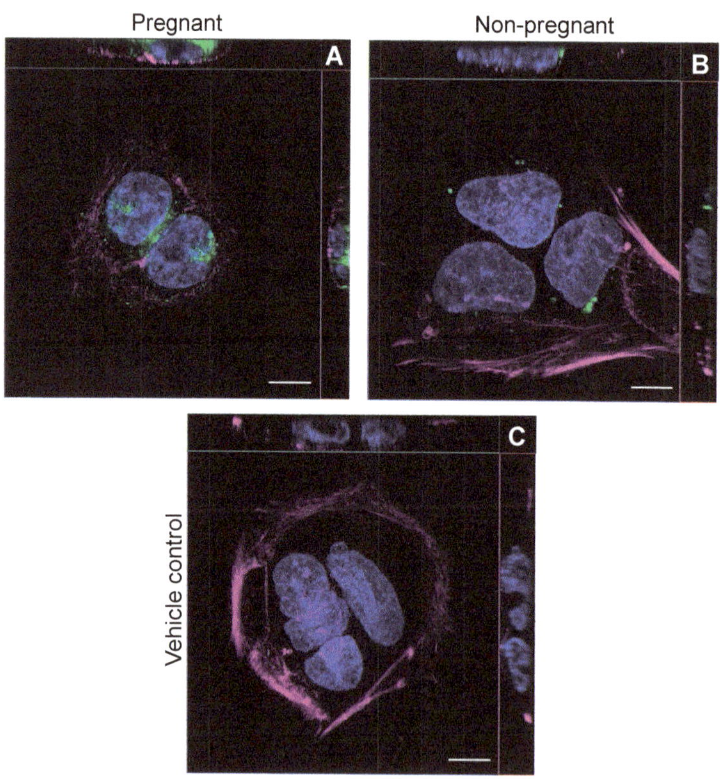

Figure 1. Exercise-associated sEVs were found within BeWo cells *in vitro*. Representative confocal microscopy images of BeWo cells after overnight (16 h) incubation with 2.5 μg/mL PKH26-labeled sEVs from pregnant (**A**) and non-pregnant (**B**) plasma post-exercise. Panel (**C**) shows a representative vehicle control image (PBS). Blue represents DAPI staining for nuclei, magenta depicts phalloidin staining, and green shows PKH26-labeled sEVs. "Magenta" and "Green" lookup tables were used to display phalloidin and sEV labeling, respectively. For each panel, orthogonal projections show the XY (main image), YZ (right of main image), and XZ (top image) planes. All images were taken using a 63× objective lens with oil immersion. Scale bar = 10 μm for all images.

3.2. BeWo Cell Proliferation Was Not Affected upon Exposure to Exercise-Associated sEVs

Immunostaining of the protein Ki67 was used to assess proliferation in BeWo cells after 24 h incubation with exercise-associated sEVs. Ki67 is a widely used marker of cell proliferation and has been used in the examination of trophoblast and BeWo cell proliferation and phenotype [36]. Exposure to sEVs obtained from pregnant participants and non-pregnant controls after exercise did not influence BeWo cell proliferation after 24 h when compared to vehicle treatment (PBS control) (Figure 2).

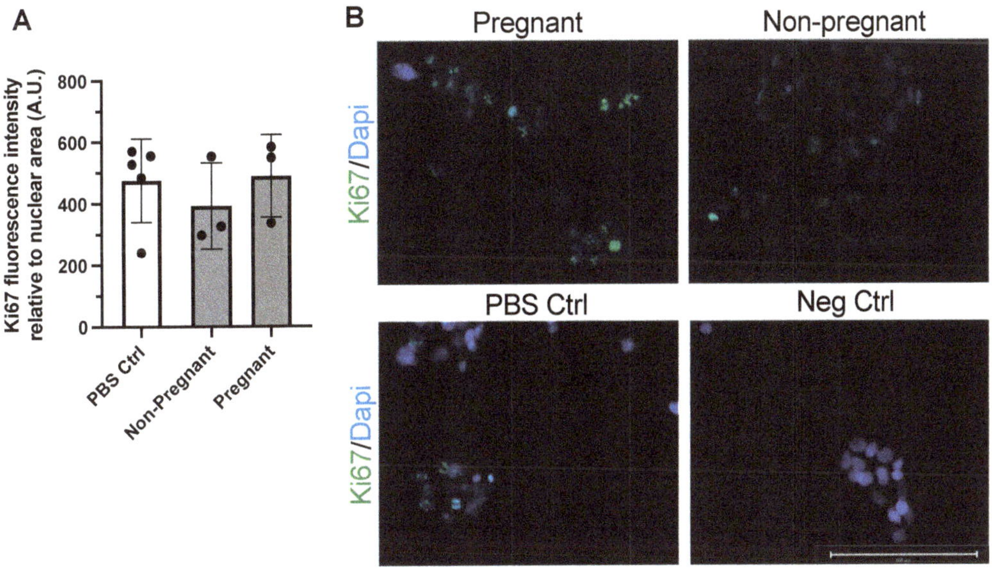

Figure 2. Exercise-associated sEVs did not affect BeWo cell proliferation. There were no differences in proliferation when no treatment (PBS Ctrl) was compared to treatment with exercise-associated sEVs from pregnant and non-pregnant individuals (F = 0.469, $p = 0.642$) (**A**). Representative merged fluorescence images of each condition (**B**) and a negative control (Neg Ctrl) where primary antibody was omitted are shown, where blue depicts DAPI staining for nuclei and green shows Ki67 positive signal. All experiments were conducted in triplicate, with sEVs obtained from $n = 3$ pregnant and $n = 3$ non-pregnant participants, with corresponding PBS controls ($n = 5$). Scale bar = 200 µm. Neg ctrl, negative control; PBS Ctrl, phosphate-buffered saline control.

3.3. Exposure to Plasma sEVs Did Not Alter the Gene Expression of Angiogenic Growth Factors in BeWo Cells

We previously reported that maternal exercise was associated with differential expression of angiogenic proteins in the placenta of individuals categorized as physically active vs. inactive during pregnancy [11]. We therefore determined whether exposure to circulating exercise-associated sEVs from pregnant or non-pregnant individuals affected gene expression of *VEGF* and *PLGF* in BeWo cells. Gene expression of both *VEGF* and *PLGF* did not differ between treatment with PBS control vs. exercise-associated sEVs obtained from both groups (F = 1.98, $p = 0.200$, and F = 0.726, $p = 0.513$, respectively) (Figure 3A,B).

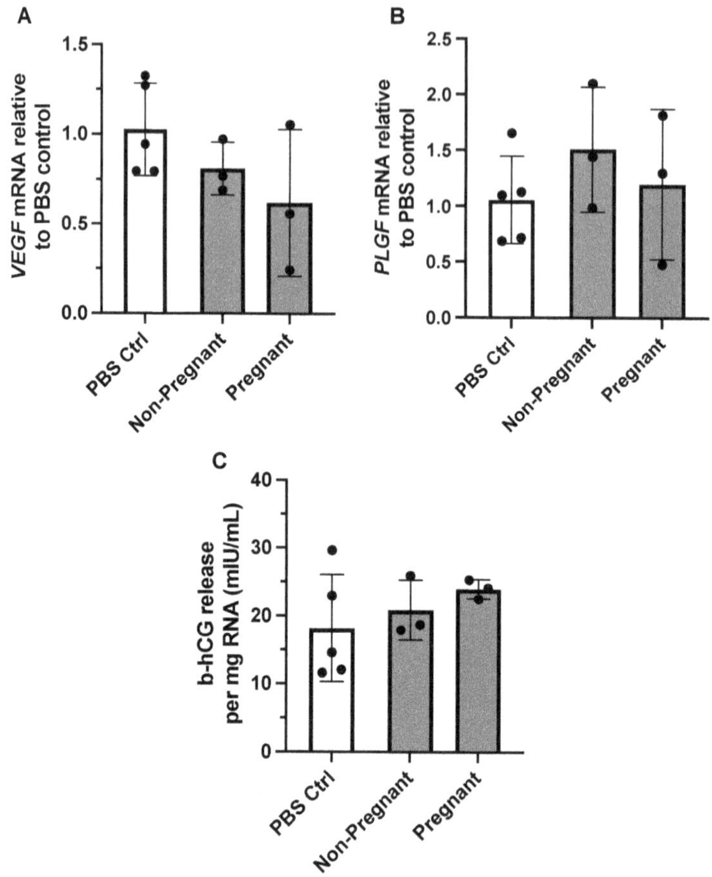

Figure 3. The effect of exercise-associated sEVs on relative gene expression of angiogenic growth factors and b-hCG production in BeWo cells. Gene expression of *VEGF* (**A**) and *PLGF* (**B**) was not altered upon exposure to circulating exercise-associated sEVs (10 µg/mL for 24 h) obtained from pregnant and non-pregnant individuals compared to PBS control (PBS Ctrl) treatment (F = 1.98, $p = 0.200$, and F = 0.726, $p = 0.513$, respectively). (**C**) There were no differences in b-hCG cell media levels when no treatment was compared to treatment with exercise-associated sEVs from pregnant and non-pregnant participants (F = 0.885, $p = 0.450$). All experiments were conducted in triplicate, with sEVs obtained from $n = 3$ pregnant and $n = 3$ non-pregnant participants, with corresponding PBS controls ($n = 5$).

3.4. Human Chorionic Gonadotropin Levels Were Not Affected upon Exposure to Exercise-Associated sEVs

The hormone b-hCG is known to be produced and released from BeWo cells *in vitro* in the process of syncytialization, an essential part of trophoblast differentiation and function [37,38]. We examined the levels of b-hCG in cell media after incubation with exercise-associated plasma sEVs from pregnant and non-pregnant participants. Exposure to exercise-associated sEVs did not result in differing levels of b-hCG in cell media when compared to no treatment (PBS control exposure) (F = 0.885, $p = 0.450$; Figure 3C).

4. Discussion

This study aimed to determine whether sEVs released after a single bout of acute moderate-intensity exercise in pregnant individuals and respective non-pregnant controls can be internalized by cells modeling placental trophoblasts *in vitro* and alter their function. We provide the first evidence that sEVs released after exercise into circulation could interact with trophoblasts *in vitro* but do not alter traditional indices of trophoblast biology, including proliferation, gene expression of angiogenic markers, or production of the pregnancy hormone b-hCG. sEVs are postulated to be an important delivery mechanism in the adaptive response to exercise on a systemic level [18,19,39]. This study provides preliminary evidence that may facilitate our understanding of how exercise is communicated from the mother to the fetus during pregnancy via the maternal–fetal interface.

Central to the hypothesis that sEVs communicate the benefits of exercise systemically is their uptake into recipient tissues and cells, or surface interactions with activating receptors. Exercise-associated sEVs from both pregnant and non-pregnant individuals were localized within BeWo cells. Few studies have evaluated whether sEVs released into circulation in response to exercise can be taken up by or interact with recipient cells. Notably, Whitham et al. (2018) showed that fluorescently labeled EVs from mouse myoblasts could be localized within mouse liver hepatocytes and that cargo of plasma EVs from exercising mice was incorporated into mouse liver hepatocytes [18]. In the context of exercise training and cardiomyocyte injury, PKH26-labeled EVs isolated from the plasma of exercising rats were found to be internalized into cardiomyocytes in vitro after a 6 h incubation period [40]. In a study conducted by Just et al. (2020), sEVs released after acute blood flow-restricted resistance exercise in healthy young men were localized within muscle stem cells and fibro-adipogenic progenitor cells in vitro [41]. Our proof-of-concept experiments show that exercise-associated sEVs can also interact with trophoblasts, specialized cells that are in direct contact with maternal blood and constitute the maternal–fetal interface. Since evidence suggests that EV uptake is not a passive process and involves a variety of energy-requiring endocytic pathways (reviewed by [42]), we postulate that exercise-associated sEVs may play a role in modifying trophoblast function in the context of maternal exercise.

Having observed that exercise-associated sEVs could interact with trophoblast-like cells *in vitro*, we sought to investigate their potential impact on trophoblast physiology. The secretion of b-hCG in cell culture media was investigated as a marker of BeWo cell and trophoblast differentiation. Impaired trophoblast differentiation and fusion are seen in pregnancy pathologies including pre-eclampsia [38], for which risk is mitigated by regular engagement in physical activity during pregnancy [2]. The release of b-hCG was not affected by exposure to exercise-associated sEVs from pregnant or non-pregnant individuals, nor was BeWo cell proliferation. Trophoblasts produce VEGF and PlGF to promote branching and non-branching placental angiogenesis, respectively [43,44]. Given that we previously reported differential expression of angiogenic growth factors VEGF, PlGF, and their respective receptors in term placenta of individuals categorized physically active or inactive [11], we aimed to determine whether gene expression of *VEGF* or *PLGF* was affected by exercise-associated sEVs. Regardless of pregnancy status, exposure to exercise-associated sEVs did not produce changes in *VEGF* or *PLGF* expression levels in BeWo cells. Our observations differ from data in human umbilical vein endothelial cells (HUVECs), where exposure to plasma sEVs isolated from pregnant and non-pregnant individuals at resting conditions was found to increase endothelial cell migration similarly to VEGF-induced migration [27]. It must be noted that Salomon et al. (2014) [27] used a concentration of sEVs that was 10-fold higher than concentrations used to expose trophoblasts in our study (i.e., 100 μg/mL vs. 10 μg/mL EV protein, respectively), and they did not examine gene expression of *VEGF*.

Relatively few studies to date have determined the physiological impact of exercise-associated sEVs on the biological functions of target cells, and none have been conducted on trophoblasts or cells constituting the maternal–fetal interface. The majority of work on the physiological consequences of exercise-associated sEVs involve animal models, where their interactions have been shown to delay prostate cancer progression [45], provide sustained cardioprotection [40], and elicit beneficial effects in ischemic stroke [46]. In humans, sEVs obtained after blood flow-restricted resistance exercise in healthy men were found to increase the proliferation of fibro-adipogenic progenitor cells [41]. The lack of biological impact on trophoblast biology demonstrated in the present study is likely due to a variety of factors. The bioactivity of sEVs is largely dependent on their diverse biological cargo, which is influenced by the cells of origin. Identifying the contents and origins of exercise-associated sEVs in pregnant and non-pregnant participants was beyond the scope of this preliminary study but represents a critical knowledge gap in this emerging field. Characterization of the biological contents and cellular origins of exercise-associated maternal sEVs will allow for the development of more targeted hypotheses regarding assessments of trophoblastic function. Exercise training status may influence the biological contents of exercise-associated sEVs, as Nair et al. (2020) reported that microRNA profiles differed in circulating sEVs obtained from sedentary vs. active older men [47]. In the present study, we were unable to objectively validate the habitual physical activity patterns of the study participants. Future studies should examine whether exercise training or chronic habitual exercise could alter the bioactivity of maternal sEVs, and evaluate their potential impact on trophoblasts. Currently, there is inconsistent evidence to suggest that exercise intensity or modality could affect sEV release and contents [19,48–50]. It is unknown whether differing exercise intensities (i.e., moderate vs. vigorous intensity) could impact sEV cargo, and whether a specific intensity or threshold is required to produce functional changes in trophoblasts.

Our study presents some strengths and limitations. As noted by others, caution must be exercised when extrapolating results obtained using transformed immortalized cell lines, including BeWo choriocarcinoma cells, in the modeling of normal trophoblast populations [51–53]. In this case, while not an exact simulation of trophoblasts, readily available and accessible BeWo cells provide invaluable insights into trophoblast function [52–54]. Future experiments deducing the potential function of sEVs in the context of maternal exercise should employ primary human trophoblasts or trophoblast populations obtained from the derivation and differentiation of trophoblast stem cells [55,56]. Another limitation relates to pitfalls associated with physical-based sEV isolation methods including differential ultracentrifugation. Lipoproteins have been reported to be isolated alongside sEVs using physical-based isolation methods, leading to the contamination of sEV isolate fractions [57,58]. Lipoproteins may also carry bioactive molecules such as miRNAs [59,60], which may have introduced potential confounders in the current preliminary study. Future studies should employ alternative sEV isolation methods (i.e., combinations of density gradient centrifugation and size-exclusion chromatography) to minimize co-isolation of contaminating non-sEV species. Further, co-isolated lipoproteins may compete with sEVs upon labeling with lipid-anchored fluorophores, including PKH26 [61–63]. Therefore, future investigations should characterize the extent to which samples may be contaminated with co-isolates that could result in the unintended labeling of non-sEV targets in uptake studies.

A strength of the sEV localization analysis stems from the use of an Airyscan detector in conjunction with confocal microscopy allowing for enhanced detection not available in traditional confocal systems [64]. However, it is important to note that the confocal imaging studies presented here are qualitative in nature. Another strength is the duration and type of exercise selected for the representation of acute exercise during pregnancy. The Canadian evidence-based physical activity guidelines throughout pregnancy recommend individuals engage in a minimum of 150 min of moderate-intensity physical activity to achieve benefits, within a recommended heart rate range based on age [1]. We therefore intentionally designed a physiologically appropriate exercise session for pregnancy, while the majority of studies to date on exercise-associated sEVs involve sustained vigorous-intensity exercise until volitional exhaustion in men (reviewed by [19]). Low sample size was a major limitation of our study, but herein we provide pilot data to support the continued exploration of maternal exercise-associated sEVs and their potential impact on placental function.

5. Conclusions

In summary, our preliminary results show that exercise-associated sEVs could be localized within trophoblast-like cells *in vitro*. Whether they can produce biological changes sufficient to improve trophoblast biology or stimulate other intercellular signaling pathways that may transmit signals to the fetus remain unknown. Since the placenta is primarily responsible for maternal–fetal communication and fetal growth, further investigation is warranted to determine the biological impact and mechanisms linking maternal sEVs to the benefits sustained from engagement in exercise during pregnancy.

Author Contributions: Conceptualization, S.M., K.A.H. and K.B.A.; data curation, S.M., V.T., M.S. and D.F.d.S.; formal analysis, S.M.; funding acquisition, K.B.A.; investigation, S.M., J.B. and V.T.; methodology, S.M., J.B., V.T. and K.A.H.; project administration, K.A.H.; resources, D.B. and K.B.A.; supervision, D.B. and K.B.A.; writing—original draft, S.M.; writing—review and editing, S.M., J.B., V.T., D.F.d.S., D.B. and K.B.A. All authors have read and agreed to the published version of the manuscript.

Funding: This research was funded by grants awarded to K.B.A. by the Canadian Institutes of Health Research, grant number MOP 142298, and the Natural Sciences and Engineering Council (NSERC), grant number RGPIN-2017-05457. S.M. was funded by the Faculty of Health Sciences uOttawa/CHEO Doctoral Fellowship for the Advancement of Biological Perspectives for Exercise Interventions Across the Lifespan and the Ontario Graduate Scholarship. K.A.H. was the recipient of the Canada Graduate Scholarships-Master's funded by NSERC.

Institutional Review Board Statement: This study was conducted in accordance with the Declaration of Helsinki and approved by the University of Ottawa Research Ethics Board (file number: H-06-18-634 approved on 23 August 2019).

Informed Consent Statement: Informed written consent was obtained from all study participants involved in the study.

Data Availability Statement: Data are available from the corresponding author upon reasonable request.

Acknowledgments: The authors acknowledge the Cell Biology and Image Acquisition (CBIA) Core funded by the University of Ottawa, Ottawa, ON, Canada, and the Canada Foundation for Innovation. We would like to specifically acknowledge the top-tier microscopy and imaging specialists at the CBIA Core, including Chloë Oostende-Triplet, Redaet Daniel, and Ian Blum. We extend our deepest gratitude to Fengxia Xiao for technical assistance with the sEV labeling experiments and ultracentrifugation. We also Tarushika Vasanthan for reviewing the manuscript. Finally, we acknowledge the gracious support provided by Shannon Bainbridge and her laboratory members during the COVID-19 pandemic.

Conflicts of Interest: The authors declare no conflict of interest or competing interests.

Sample Availability: Samples from this study are not available.

References

1. Mottola, M.F.; Davenport, M.H.; Ruchat, S.M.; Davies, G.A.; Poitras, V.J.; Gray, C.E.; Garcia, A.J.; Barrowman, N.; Adamo, K.B.; Duggan, M.; et al. 2019 Canadian guideline for physical activity throughout pregnancy. *Br. J. Sport. Med.* **2018**, *52*, 1339–1346. [CrossRef] [PubMed]
2. Davenport, M.H.; Ruchat, S.M.; Poitras, V.J.; Garcia, A.J.; Gray, C.E.; Barrowman, N.; Skow, R.J.; Meah, V.L.; Riske, L.; Sobierajski, F.; et al. Prenatal exercise for the prevention of gestational diabetes mellitus and hypertensive disorders of pregnancy: A systematic review and meta-analysis. *Br. J. Sport. Med.* **2018**, *52*, 1367. [CrossRef]
3. Davenport, M.H.; McCurdy, A.P.; Mottola, M.F.; Skow, R.J.; Meah, V.L.; Poitras, V.J.; Garcia, A.J.; Gray, C.E.; Barrowman, N.; Riske, L.; et al. Impact of prenatal exercise on both prenatal and postnatal anxiety and depressive symptoms: A systematic review and meta-analysis. *Br. J. Sport. Med.* **2018**, *52*, 1376. [CrossRef] [PubMed]
4. Davenport, M.H.; Sobierajski, F.; Mottola, M.F.; Skow, R.J.; Meah, V.L.; Poitras, V.J.; Gray, C.E.; Garcia, A.J.; Barrowman, N.; Riske, L.; et al. Glucose responses to acute and chronic exercise during pregnancy: A systematic review and meta-analysis. *Br. J. Sport. Med.* **2018**, *52*, 1357. [CrossRef] [PubMed]
5. Davenport, M.H.; Meah, V.L.; Ruchat, S.M.; Davies, G.A.; Skow, R.J.; Barrowman, N.; Adamo, K.B.; Poitras, V.J.; Gray, C.E.; Garcia, A.J.; et al. Impact of prenatal exercise on neonatal and childhood outcomes: A systematic review and meta-analysis. *Br. J. Sport. Med.* **2018**, *52*, 1386. [CrossRef]

6. Clapp, J.F., 3rd. Morphometric and neurodevelopmental outcome at age five years of the offspring of women who continued to exercise regularly throughout pregnancy. *J. Pediatr.* **1996**, *129*, 856–863. [CrossRef]
7. Bhattacharjee, J.; Mohammad, S.; Adamo, K.B. Does exercise during pregnancy impact organs or structures of the maternal-fetal interface? *Tissue Cell* **2021**, *72*, 101543. [CrossRef]
8. Ramírez-Vélez, R.; Bustamante, J.; Czerniczyniec, A.; Aguilar de Plata, A.C.; Lores-Arnaiz, S. Effect of exercise training on eNOS expression, NO production and oxygen metabolism in human placenta. *PLoS ONE*. **2013**, *8*, e80225. [CrossRef]
9. Hutchinson, K.A.; Vuong, N.H.; Mohammad, S.; Everest, C.; Leung, M.L.; Bhattacharjee, J.; Adamo, K.B. Physical Activity During Pregnancy Is Associated with Increased Placental FATP4 Protein Expression. *Reprod. Sci.* **2020**, *27*, 1909–1919. [CrossRef]
10. Brett, K.E.; Ferraro, Z.M.; Holcik, M.; Adamo, K.B. Prenatal physical activity and diet composition affect the expression of nutrient transporters and mTOR signaling molecules in the human placenta. *Placenta* **2015**, *36*, 204–212. [CrossRef] [PubMed]
11. Bhattacharjee, J.; Mohammad, S.; Goudreau, A.D.; Adamo, K.B. Physical activity differentially regulates VEGF, PlGF, and their receptors in the human placenta. *Physiol. Rep.* **2021**, *9*, e14710. [CrossRef] [PubMed]
12. Hardy, D.B.; Mu, X.; Marchiori, K.S.; Mottola, M.F. Exercise in Pregnancy Increases Placental Angiogenin without Changes in Oxidative or Endoplasmic Reticulum Stress. *Med. Sci. Sport. Exerc.* **2021**, *53*, 1846–1854. [CrossRef] [PubMed]
13. Clapp, J.F., 3rd; Kim, H.; Burciu, B.; Lopez, B. Beginning regular exercise in early pregnancy: Effect on fetoplacental growth. *Am. J. Obstet. Gynecol.* **2000**, *183*, 1484–1488. [CrossRef]
14. Jackson, M.R.; Gott, P.; Lye, S.J.; Ritchie, J.W.; Clapp, J.F., 3rd. The effects of maternal aerobic exercise on human placental development: Placental volumetric composition and surface areas. *Placenta* **1995**, *16*, 179–191. [CrossRef]
15. Bergmann, A.; Zygmunt, M.; Clapp, J.F., 3rd. Running throughout pregnancy: Effect on placental villous vascular volume and cell proliferation. *Placenta* **2004**, *25*, 694–698. [CrossRef] [PubMed]
16. Pedersen, B.K. Muscles and their myokines. *J. Exp. Biol.* **2011**, *214 Pt 2*, 337–346. [CrossRef] [PubMed]
17. Pedersen, B.K.; Steensberg, A.; Fischer, C.; Keller, C.; Ostrowski, K.; Schjerling, P. Exercise and cytokines with particular focus on muscle-derived IL-6. *Exerc. Immunol. Rev.* **2001**, *7*, 18–31. [PubMed]
18. Whitham, M.; Parker, B.L.; Friedrichsen, M.; Hingst, J.R.; Hjorth, M.; Hughes, W.E.; Egan, C.L.; Cron, L.; Watt, K.I.; Kuchel, R.P.; et al. Extracellular Vesicles Provide a Means for Tissue Crosstalk during Exercise. *Cell Metab.* **2018**, *27*, 237–251.e4. [CrossRef]
19. Nederveen, J.P.; Warnier, G.; Di Carlo, A.; Nilsson, M.I.; Tarnopolsky, M.A. Extracellular Vesicles and Exosomes: Insights From Exercise Science. *Front Physiol.* **2020**, *11*, 604274. [CrossRef]
20. Witwer, K.W.; Théry, C. Extracellular vesicles or exosomes? On primacy, precision, and popularity influencing a choice of nomenclature. *J. Extracell. Vesicles.* **2019**, *8*, 1648167. [CrossRef]
21. Raposo, G.; Stoorvogel, W. Extracellular vesicles: Exosomes, microvesicles, and friends. *J. Cell Biol.* **2013**, *200*, 373–383. [CrossRef]
22. Valadi, H.; Ekström, K.; Bossios, A.; Sjöstrand, M.; Lee, J.J.; Lötvall, J.O. Exosome-mediated transfer of mRNAs and microRNAs is a novel mechanism of genetic exchange between cells. *Nat. Cell Biol.* **2007**, *9*, 654–659. [CrossRef] [PubMed]
23. Simons, M.; Raposo, G. Exosomes—vesicular carriers for intercellular communication. *Curr. Opin. Cell Biol.* **2009**, *21*, 575–581. [CrossRef] [PubMed]
24. Mathieu, M.; Martin-Jaular, L.; Lavieu, G.; Théry, C. Specificities of secretion and uptake of exosomes and other extracellular vesicles for cell-to-cell communication. *Nat. Cell Biol.* **2019**, *21*, 9–17. [CrossRef]
25. Mohammad, S.; Hutchinson, K.A.; da Silva, D.F.; Bhattacharjee, J.; McInnis, K.; Burger, D.; Adamo, K.B. Circulating small extracellular vesicles increase after an acute bout of moderate-intensity exercise in pregnant compared to non-pregnant women. *Sci. Rep.* **2021**, *11*, 12615. [CrossRef]
26. Tannetta, D.; Dragovic, R.; Alyahyaei, Z.; Southcombe, J. Extracellular vesicles and reproduction-promotion of successful pregnancy. *Cell. Mol. Immunol.* **2014**, *11*, 548–563. [CrossRef]
27. Salomon, C.; Torres, M.J.; Kobayashi, M.; Scholz-Romero, K.; Sobrevia, L.; Dobierzewska, A.; Illanes, S.E.; Mitchell, M.D.; Rice, G.E. A gestational profile of placental exosomes in maternal plasma and their effects on endothelial cell migration. *PLoS ONE* **2014**, *9*, e98667. [CrossRef] [PubMed]
28. Hutchinson, K.A.; Mohammad, S.; Garneau, L.; McInnis, K.; Aguer, C.; Adamo, K.B. Examination of the Myokine Response in Pregnant and Non-pregnant Women Following an Acute Bout of Moderate-Intensity Walking. *Front. Physiol.* **2019**, *10*, 1188. [CrossRef]
29. American College of Sports Medicine Position Stand. The recommended quantity and quality of exercise for developing and maintaining cardiorespiratory and muscular fitness, and flexibility in healthy adults. *Med. Sci. Sport. Exerc.* **1998**, *30*, 975-91.
30. Davenport, M.H.; Ruchat, S.M.; Mottola, M.F.; Davies, G.A.; Poitras, V.J.; Gray, C.E.; Garcia, A.J.; Barrowman, N.; Adamo, K.B.; Duggan, M.; et al. 2019 Canadian Guideline for Physical Activity Throughout Pregnancy: Methodology. *J. Obstet. Gynaecol. Can. JOGC = J. D'obstet. Gynecol. Can. JOGC* **2018**, *40*, 1468–1483. [CrossRef]
31. Karvonen, M.J.; Kentala, E.; Mustala, O. The effects of training on heart rate; a longitudinal study. *Ann. Med. Exp. Biol. Fenn.* **1957**, *35*, 307–315. [PubMed]
32. Munkonda, M.N.; Akbari, S.; Landry, C.; Sun, S.; Xiao, F.; Turner, M.; Holterman, C.E.; Nasrallah, R.; Hébert, R.L.; Kennedy, C.R.; et al. Podocyte-derived microparticles promote proximal tubule fibrotic signaling via p38 MAPK and CD36. *J. Extracell. Vesicles* **2018**, *7*, 1432206. [CrossRef]

33. Burger, D.; Viñas, J.L.; Akbari, S.; Dehak, H.; Knoll, W.; Gutsol, A.; Carter, A.; Touyz, R.M.; Allan, D.S.; Burns, K.D. Human endothelial colony-forming cells protect against acute kidney injury: Role of exosomes. *Am. J. Pathol.* **2015**, *185*, 2309–2323. [CrossRef]
34. Shelke, G.V.; Lässer, C.; Gho, Y.S.; Lötvall, J. Importance of exosome depletion protocols to eliminate functional and RNA-containing extracellular vesicles from fetal bovine serum. *J. Extracell. Vesicles* **2014**, *3*, 24783. [CrossRef] [PubMed]
35. Livak, K.J.; Schmittgen, T.D. Analysis of relative gene expression data using real-time quantitative PCR and the 2(-Delta Delta C(T)) Method. *Methods* **2001**, *25*, 402–408. [CrossRef]
36. Lu, X.; Wang, R.; Zhu, C.; Wang, H.; Lin, H.Y.; Gu, Y.; Cross, J.C.; Wang, H. Fine-Tuned and Cell-Cycle-Restricted Expression of Fusogenic Protein Syncytin-2 Maintains Functional Placental Syncytia. *Cell Rep.* **2017**, *21*, 1150–1159. [CrossRef] [PubMed]
37. Huppertz, B.; Borges, M. Placenta Trophoblast Fusion. In *Cell Fusion: Overviews and Methods*; Chen, E.H., Ed.; Humana Press: Totowa, NJ, USA, 2008; pp. 135–147.
38. Huppertz, B.; Bartz, C.; Kokozidou, M. Trophoblast fusion: Fusogenic proteins, syncytins and ADAMs, and other prerequisites for syncytial fusion. *Micron* **2006**, *37*, 509–517. [CrossRef]
39. Trovato, E.; Di Felice, V.; Barone, R. Extracellular Vesicles: Delivery Vehicles of Myokines. *Front. Physiol.* **2019**, *10*, 522. [CrossRef] [PubMed]
40. Hou, Z.; Qin, X.; Hu, Y.; Zhang, X.; Li, G.; Wu, J.; Li, J.; Sha, J.; Chen, J.; Xia, J.; et al. Longterm Exercise-Derived Exosomal miR-342-5p: A Novel Exerkine for Cardioprotection. *Circ. Res.* **2019**, *124*, 1386–1400. [CrossRef]
41. Just, J.; Yan, Y.; Farup, J.; Sieljacks, P.; Sloth, M.; Venø, M.; Gu, T.; de Paoli, F.V.; Nyengaard, J.R.; Bæk, R.; et al. Blood flow-restricted resistance exercise alters the surface profile, miRNA cargo and functional impact of circulating extracellular vesicles. *Sci. Rep.* **2020**, *10*, 5835. [CrossRef]
42. Mulcahy, L.A.; Pink, R.C.; Carter, D.R. Routes and mechanisms of extracellular vesicle uptake. *J. Extracell. Vesicles* **2014**, *3*, 24641. [CrossRef]
43. Shore, V.H.; Wang, T.H.; Wang, C.L.; Torry, R.J.; Caudle, M.R.; Torry, D.S. Vascular endothelial growth factor, placenta growth factor and their receptors in isolated human trophoblast. *Placenta* **1997**, *18*, 657–665. [CrossRef]
44. Kingdom, J.; Huppertz, B.; Seaward, G.; Kaufmann, P. Development of the placental villous tree and its consequences for fetal growth. *Eur. J. Obstet. Gynecol. Reprod. Biol.* **2000**, *92*, 35–43. [CrossRef] [PubMed]
45. Sadovska, L.; Auders, J.; Keiša, L.; Romanchikova, N.; Silamiķele, L.; Kreišmane, M.; Zayakin, P.; Takahashi, S.; Kalniņa, Z.; Linē, A. Exercise-Induced Extracellular Vesicles Delay the Progression of Prostate Cancer. *Front. Mol. Biosci.* **2021**, *8*, 784080. [CrossRef]
46. Wang, J.; Liu, H.; Chen, S.; Zhang, W.; Chen, Y.; Yang, Y. Moderate exercise has beneficial effects on mouse ischemic stroke by enhancing the functions of circulating endothelial progenitor cell-derived exosomes. *Exp. Neurol.* **2020**, *330*, 113325. [CrossRef]
47. Nair, V.D.; Ge, Y.; Li, S.; Pincas, H.; Jain, N.; Seenarine, N.; Amper, M.A.; Goodpaster, B.H.; Walsh, M.J.; Coen, P.M.; et al. Sedentary and Trained Older Men Have Distinct Circulating Exosomal microRNA Profiles at Baseline and in Response to Acute Exercise. *Front. Physiol.* **2020**, *11*, 605. [CrossRef] [PubMed]
48. Frühbeis, C.; Helmig, S.; Tug, S.; Simon, P.; Krämer-Albers, E.M. Physical exercise induces rapid release of small extracellular vesicles into the circulation. *J. Extracell. Vesicles* **2015**, *4*, 28239. [CrossRef]
49. Oliveira, G.P., Jr.; Porto, W.F.; Palu, C.C.; Pereira, L.M.; Petriz, B.; Almeida, J.A.; Viana, J.; Filho, N.N.; Franco, O.L.; Pereira, R.W. Effects of Acute Aerobic Exercise on Rats Serum Extracellular Vesicles Diameter, Concentration and Small RNAs Content. *Front. Physiol.* **2018**, *9*, 532. [CrossRef] [PubMed]
50. Brahmer, A.; Neuberger, E.W.I.; Simon, P.; Krämer-Albers, E.M. Considerations for the Analysis of Small Extracellular Vesicles in Physical Exercise. *Front. Physiol.* **2020**, *11*, 576150. [CrossRef]
51. Al-Nasiry, S.; Spitz, B.; Hanssens, M.; Luyten, C.; Pijnenborg, R. Differential effects of inducers of syncytialization and apoptosis on BeWo and JEG-3 choriocarcinoma cells. *Hum. Reprod.* **2006**, *21*, 193–201. [CrossRef]
52. Renaud, S.J. Chapter 66—Strategies for Investigating Hemochorial Placentation. In *Reproductive and Developmental Toxicology*, 2nd ed.; Gupta, R.C., Ed.; Academic Press: Cambridge, MA, USA, 2017; pp. 1259–1273.
53. Bischof, P.; Irminger-Finger, I. The human cytotrophoblastic cell, a mononuclear chameleon. *Int. J. Biochem. Cell Biol.* **2005**, *37*, 1–16. [CrossRef]
54. Rothbauer, M.; Patel, N.; Gondola, H.; Siwetz, M.; Huppertz, B.; Ertl, P. A comparative study of five physiological key parameters between four different human trophoblast-derived cell lines. *Sci. Rep.* **2017**, *7*, 5892. [CrossRef]
55. Okae, H.; Toh, H.; Sato, T.; Hiura, H.; Takahashi, S.; Shirane, K.; Kabayama, Y.; Suyama, M.; Sasaki, H.; Arima, T. Derivation of Human Trophoblast Stem Cells. *Cell Stem Cell* **2018**, *22*, 50–63.e6. [CrossRef] [PubMed]
56. Haider, S.; Meinhardt, G.; Saleh, L.; Kunihs, V.; Gamperl, M.; Kaindl, U.; Ellinger, A.; Burkard, T.R.; Fiala, C.; Pollheimer, J.; et al. Self-Renewing Trophoblast Organoids Recapitulate the Developmental Program of the Early Human Placenta. *Stem Cell Rep.* **2018**, *11*, 537–551. [CrossRef]
57. Yuana, Y.; Levels, J.; Grootemaat, A.; Sturk, A.; Nieuwland, R. Co-isolation of extracellular vesicles and high-density lipoproteins using density gradient ultracentrifugation. *J. Extracell. Vesicles* **2014**, *3*, 23262. [CrossRef] [PubMed]
58. Sódar, B.W.; Kittel, Á.; Pálóczi, K.; Vukman, K.V.; Osteikoetxea, X.; Szabó-Taylor, K.; Németh, A.; Sperlágh, B.; Baranyai, T.; Giricz, Z.; et al. Low-density lipoprotein mimics blood plasma-derived exosomes and microvesicles during isolation and detection. *Sci. Rep.* **2016**, *6*, 1–2. [CrossRef] [PubMed]

59. Wagner, J.; Riwanto, M.; Besler, C.; Knau, A.; Fichtlscherer, S.; Röxe, T.; Zeiher, A.M.; Landmesser, U.; Dimmeler, S. Characterization of levels and cellular transfer of circulating lipoprotein-bound microRNAs. *Arterioscler. Thromb. Vasc. Biol.* **2013**, *33*, 1392–1400. [CrossRef] [PubMed]
60. Vickers, K.C.; Palmisano, B.T.; Shoucri, B.M.; Shamburek, R.D.; Remaley, A.T. MicroRNAs are transported in plasma and delivered to recipient cells by high-density lipoproteins. *Nat. Cell Biol.* **2011**, *13*, 423–433. [CrossRef] [PubMed]
61. Takov, K.; Yellon, D.M.; Davidson, S.M. Confounding factors in vesicle uptake studies using fluorescent lipophilic membrane dyes. *J. Extracell. Vesicles* **2017**, *6*, 1388731. [CrossRef]
62. Dominkuš, P.P.; Stenovec, M.; Sitar, S.; Lasič, E.; Zorec, R.; Plemenitaš, A.; Žagar, E.; Kreft, M.; Lenassi, M. PKH26 labeling of extracellular vesicles: Characterization and cellular internalization of contaminating PKH26 nanoparticles. *Biochim. Biophys. Acta (BBA)-Biomembr.* **2018**, *1860*, 1350–1361. [CrossRef] [PubMed]
63. Simonsen, J.B. Pitfalls associated with lipophilic fluorophore staining of extracellular vesicles for uptake studies. *J. Extracell. Vesicles* **2019**, *8*, 1582237. [CrossRef] [PubMed]
64. Wu, X.; Hammer, J.A. ZEISS Airyscan: Optimizing Usage for Fast, Gentle, Super-Resolution Imaging. *Methods Mol. Biol.* **2021**, *2304*, 111–130. [PubMed]

biomedicines

MDPI

Article

Antimicrobial and Immunomodulatory Potential of Cow Colostrum Extracellular Vesicles (ColosEVs) in an Intestinal In Vitro Model

Samanta Mecocci [1,†], Livia De Paolis [2,†], Roberto Zoccola [3], Floriana Fruscione [2,*], Chiara Grazia De Ciucis [2], Elisabetta Chiaradia [1], Valentina Moccia [4], Alessia Tognoloni [1], Luisa Pascucci [1], Simona Zoppi [5], Valentina Zappulli [4], Giovanni Chillemi [6], Maria Goria [3], Katia Cappelli [1,*,‡] and Elisabetta Razzuoli [2,‡]

1 Department of Veterinary Medicine, University of Perugia, 06123 Perugia, Italy
2 National Reference Center of Veterinary and Comparative Oncology (CEROVEC), Istituto Zooprofilattico Sperimentale del Piemonte, Liguria e Valle d'Aosta, Piazza Borgo Pila 39-24, 16129 Genova, Italy
3 S.C. Biotecnologie Applicate alle Produzioni, Istituto Zooprofilattico Sperimentale del Piemonte, Liguria e Valle d'Aosta, via Bologna 148, 10154 Torino, Italy
4 Department of Comparative Biomedicine and Food Science, University of Padova, 35020 Legnaro, Italy
5 S.C. Diagnostica Generale, Istituto Zooprofilattico Sperimentale del Piemonte, Liguria e Valle d'Aosta, via Bologna 148, 10154 Torino, Italy
6 Department for Innovation in Biological, Agro-Food and Forest Systems (DIBAF), University of Tuscia, 01100 Viterbo, Italy
* Correspondence: floriana.fruscione@izsto.it (F.F.); katia.cappelli@unipg.it (K.C.); Tel.: +39-010-542274 (F.F.); +39-075-5857722 (K.C.)
† These authors contributed equally to this work.
‡ These authors contributed equally as last authors.

Abstract: Extracellular Vesicles (EVs) are nano-sized double-lipid-membrane-bound structures, acting mainly as signalling mediators between distant cells and, in particular, modulating the immune response and inflammation of targeted cells. Milk and colostrum contain high amounts of EVs that could be exploited as alternative natural systems in antimicrobial fighting. The aim of this study is to evaluate cow colostrum-derived EVs (colosEVs) for their antimicrobial, anti-inflammatory and immunomodulating effects in vitro to assess their suitability as natural antimicrobial agents as a strategy to cope with the drug resistance problem. ColosEVs were evaluated on a model of neonatal calf diarrhoea caused by *Escherichia coli* infection, a livestock disease where antibiotic therapy often has poor results. Colostrum from Piedmontese cows was collected within 24 h of calving and colosEVs were immediately isolated. IPEC-J2 cell line was pre-treated with colosEVs for 48 h and then infected with EPEC/NTEC field strains for 2 h. Bacterial adherence and IPEC-J2 gene expression analysis (RT-qPCR) of *CXCL8*, *DEFB1*, *DEFB4A*, *TLR4*, *TLR5*, *NFKB1*, *MYD88*, *CGAS*, *RIGI* and *STING* were evaluated. The colosEVs pre-treatment significantly reduced the ability of EPEC/NTEC strains to adhere to cell surfaces ($p = 0.006$), suggesting a role of ColosEVs in modulating host–pathogen interactions. Moreover, our results showed a significant decrease in *TLR5* ($p < 0.05$), *CGAS* ($p < 0.05$) and *STING* ($p < 0.01$) gene expression in cells that were pre-treated with ColosEVs and then infected, thus highlighting a potential antimicrobial activity of ColosEVs. This is the first preliminarily study investigating ColosEV immunomodulatory and anti-inflammatory effects on an in vitro model of neonatal calf diarrhoea, showing its potential as a therapeutic and prophylactic tool.

Keywords: colostrum; Extracellular Vesicles; colibacillosis; coloEVs; antimicrobial

1. Introduction

Colostrum is the first unique nutrition source for the mammalian newborn, giving nutritive elements and playing an important role in health protection and the development of the immune system. Cow's colostrum, compared with milk, is enriched in fat, proteins, peptides, non-protein nitrogen, ash, vitamins and minerals, hormones, growth factors, cytokines and nucleotides, which influence metabolism, endocrine systems and the nutritional state of neonatal calves. Moreover, it contains enzymes with antimicrobial functions and immunoglobulins conferring passive immunity, and it stimulates the development and function of the gastrointestinal tract [1]. The sophisticated signalling system of maternal messages to promote postnatal health is also composed of transcription modulatory elements, such as small RNAs, derived from various cell sources of the mammary gland and present in different milk fractions (cells, lipids, and the skim milk) [2]. Small RNAs can be found as free molecules or packed in vesicles that confer protection to these labile molecules, allowing to overcome the harsh conditions of the gastrointestinal tract [3].

Extracellular Vesicles (EVs) are micro- and nano-sized phospholipidic double-layer-enclosed systems, mainly functioning as message delivery vectors of molecules, such as proteins, antigens, lipids, metabolites, RNAs and, as recently found, DNA fragments [4–6]. Being produced by all cell types, EVs can be taken-up by receiving cells, inducing the regulation of biological processes though the molecular cargo delivery [7]. EVs can be classified as: exosomes, released from the fusion of multi-vesicular bodies and cell membrane, generated through the late endosomal pathway and characterized by the smallest size (30–150 nm); microvesicles (ectosomes or shedding vesicles), released for exocytosis and ranging from 100 to 1000 nm; and the biggest apoptotic bodies (generally greater than 1000 nm) [5,7–11]. However, the impossibility to distinguish the different types merely on the basis of their size induced the International Society of Extracellular Vesicles (ISEV) to adopt and suggest the use of a size-based nomenclature, namely small, medium/large EVs and apoptotic bodies [12]. Being released in the extracellular environment, EVs can be recovered from every biological fluid, including milk (mEVs) and colostrum (colosEVs) [13–17].

The amount of EVs and dimension-based subtypes within colostrum/milk depend on the lactation period, characterized by a dilution in the EVs concentration going through the lactation stages and an enrichment in small EVs in colostrum [18]. The lactation stage also influences the cargo composition and function, with colosEVs particularly characterized by proteins and transcripts that could be related to the regulation of homeostasis and the immune system at a protein–protein interaction functional analysis, although further studies are needed to prove this hypothesis [19]. ColosEVs have been found to induce apoptosis in cultured cells [20] and liver cancer cells and to decrease the gene expression of inflammatory and angiogenetic genes [21]. Similar to bovine mEVs, colosEVs showed a positive effect on inflammation and immune regulation in colitis [22] and were able to shift the inflammatory process to the fibroblast proliferation, migration and endothelial tube formation, accelerating wound recovery [23]. A role in shaping microbiota was found for cow colosEVs, which correlates with bone remodelling and partial recovery in a osteoporosis mouse model [24]. Bovine transcriptomic analysis shows differences between the colosEVs of two breeds, thus highlighting variability among individual features and the need for deeper investigations into these important natural signalling systems [25].

Neonatal calf diarrhoea represents a relevant livestock disease caused by different types of *Escherichia coli* (*E. coli*), for which antibiotic therapy often has poor results due to the high rates of multi- and extensively drug-resistant isolates [26,27]. To date, it represents one of the major health challenges for livestock production, since it can lead to an increased death rate and, subsequently, to serious economic losses [28]. In this context, colosEV features can be exploited for alternative strategies in fighting infections, assisting or replacing the action of conventional antimicrobials [29] when trying to cope with the multi-drug resistance problem [30]. Antimicrobial properties have been found for EVs deriving from different human cells but also from plant and animal products, such as honey [31–33]. This study aimed to investigate the protective potential of colosEVs using an in vitro model of neonatal calf diarrhoea. In detail, we evaluated the immunomodulatory, anti-inflammatory and antimicrobial effects of ColosEV pre-treatment on porcine intestinal epithelial cells (IPEC-J2) infected with wildtype *E. coli* isolates. According to previous studies, IPEC-J2 was proven to be an effective in vitro model for investigating host–pathogen interactions [34] since it is able to express and produce cytokines, toll-like receptors (TLRs) and mucins [35]. By infecting ColosEV-pre-treated IPEC-J2 cells, we intended to highlight the effect of ColosEV on bacterial adhesion and immune-related gene expression and, thus, to preliminarily investigate the feasibility of ColosEV application as prophylaxis against infectious disease in cattle herds.

2. Materials and Methods

2.1. Farm and Animals Selection

In order to minimize variables capable of influencing the EV composition (stress, nutrition, genetics, age), selection criteria allowing to have a homogeneous study group of cows were adopted. Five heifers (primiparous cows) were selected from a closed-cycle farm consisting solely of Piedmontese cattle with the presence of newborn calves affected by neonatal diarrhoea attributable to ETEC. Selected animals were fed in the pre-calving period with a homogeneous diet.

2.2. Strains Isolation and Characterization

Following episodes of diarrhoea in new-born calves, stool samples and deceased subjects were transferred to the laboratories for strain isolation. A total of 1 g of faeces was diluted in 10 mL of buffered peptone water BPW (Biolife, Monza, Italy) and then submitted to serial 10-fold dilution in the same medium until reaching the fifth dilution. The last three dilutions were streaked by a 10 μL loop onto McConkey agar plates (MCK) (Microbiol, Macchiareddu, Italy) and incubated overnight at 37 °C. Thirty suspected *E. coli* colonies (relatively big, rounded, convex and pink colonies on purple-turned medium) were selected from the three MCK plates, sub-cultured on blood agar plate (BA) and MCK, then incubated overnight at 37 °C and 42 °C, respectively. Identification procedures based on growth on MCK at 42 °C, indole production and Gram staining suggestive of *E. coli* were performed before the preparation of six pooled samples with selected colonies. The pooled samples were inactivated by heat and submitted to molecular test aimed to highlight presence of some pathogenic factors specific for: enteropathogenic *E. coli* (EPEC) intimin-coding gene (*eae*); ETEC adhesin (K99) and shigatoxin genes (*STa*, *STb*); and/or necrotoxigenic *E. coli* (NTEC) cytotoxic necrotizing factor 1 (*CNF1*). Colonies selected for biomolecular analyses were diluted in 200 μL of ultrapure water and subjected to DNA extraction by thermal lysis (boiling for 15 min on heating mantle). The extracted DNA was subjected to qualitative–quantitative analysis by BioSpectrometer® (Eppendorf, De). The determination of *eae* presence was performed by a multiplex PCR according to ISO/TS 13136 [36], while the identification of *K99*, *STa* and *STb* was carried out with a multiplex PCR described by Casey et al. (2009) [37]. Moreover, *CNF1* was detected in simplex PCR. Primers, amplicon sizes and thermal profiles are summarized in Table S1. When the pooled samples gave positive results for target pathogenic factors, the single colonies constituting the positive pool [38] were submitted to the cited molecular test in order to confirm the results and obtain the strain eligible for drug susceptibility test. Drug susceptibility was tested using the minimum inhibitory concentrations (MICs) method according to the guidelines of the Clinical and Laboratory Standards Institute (CLSI). Quality controls of the plates used for MIC were performed according to the CLSI VET01S supplement (CLSI, 2020) [39]. MIC breakpoints (expressed in μg/mL) were evaluated and interpretative criteria were retrieved from both human (M100) [39] and veterinary CLSI Standards (VET08) [40] from the European Committee on Antimicrobial Susceptibility Testing (EUCAST) [41] and from the guidelines of the Committee for the Antibiotic Susceptibility testing of the Société Française de Microbiologie Comité de l'Antibiogramme (CA-SFM) [42] (Table S2).

Collected *E.coli* strains were used for further in vitro assays (see Sections 2.5.2 and 2.6).

2.3. Colostrum Collection and ColosEV Isolation

From each of the five heifers, three samples of colostrum collected within 24 h of calving were pooled to reach a final quantity of 500 mL and stored at 4 °C for less than 24 h before processing, avoiding cryo-preservation to minimize artifacts. ColosEVs were isolated by serial differential centrifugations (DC) and a step using ethylenediaminetetraacetic acid tetrasodium salt dihydrate (EDTA) before an ultracentrifugation at 35,000× g for 1 h at 4 °C. The resulted supernatant was submitted to ultracentrifugation at 200,000× g for 90 min at 4 °C using a Beckman Coulter Optima L-100 XP with a 45 Ti rotor following the protocol of Mecocci et al. [43]. Collected colosEV pellets were used for morphological analysis and in vitro assays.

2.4. ColosEV Morphological Characterization

2.4.1. Western Blotting

To extract proteins, colosEVs were lysed in RIPA Buffer (25 mM Tris-HCl pH 7.6, 150 mM NaCl, 1% NP-40, 1% sodium deoxycholate, 0.1% SDS). Total protein concentration was measured using Bradford assay. A quantity of 25 µg of total proteins were separated using 12% T sodium dodecyl sulfate–polyacrylamide gel electrophoresis and transferred to polyvinylidene fluoride membranes. Blotted membranes were saturated and incubated overnight with primary antibodies against CD81 (1:500; Bioss Antibodies, Woburn, MA, USA), TSG-101 (1:400, Santa Cruz Biotechnology, Santa Cruz, CA, USA) and calnexin (1:400 sc-23954, Santa Cruz Biotechnology, Santa Cruz, CA, USA). Anti-rabbit HRP-conjugated IgG (1:3000, Cell Signaling Technology, Danvers, MA, USA) and anti-mouse HRP-conjugated IgG (1:3000, Cell Signaling Technology) were used as secondary antibody. Clarity Western ECL Substrate (Bio-Rad) was used to evidence protein bands, and the images were acquired using a GS-800 imaging systems scanner (Bio-Rad, Hercules, CA, USA).

2.4.2. Transmission Electron Microscopy (TEM)

Few drops of colosEV suspension were deposited on Parafilm. Formvar-coated copper grids (Electron Microscopy Sciences) were gently placed on the drops with the coated side towards the suspension and colosEVs were allowed to adhere to the grids for about 20 min. Grids were contrasted with 2% uranyl acetate for 5 min after being rinsed in PBS and distilled water. The observation was performed using a Philips EM208 transmission electron microscope equipped with a digital camera (University Centre of Electron and Fluorescence Microscopy—CUMEF).

2.4.3. Nanoparticle Tracking Analysis (NTA)

A Malvern Panalytical NanoSight NS300 nanoparticle tracking analysis (NTA) system (Malvern, Worcestershire, UK) was used to assess the concentration and size distribution of isolated colosEVs. One colosEV pellet, derived approximately from 15 mL of colostrum, was resuspended and diluted in filtered (0.22 µm pore size) phosphate-buffered saline (PBS) (Sigma, St. Louis, MO, USA) to be suitable for the NTA system's working concentration range, and five measurements were performed. Concentration and diameter results are reported as mean ± 1 standard error of the mean.

2.5. Cell Cultures

IPEC-J2 cells (porcine jejunal epithelial cells, IZSLER Cell Bank code BS CL 205) were grown in a mixture (1:1) of Dulbecco's Modified Eagle (DMEM) (Euroclone, Milan, Italy) and Nutrient Mixture F-12 (F12) (Euroclone, Milan, Italy) enriched with 10% Fetal Bovine Serum (FBS, GIBCO™, Thermofisher scientific, Milan, Italy), 1% L-glutamine solution (Carlo Erba Reagents s.r.l., Milan, Italy) and 1% penicillin/streptomycin solution (Carlo Erba Reagents s.r.l., Milan, Italy). We decided to use these cells because they spontaneously secrete IL-8 and were previously employed in studies on bacterial and virus pathogenicity and on the intestinal inflammatory response [44].

2.5.1. Cell Viability Assay

Firstly, in order to determine the most suitable vesicle concentration to be used for the in vitro assay, we tested different colosEV quantities at scalar concentrations in terms of protein weight (0.015 μg, 0.15 μg, 1.5 μg, 15 μg, 150 μg). A 2,3-bis-(2-methoxy-4-nitro-5-sulfophenyl)-2H-tetrazolium-5-carboxanilide (XTT) assay was performed according to the manufacturer's instructions (XTT Cell Viability Kit, Cell Signaling Technology Inc., Danvers, MA, USA). In brief, IPEC-J2 cells were plated on a 96-well plate (100 μL per well, 0.1×10^5) in DMEM/F12 medium, 10% FBS, 1% L-glutamine and 1% penicillin/streptomycin and incubated for 24 h at 37 °C until confluence. The day after, the 96-well plates' seeding cells were exposed to a scalar concentration of colosEVs and then incubated again for 48 h at 37 °C, 5% CO_2. Untreated cells were used as controls. XTT assay was performed at selected time points (24 h and 48 h). On the day of the assay, cell culture medium was removed and replaced with 100 μL of fresh DMEM/F12 medium supplemented with XTT detection solution (1:50). The plates were then incubated again at 37 °C, 5% CO_2 for 2 h, and the absorbance was measured at 450 nm using a multimode microplate reader (Glomax®, Promega™, Milan, Italy). This assay was performed three times for each colostrum at scalar concentrations, setting up four technical replicas each.

2.5.2. ColosEV and *E. coli* Cell Treatments

Cells were seeded into 12-well culture plates (1 mL per well, 1.5×10^5 cells/mL), as stated in Section 2.5, and exposed to 1.5 μg (protein weight) colosEVs, incubated at 37 °C, 5% CO_2. After 48 h, 1 mL of *E. coli* suspension was added to the cultures and incubated at 37 °C in 5% CO_2 for 2 h. For *E. coli* stimulation, a pool of two different *E. coli* strains (EPEC, NTEC) was used. Briefly, bacteria were grown in brain heart infusion (BHI) medium at 37 °C for 12–18 h. Subsequently, 200 μL of overnight cultures were inoculated into fresh BHI and incubated for 1–2 h at 37 °C in order to obtain mid-log-phase cultures. *E. coli* strains were pelleted and resuspended as 10^8 colony-forming units (CFU)/mL in DMEM/F12, 1% L-glutamine solution.

At 2 h post-stimulation bacteria were removed and cell monolayers were gently washed five times with DMEM/F12, 1% L-glutamine solution. Untreated cells were used as control. The experiment was performed three times with three technical replicates each.

For each experiment, we have untreated cells ("Control" in the graphs), cells infected with *E. coli* strains ("*E. coli*" in the graphs) and cells pre-treated with 1.5 μg (protein weight) colosEVs and subsequently infected with *E. coli* ("*E. coli* + colosEVs" in the graphs).

2.6. *Bacterial Adhesion Assay*

For the experimental point reported in Section 2.5.2, cells were lysed by adding 200 μL of 1% Triton X-100 in PBS at room temperature for 5 min [44–46]. After cell lysis, 800 μL of PBS was added to each well; the resulting cell suspension was vortexed, serially diluted and seeded on Tryptone Bile X-GLUC (TBX) agar plates.

2.7. *Gene Expression Assay*

Cells of the experimental points reported in Section 2.5.2 were also tested for gene expression. After removing supernatants, cells were washed three times and again incubated in their medium for 3 h. Cells were lysed with 400 μL of RLT buffer (Qiagen, Hilden, Germany) and, after incubation for 10 min at room temperature, they were collected and stored at −80 °C until analysis. Untreated cells were used as controls.

Total RNA was extracted from IPEC-J2 cells using RNeasy Mini Kit (Qiagen s.r.l., Milan, Italy) following manufacturer's instructions and eluted in 50 μL of ultrapure RNase-free water. RNA extracted was quantified through Qubit 3.0 Fluorometer (Thermo Fisher Scientific, Waltham, MA, USA).

From each sample, 250 ng of RNA was reverse-transcribed into cDNA, using iScript® cDNASyntesis Kit (Bio-Rad, Milan, Italy). Real-time PCR amplification was performed on

CFX96™ Real-Time System (Bio-Rad, Milan, Italy) in accordance to a protocol previously described [47,48].

Primers of target and reference genes were derived from previous studies [49,50] or designed according to the sequences available on the Primer-BLAST online design platform (https://www.ncbi.nlm.nih.gov/tools/primerblast/, accessed on 31 July 2021). Primer pairs were placed in different exons or at exon–exon junctions to avoid biases due to genomic DNA amplification. Specific primer pairs for the reference genome were verified in silico using in silico PCR software (https://genome.ucsc.edu/cgi-bin/hgPcr, accessed on 31 December 2021) to confirm their specificity for targeting. Primer sequences of target genes and gene reference are reported in Table 1.

Table 1. Primer set sequences for target genes and reference.

Gene	Primer Sequences	Amplicon Length	Source
CXCL8	For—5′-TTCGATGCCAGTGCATAAATA -3′ Rev—5′-CTGTACAACCTTCTGCACCCA-3′	175	[44]
NFKB1	For—5′-CGAGAGGAGCACGGATACCA-3′ Rev—5′-GCCCCGTGTAGCCATTGA-3′	61	[44]
TLR4	For—5′-TGGCAGTTTCTGAGGAGTCATG-3′ Rev—5′-CCGCAGCAGGGACTTCTC-3′	71	[44]
TLR5	For—5′-TCAAAGATCCTGACCATCACA– 3′ Rev—5′-CCAGCTGTATCAGGGAGCTT-3′	59	[44]
IFNB	For-5′-AGTTGCCTGGGACTCCTCAA-3′ Rev-5′-CCTCAGGGACCTCGAAGTTCAT-3′	59	[44]
DEFB1	For—5′-CTGTTAGCTGCTTAAGGAATAAAGGC-3′ Rev—5′-TGCCACAGGTGCCGATCT-3′	80	[44]
DEFB4A	For—5′-CCAGAGGTCCGACCACTA-3′ Rev—5′-GGTCCCTTCAATCCTGTT-3′	87	[44]
CGAS	For—5′-TGGAGTGAAATGTTGCAGGAAAGA-3′ Rev—5′-GGGTCCTGGGTACAGACGTG-3′	149	XM_013985148
STING	For—5′-GCCTGCATCCATCCATCCCA-3′ Rev—5′-GCTGCTCTGGTACCTGGAGTG-3′	226	MK302493.1
RIGI	For—5′-GAATCTGCACGCTTTCGGGG-3′ Rev—5′-CTGCACCTCATCGTCCCTA-3′	96	NM_213804.2
GAPDH	For—5′-ATGGTGAAGGTCGGAGTGAA-3′ Rev—5′-AGTGGAGGTCAATGAAGGGG -3′	61	NM_001206359.1

2.8. Statystical Analysis

A Kolmogorov–Smirnov test was carried out to check Gaussian distributions in the data sets concerning viability assay, gene expression and bacterial adhesion.

All the results failed the Kolmogorov–Smirnov test; therefore, statistically significant differences were checked through the non-parametric Kruskal–Wallis test, followed by a Dunn's post hoc test for viability assay and gene expression. For the bacterial adhesion assay, CFU data were converted into log10 values and a Student's *t*-test was performed. The significance threshold was set at $p < 0.05$ (Prism 5, GraphPad Software, GraphPad Software Inc., San Diego, CA, USA).

3. Results

3.1. Strains Isolation and Characterization

Two different *E. coli* strains were isolated from stool samples. The strain n.1, which resulted positive for the presence of the intimin-coding gene (*eae*), was identified as EPEC; differently, the strain n.2 was classified as a chimeric NTEC since it resulted positive for *eae* and the *CFN1* gene (Table S3). Results obtained from antimicrobial characterization through MIC are summarized in Table S4. Isolated *E. coli* strains were used for further in vitro assays.

3.2. ColosEVs Morphologic Characterization

The presence and purity of colosEVs in the pellet generated from the colostrum along with the size range and shape assessment were determined, respectively, by Western blotting and TEM. At TEM, colosEVs appeared rather homogeneous in shape. They ranged from 30 to 120 nm and were single or arranged in aggregates. The absence of cell debris and background confirmed the efficiency of purification procedure (Figure 1A,B). Western blot assay proved the EVs presence, showing a positive reaction for Tumor Susceptibility Gene 101 protein (TSG101) and Cluster of Differentiation 81 (CD81). One vesicle-negative antigen, the calnexin, was used to evaluate the presence/absence of cellular contaminants (Figure 1C). Based on the NTA data, the colosEV mean (±standard error) diameter was 177.4 ± 2.4 nm (Figure 1D). The distribution of colosEV populations showed three main picks at different diameters (110 nm, 172 nm and 253 nm) and a mode of 117.5 ± 5.3 nm (D10 = 105.0 ± 0.9 nm and D90 = 269.7 ± 4.8 nm). NTA also determines nanoparticle densities, reporting the mean concentration (particles/mL) (±standard deviation) of five measurements after a pellet resuspension in 400 µL of PBS that resulted in 1.02×10^{12} ($\pm 4.88 \times 10^{10}$).

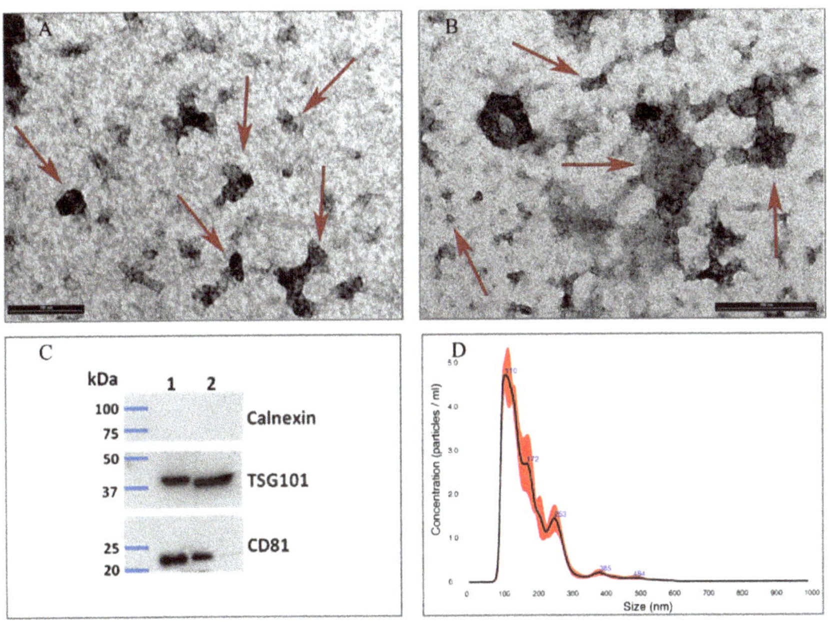

Figure 1. Morphological characterization of isolated colosEVs: Transmission electron microscopy low (**A**) and high (**B**) magnification micrographs showing single and clustered colosEVs indicated by red arrows. Scale bar: A. 100 nm; B. 200 nm; (**C**) Western blot images obtained using Ab against Tsg101 (Tumor Susceptibility Gene 101 protein) and CD81 (Cluster of Differentiation 81) that are both mEV antigens and calnexin as negative cellular debris control of two colosEV samples (1 and 2); (**D**) nanoparticle tracking analysis graph indicating colosEV size distribution.

3.3. Cell Viability

The IPEC-J2 cells cultured in 96-well plates and treated with scalar concentrations of colosEVs (see Section 2.5.1) were analysed by measuring the absorbance at 450 nm using a microplate reader. As shown in Figure 2, 150 µg (protein weight) colosEVs at 48 h determined a significant reduction in cell viability with respect to controls ($p < 0.0001$). No significant effect in terms of cell viability was observed at 24 h (Figure S1).

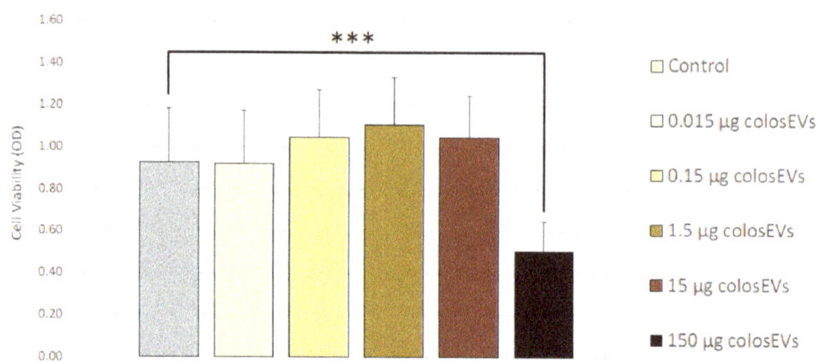

Figure 2. Viability of IPEC-J2 after colosEVs exposure at 48 h. The different concentrations of colosEVs did not determine a significant difference in terms of cell viability after 24 h (see Figure S1), whereas 150 µg colosEVs determined a significant reduction in IPECJ2 vitality at 48 h ($p < 0.0001$, indicated by *** in the graph). Data are expressed as optical density (OD) ± SD. Differences were evaluated through the Kruskal–Wallis test and applying the post hoc Dunn's multiple comparison test.

3.4. Gene Expression Assay

In order to determine the effect of colosEVs on cells infected with *E. coli* strains, we compared IPECJ2 gene expression in *E. coli*-inflamed cells, pre-treated cells with 1.5 µg colosEVs and then infected with *E. coli* and untreated ones (control). According to the results obtained, a significant upregulation of *CXCL8* ($p < 0.001$), *NFKB1* ($p < 0.001$), *DEFB1* ($p < 0.001$), *DEFB4A* ($p < 0.001$), *RIGI* ($p < 0.01$) and down-regulation of *IFNB* ($p < 0.05$) was highlighted in *E. coli*-inflamed cells compared with control (Figure 3).

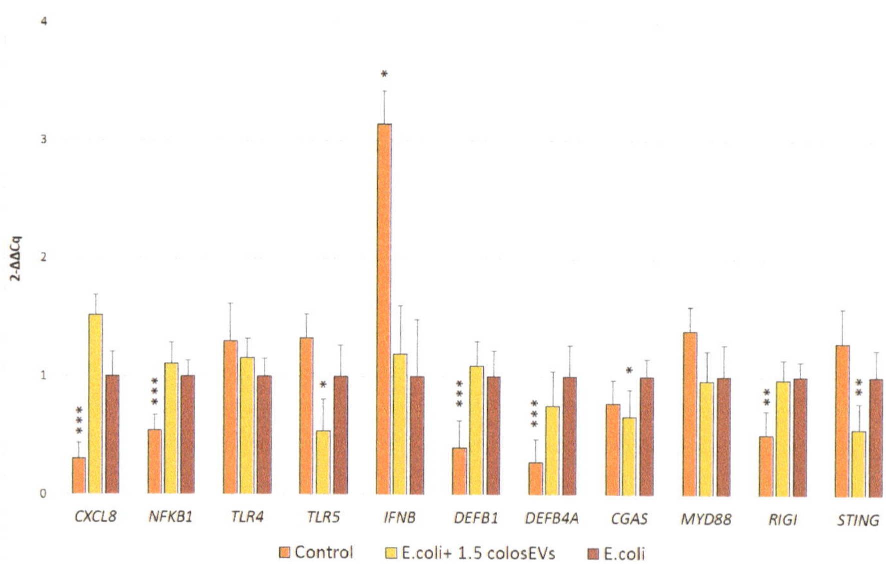

Figure 3. Effect of 48 h +1.5 µg colosEVs on *E. Coli*-inflamed IPEC-J2 cells. IPEC-J2-tested conditions were: inflamed (*E. coli*, pink), inflamed 1.5 µg colosEVs (*E. coli* + 1.5 µg colosEVs, light yellow), untreated (control, dark yellow). Significant differences are reported with respect to infected cells with *E. coli*. Differences were evaluated through the Kruskal–Wallis test and applying the post hoc Dunn's multiple comparison test. The asterisks indicate the statistical significance: * $p < 0.05$, ** $p < 0.01$ and *** $p < 0.001$.

Concerning cells pre-treated with colosEVs and then infected, our results highlighted a significant decrease in *TLR5* ($p < 0.05$), *CGAS* ($p < 0.05$) and *STING* ($p < 0.01$) gene expression compared with *E. coli*-inflamed cells, while no significant modulation was proved for the other tested genes (Figure 3).

3.5. Bacterial Adhesion

Since NTEC/EPEC strains are associated to neonatal calf diarrhoea in cattle [27], we performed our in vitro bacterial adhesion assay by using previously isolated *E. coli* strains (see Section 3.1). In detail, our aim was to investigate the ColosEV effect on host–pathogen interactions and, more specifically, to evaluate if ColosEV pre-treatment could modulate *E. coli* in vitro adhesion. Based on our results, the pools of strains under study were able to adhere to IPECJ2 cells. Our results highlighted greater adhesion of *E. coli* strains on untreated IPEC-J2 (7.5 ± 0.06 SD log10 CFU/5×10^5) compared with cells pre-treated with 1.5 μg colosEVs cells (7.3 ± 0.09 SD log10 CFU/5×10^5) ($p = 0.006$) (Figure 4). In particular, exposure to 1.5 μg colosEVs cells determined a decrease in bacterial adhesion of 0.2 log10 CFU/10^5 cells.

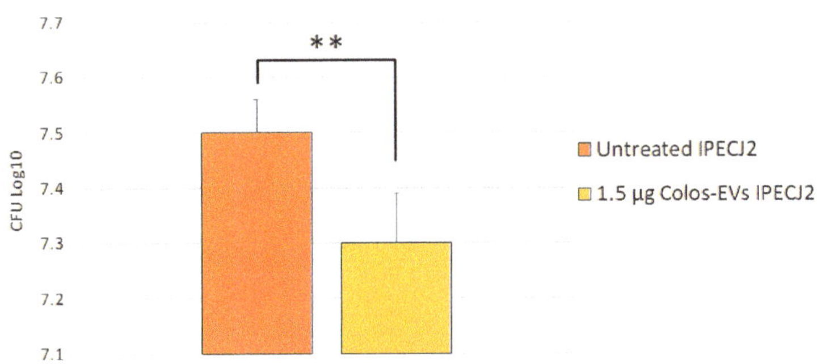

Figure 4. Adhesion of *E. coli* strains on 1.5 μg colosEVs pre-treated cells compared with untreated ones. Data are expressed as log10 CFU of adherent, *E. coli*/5×10^5 cells and mean value of 3 experiments $\pm$ 1 standard deviation. Differences were evaluated through the Student's *t*-test. The asterisks indicate the statistical significance: ** $p < 0.01$.

4. Discussion

In order to reduce the use of bactericidal and bacteriostatic chemotherapeutic agents in animals, which is necessary to also fight the spread of antibiotic resistance in humans, an increasing attention to research aimed at clarifying the mechanisms of action underlying both innate and acquired immunity should be considered strategic, since there is a need to obtain new tools capable of enhancing current prophylactic and therapeutic protocols.

Calf neonatal diarrhoea infections, caused by several strains of *E. coli*, are among the livestock diseases where the use of chemotherapeutic agents is the most common treatment practice [27,51]. However, antimicrobial-based therapeutic protocols achieve poor results due to the widespread of antibiotic resistance; the immunization of the calves takes place through the intake of colostrum and failure of transfer of passive immunity to the calf entails a high risk of mortality.

This study provides insights into the interaction between pathogens–hosts and the possibility to provide potential therapeutic and prophylactic support using colosEVs that are known to contain a miRNA cargo capable of modifying the responses of the calf's innate immunity, as described by Hata and collaborators [52]. In this study, the presence of RNA capable of modulating the early differentiation of lymphocytes and regulating inflammatory processes was found for milk and, even more so, for colostrum EVs.

Our results evidenced how the cellular adhesion of *E. coli* induces modifications of inflammation-related gene expression. Indeed *CXCL8* and *NFKB1* were significantly up-regulated after bacterial incubation, while *IFNB* was down-regulated [53]. These data are in agreement with previous studies on *E. coli* infection. In particular, Tsai and co-workers demonstrated that *E. coli* adhesion determines the increase in *CXCL8* expression by the activation of MAPK and NF-kB pathways [54]. Our results highlighted the increased expression of the RIGI gene, which is one of the molecules responsible for the transcription factor NFKB1 pathway activation in *E. coli* infections [55]. *E. coli* infection also induces the inhibition of IFN-β production, promoting inflammation and barrier disruption [56], a condition that seems to be also established in our experiment.

Moreover, the *E. coli* adhesion of our model determines the up-regulation of *DEFB1* and *DEFB4A* transcripts whose encoded proteins may function as important regulators of host defence against exogenous pathogens. Indeed, these cationic antimicrobial peptides have broad-spectrum antibacterial activity, inhibiting the growth of *E. coli* and modulating the innate immune response [57].

Conversely, an antimicrobial reaction through the down-regulation of *TLR5*, *CGAS* and *STING* genes was seen in *E. coli*-infected cells pre-treated with colosEVs. It is worth noting that *TLR5* is the host molecule that recognizes *E. coli* flagellin and activates the immune response [58]. Indeed, the *E. coli* infection modifies *TLR5* distribution and increases its presence on the cell surface through EPEC flagellum, translocation of effectors and intimate adherence; in turn, the modulation of *TLR5* leads the intimate adherence that alters the proinflammatory response [59]. In our study, *TLR5* was up-regulated after *E. coli* infection as a consequence of both *NFKB1* and *CXCL8* increases; furthermore, 48 h of colosEV incubation significantly down-regulated *TLR5*, demonstrating the capabilities of these vesicles to interact with the molecular mechanism behind the *E. coli* intimate adhesion.

Beyond *TLR5* activation, innate cytosolic sensing of foreign nucleic acids represents an important trigger of innate immune responses in several microbial infections. There are mechanisms of crosstalk between the cytosolic RIG-1 and cGAS–STING nucleic acid-sensing pathways that amplify the innate antimicrobial responses against both RNA and DNA [60]. Indeed, a central regulator of cytosolic DNA sensing is cyclic GMP-AMP (cGAMP) synthase (cGAS), and cGAMP binds to an essential cytosolic sensor stimulator of interferon genes (STINGs). STINGs, moreover, antagonize RIG-1 by binding its N-terminus, probably to avoid the overactivation of RIG-1 signalling and the associated autoimmunity [61]. Nevertheless, most studies have focused on viruses' infections, and only a few studies evaluated the interaction between bacteria, especially *E. coli*. To date, the cGAS–STING signalling pathway has emerged as a key mediator of inflammation in the settings of infection, cellular stress and tissue damage, and has recently emerged as a nodal player in immunity that is currently being explored as a potential therapeutic target [62].

In this contest, in our experimental study, *CGAS* and *STING* genes were up-regulated after *E. coli* incubation, as expected, and, interestingly, down-regulated in cultures pre-treated with colosEVs for 48 h and then infected. This suggests the colosEVs and the molecular cargo may be inhibitors of the cGAS-STING pathway and therefore responsible for the decreased bacterial adhesion observed in our experiments after vesicle treatment (Figure 4). Nevertheless, epithelial cells participate actively in the innate immune response in the gut. Thus, we may speculate that their stimulation, for example by the EV cargo, might result in the generation of antibacterial bioactive molecules to eliminate E. *coli*. Our findings are particularly relevant considering that recent studies have linked STING and type I IFNs to necroptosis, a highly pro-inflammatory form of cell death [63,64]. The down-regulation of this pathway by colosEVs suggests their anti-inflammatory activity.

Concerning host–pathogen interaction, as mentioned above, colosEV pre-treatment determines the reduction in *E. coli* adhesion, probably due to the decrease in *TLR5* expression and the down-regulation of the cGAS/STING pathway. In this way, we can speculate that adhesion reduction could be due to the modulation of cellular receptor expression. It is worth noting that the strains isolated in this study showed multi-antimicrobial resistance; therefore, the evidence that colosEV treatment altered the host–pathogen interaction suggests the possibility of using them as an alternative to antibiotic treatment.

5. Conclusions

The results obtained from our study highlighted the capacity of colosEVs to modulate host–pathogen interactions. In particular, our data showed a significant reduction in the ability of *E. coli* to adhere to cells pre-treated with 1.5 μg colosEVs when compared with untreated IPEC-J2. Furthermore, a significant decrease in *TLR5, CGAS* and *STING* gene expression was detected, suggesting that ColosEV molecular cargo could exert an antimicrobial activity by modulating the cGAS/STING pathway, a key player in inflammation, tissue damage and cellular response. This is a preliminary but promising result that highlights a possible mechanism of action of the molecular cargo against microbial infections. It represents a starting point for future studies to further evaluate the feasibility of colosEV application as a natural antimicrobial agent to cope with the drug resistance problem.

Supplementary Materials: The following supporting information can be downloaded at: https://www.mdpi.com/article/10.3390/biomedicines10123264/s1, Figure S1: Viability of IPEC-J2 after 24 h colosEVs exposure; Table S1: Primers, amplicon sizes and thermal profiles used for Multiplex and Simplex PCR; Table S2: Classes of antibiotic drugs employed for antimicrobial characterization and related clinical breakpoints; Table S3: Results obtained from Multiplex PCR and Simplex PCR; Table S4: MIC values (μg/mL) and related SIR results of antimicrobial agents tested against *E. coli* strains.

Author Contributions: Conceptualization, E.R., K.C. and M.G.; methodology, E.R., K.C., S.M., E.C., L.P., M.G., S.Z., V.M. and V.Z.; formal analysis, L.D.P., S.M., R.Z., S.Z., G.C. and F.F.; investigation, L.D.P., S.M., R.Z., F.F., C.G.D.C., A.T., L.P. and V.M.; resources, E.R., M.G., K.C., E.C., L.P., G.C. and V.Z.; data curation, L.D.P. and S.M.; writing—original draft preparation, S.M., L.D.P., K.C., E.R. and S.Z.; writing—review and editing, E.C., L.P., G.C., F.F. and C.G.D.C.; supervision, K.C. and E.R.; project administration, E.R. and M.G.; funding acquisition, M.G. All authors have read and agreed to the published version of the manuscript.

Funding: This research was funded by the Italian Ministry of Health, Grant Number IZS PLV 08/19 RC; the APC was funded by IZS PLV08/19 RC.

Institutional Review Board Statement: This project was approved on the basis of D.Lgs.vo 26/14 (implementing of CE 63/2010).

Informed Consent Statement: Not applicable.

Data Availability Statement: Not applicable.

Acknowledgments: The authors would like to thank Flavia Ferlisi for her technical support.

Conflicts of Interest: The authors declare no conflict of interest.

References

1. McGrath, B.A.; Fox, P.F.; McSweeney, P.L.H.; Kelly, A.L. Composition and Properties of Bovine Colostrum: A Review. *Dairy Sci. Technol.* **2016**, *96*, 133–158. [CrossRef]
2. Van Hese, I.; Goossens, K.; Vandaele, L.; Opsomer, G. Invited Review: MicroRNAs in Bovine Colostrum—Focus on Their Origin and Potential Health Benefits for the Calf. *J. Dairy Sci.* **2020**, *103*, 1–15. [CrossRef] [PubMed]
3. Ma, T.; Li, W.; Chen, Y.; Cobo, E.R.; Windeyer, C.; Gamsjäger, L.; Diao, Q.; Tu, Y.; Guan, L.L. Assessment of MicroRNA Profiles in Small Extracellular Vesicles Isolated from Bovine Colostrum with Different Immunoglobulin G Concentrations. *JDS Commun.* **2022**, *3*, 328–333. [CrossRef] [PubMed]
4. Kalluri, R.; LeBleu, V.S. The Biology, Function, and Biomedical Applications of Exosomes. *Science* **2020**, *367*, eaau6977. [CrossRef] [PubMed]
5. El Andaloussi, S.; Mäger, I.; Breakefield, X.O.; Wood, M.J.A. Extracellular Vesicles: Biology and Emerging Therapeutic Opportunities. *Nat. Rev. Drug Discov.* **2013**, *12*, 347–357. [CrossRef]
6. Malkin, E.Z.; Bratman, S.V. Bioactive DNA from Extracellular Vesicles and Particles. *Cell Death Dis.* **2020**, *11*, 584. [CrossRef]
7. Zhang, Y.; Liu, Y.; Liu, H.; Tang, W.H. Exosomes: Biogenesis, Biologic Function and Clinical Potential. *Cell Biosci.* **2019**, *9*, 19. [CrossRef]
8. Lee, Y.; El Andaloussi, S.; Wood, M.J.A. Exosomes and Microvesicles: Extracellular Vesicles for Genetic Information Transfer and Gene Therapy. *Hum. Mol. Genet.* **2012**, *21*, R125–R134. [CrossRef]
9. Cocucci, E.; Meldolesi, J. Ectosomes and Exosomes: Shedding the Confusion between Extracellular Vesicles. *Trends Cell Biol.* **2015**, *25*, 364–372. [CrossRef]

10. Caruso, S.; Poon, I.K.H. Apoptotic Cell-Derived Extracellular Vesicles: More Than Just Debris. *Front. Immunol.* **2018**, *9*, 1486. [CrossRef]
11. Raposo, G.; Stoorvogel, W. Extracellular Vesicles: Exosomes, Microvesicles, and Friends. *J. Cell Biol.* **2013**, *200*, 373–383. [CrossRef]
12. Théry, C.; Witwer, K.W.; Aikawa, E.; Alcaraz, M.J.; Anderson, J.D.; Andriantsitohaina, R.; Antoniou, A.; Arab, T.; Archer, F.; Atkin-Smith, G.K.; et al. Minimal Information for Studies of Extracellular Vesicles 2018 (MISEV2018): A Position Statement of the International Society for Extracellular Vesicles and Update of the MISEV2014 Guidelines. *J. Extracell. Vesicles* **2018**, *7*, 1535750. [CrossRef]
13. Ogawa, Y.; Miura, Y.; Harazono, A.; Kanai-Azuma, M.; Akimoto, Y.; Kawakami, H.; Yamaguchi, T.; Toda, T.; Endo, T.; Tsubuki, M.; et al. Proteomic Analysis of Two Types of Exosomes in Human Whole Saliva. *Biol. Pharm. Bull.* **2011**, *34*, 13–23. [CrossRef]
14. Masyuk, A.I.; Huang, B.Q.; Ward, C.J.; Gradilone, S.A.; Banales, J.M.; Masyuk, T.V.; Radtke, B.; Splinter, P.L.; LaRusso, N.F. Biliary Exosomes Influence Cholangiocyte Regulatory Mechanisms and Proliferation through Interaction with Primary Cilia. *Am. J. Physiol. Gastrointest. Liver Physiol.* **2010**, *299*, G990–G999. [CrossRef]
15. Admyre, C.; Grunewald, J.; Thyberg, J.; Gripenbäck, S.; Tornling, G.; Eklund, A.; Scheynius, A.; Gabrielsson, S. Exosomes with Major Histocompatibility Complex Class II and Co-Stimulatory Molecules Are Present in Human BAL Fluid. *Eur. Respir. J.* **2003**, *22*, 578–583. [CrossRef]
16. Dear, J.W.; Street, J.M.; Bailey, M.A. Urinary Exosomes: A Reservoir for Biomarker Discovery and Potential Mediators of Intrarenal Signalling. *Proteomics* **2013**, *13*, 1572–1580. [CrossRef]
17. Admyre, C.; Johansson, S.M.; Qazi, K.R.; Filen, J.-J.; Lahesmaa, R.; Norman, M.; Neve, E.P.A.; Scheynius, A.; Gabrielsson, S. Exosomes with Immune Modulatory Features Are Present in Human Breast Milk. *J. Immunol.* **2007**, *179*, 1969–1978. [CrossRef]
18. Santoro, J.; Mukhopadhya, A.; Oliver, C.; Brodkorb, A.; Giblin, L.; O'Driscoll, L. An Investigation of Extracellular Vesicles in Bovine Colostrum, First Milk and Milk over the Lactation Curve. *Food Chem.* **2023**, *401*, 134029. [CrossRef]
19. Ferreira, R.F. Comparative Proteome Profiling in Exosomes Derived from Porcine Colostrum versus Mature Milk Reveals Distinct Functional Proteomes. *J. Proteom.* **2021**, *249*, 104338. [CrossRef]
20. Ross, M. The Bioactivity of Colostrum and Milk Exosomes of High, Average, and Low Immune Responder Cows on Human Intestinal Epithelial Cells. *J. Dairy Sci.* **2021**, *104*, 2499–2510. [CrossRef]
21. El-kattawy, A.M.; Algezawy, O.; Alfaifi, M.Y.; Noseer, E.A.; Hawsawi, Y.M.; Alzahrani, O.R.; Algarni, A.; Kahilo, K.A.; El-Magd, M.A. Therapeutic Potential of Camel Milk Exosomes against HepaRG Cells with Potent Apoptotic, Anti-Inflammatory, and Anti-Angiogenesis Effects for Colostrum Exosomes. *Biomed. Pharmacother.* **2021**, *143*, 112220. [CrossRef] [PubMed]
22. Han, G.; Cho, H.; Kim, H.; Jang, Y.; Jang, H.; Kim, D.E.; Kim, E.S.; Kim, E.H.; Hwang, K.Y.; Kim, K.; et al. Bovine Colostrum Derived-Exosomes Prevent Dextran Sulfate Sodium-Induced Intestinal Colitis via Suppression of Inflammation and Oxidative Stress. *Biomater. Sci.* **2022**, *10*, 2076–2087. [CrossRef] [PubMed]
23. Kim, H.; Kim, D.E.; Han, G.; Lim, N.R.; Kim, E.H.; Jang, Y.; Cho, H.; Jang, H.; Kim, K.H.; Kim, S.H.; et al. Harnessing the Natural Healing Power of Colostrum: Bovine Milk-Derived Extracellular Vesicles from Colostrum Facilitating the Transition from Inflammation to Tissue Regeneration for Accelerating Cutaneous Wound Healing. *Adv. Healthc. Mater.* **2022**, *11*, 2102027. [CrossRef] [PubMed]
24. Yun, B.; Maburutse, B.E.; Kang, M.; Park, M.R.; Park, D.J.; Kim, Y.; Oh, S. Short Communication: Dietary Bovine Milk–Derived Exosomes Improve Bone Health in an Osteoporosis-Induced Mouse Model. *J. Dairy Sci.* **2020**, *103*, 7752–7760. [CrossRef] [PubMed]
25. Özdemir, S. Identification and Comparison of Exosomal MicroRNAs in the Milk and Colostrum of Two Different Cow Breeds. *Gene* **2020**, *743*, 144609. [CrossRef]
26. Feuerstein, A.; Scuda, N.; Klose, C.; Hoffmann, A.; Melchner, A.; Boll, K.; Rettinger, A.; Fell, S.; Straubinger, R.K.; Riehm, J.M. Antimicrobial Resistance, Serologic and Molecular Characterization of *E. Coli* Isolated from Calves with Severe or Fatal Enteritis in Bavaria, Germany. *Antibiotics* **2021**, *11*, 23. [CrossRef]
27. Naylor, J.M. Neonatal Calf Diarrhea. In *Food Animal Practice*, 5th ed.; Anderson, D.E., Rings, D.M., Eds.; W.B. Saunders: Saint Louis, MO, USA, 2009; Chapter 21; pp. 70–77. ISBN 978-1-4160-3591-6.
28. Mohammed, S.A.E.-M.; Marouf, S.A.E.-M.; Erfana, A.M.; El-Jakee, J.K.A.E.-H.; Hessain, A.M.; Dawoud, T.M.; Kabli, S.A.; Moussa, I.M. Risk Factors Associated with *E. Coli* Causing Neonatal Calf Diarrhea. *Saudi J. Biol. Sci.* **2019**, *26*, 1084–1088. [CrossRef]
29. Lu, L.; Hu, W.; Tian, Z.; Yuan, D.; Yi, G.; Zhou, Y.; Cheng, Q.; Zhu, J.; Li, M. Developing Natural Products as Potential Anti-Biofilm Agents. *Chin. Med.* **2019**, *14*, 11. [CrossRef]
30. Vivas, R.; Barbosa, A.A.T.; Dolabela, S.S.; Jain, S. Multidrug-Resistant Bacteria and Alternative Methods to Control Them: An Overview. *Microb. Drug Resist.* **2019**, *25*, 890–908. [CrossRef]
31. He, B.; Hamby, R.; Jin, H. Plant Extracellular Vesicles: Trojan Horses of Cross-kingdom Warfare. *FASEB Bioadv.* **2021**, *3*, 657–664. [CrossRef]
32. Brakhage, A.A.; Zimmermann, A.-K.; Rivieccio, F.; Visser, C.; Blango, M.G. Host-Derived Extracellular Vesicles for Antimicrobial Defense. *microLife* **2021**, *2*, uqab003. [CrossRef]
33. Leiva-Sabadini, C.; Alvarez, S.; Barrera, N.P.; Schuh, C.M.A.P.; Aguayo, S. Antibacterial Effect of Honey-Derived Exosomes Containing Antimicrobial Peptides Against Oral Streptococci. *Int. J. Nanomed.* **2021**, *16*, 4891–4900. [CrossRef]
34. Razzuoli, E.; Villa, R.; Amadori, M. IPEC-J2 Cells as Reporter System of the Anti-Inflammatory Control Actions of Interferon-Alpha. *J. Interferon Cytokine Res.* **2013**, *33*, 597–605. [CrossRef]

35. Mariani, V.; Palermo, S.; Fiorentini, S.; Lanubile, A.; Giuffra, E. Gene Expression Study of Two Widely Used Pig Intestinal Epithelial Cell Lines: IPEC-J2 and IPI-2I. *Vet. Immunol. Immunopathol.* **2009**, *131*, 278–284. [CrossRef]
36. Nielsen, E.M.; Andersen, M.T. Detection and Characterization of Verocytotoxin-Producing *Escherichia Coli* by Automated 5′ Nuclease PCR Assay. *J. Clin. Microbiol.* **2003**, *41*, 2884–2893. [CrossRef]
37. Casey, T.A.; Bosworth, B.T. Design and Evaluation of a Multiplex Polymerase Chain Reaction Assay for the Simultaneous Identification of Genes for Nine Different Virulence Factors Associated with *Escherichia Coli* That Cause Diarrhea and Edema Disease in Swine. *J. Vet. Diagn. Investig.* **2009**, *21*, 25–30. [CrossRef]
38. de Brito, B.G.; da Silva Leite, D.; Linhares, R.E.C.; Vidotto, M.C. Virulence-Associated Factors of Uropathogenic Escherichia Coli Strains Isolated from Pigs. *Vet. Microbiol.* **1999**, *65*, 123–132. [CrossRef]
39. *Performance Standards for Antimicrobial Disk and Dilution Susceptibility Tests for Bacteria Isolated from Animals*, 5th ed.; Clinical and Laboratory Standards Institute: Wayne, PA, USA, 2020; ISBN 978-1-68440-092-8.
40. *Performance Standards for Antimicrobial Disk and Dilution Susceptibility Tests for Bacteria Isolated from Animals*, 4th ed.; VET08; Lubbers, B.V. (Ed.) Clinical and Laboratory Standards Institute: Wayne, PA, USA, 2018; ISBN 978-1-68440-010-2.
41. The European Committee on Antimicrobial Susceptibility Testing. Breakpoint Tables for Interpretation of MICs for Antifungal Agents, Version 10.0. 2020. Available online: http://www.policlinico.pa.it/portal/pdf/news/CIO/Breakpoint%20EUCAST%20per%20l_interpretazione%20delle%20MIC%20per%20farmaci%20antimicotici%202022.pdf (accessed on 14 December 2021).
42. Teale, C.; Borriello, P. A Proposed Scheme for the Monitoring of Antibiotic Resistance in Veterinary Pathogens of Food Animals in the UK. *Vet. Rec.* **2021**, *189*, e201. [CrossRef]
43. Mecocci, S.; Pietrucci, D.; Milanesi, M.; Pascucci, L.; Filippi, S.; Rosato, V.; Chillemi, G.; Capomaccio, S.; Cappelli, K. Transcriptomic Characterization of Cow, Donkey and Goat Milk Extracellular Vesicles Reveals Their Anti-Inflammatory and Immunomodulatory Potential. *Int. J. Mol. Sci.* **2021**, *22*, 12759. [CrossRef]
44. Razzuoli, E.; Amadori, M.; Lazzara, F.; Bilato, D.; Ferraris, M.; Vito, G.; Ferrari, A. Salmonella Serovar-Specific Interaction with Jejunal Epithelial Cells. *Vet. Microbiol.* **2017**, *207*, 219–225. [CrossRef]
45. Schmidt, L.D.; Kohrt, L.J.; Brown, D.R. Comparison of Growth Phase on Salmonella Enterica Serovar Typhimurium Invasion in an Epithelial Cell Line (IPEC J2) and Mucosal Explants from Porcine Small Intestine. *Comp. Immunol. Microbiol. Infect. Dis.* **2008**, *31*, 63–69. [CrossRef] [PubMed]
46. Razzuoli, E.; Vencia, W.; Modesto, P.; Franzoni, G.; Giudici, S.D.; Parisi, E.; Ferrari, A.; Amadori, M. Yersinia Enterocolitica-Specific Modulation of Innate Immune Responses in Jejunal Epithelial Cells. *Vet. Microbiol.* **2020**, *242*, 108596. [CrossRef]
47. Mecocci, S.; Ottaviani, A.; Razzuoli, E.; Fiorani, P.; Pietrucci, D.; De Ciucis, C.G.; Dei Giudici, S.; Franzoni, G.; Chillemi, G.; Cappelli, K. Cow Milk Extracellular Vesicle Effects on an In Vitro Model of Intestinal Inflammation. *Biomedicines* **2022**, *10*, 570. [CrossRef]
48. Mecocci, S.; De Paolis, L.; Fruscione, F.; Pietrucci, D.; De Ciucis, C.G.; Giudici, S.D.; Franzoni, G.; Chillemi, G.; Cappelli, K.; Razzuoli, E. In Vitro Evaluation of Immunomodulatory Activities of Goat Milk Extracellular Vesicles (MEVs) in a Model of Gut Inflammation. *Res. Vet. Sci.* **2022**, *152*, 546–556. [CrossRef] [PubMed]
49. Razzuoli, E.; Villa, R.; Sossi, E.; Amadori, M. Reverse Transcription Real-Time PCR for Detection of Porcine Interferon α and β Genes: RT Real-Time PCR for Pig Interferon Genes. *Scand. J. Immunol.* **2011**, *74*, 412–418. [CrossRef] [PubMed]
50. Veldhuizen, E.J.A.; Koomen, I.; Ultee, T.; van Dijk, A.; Haagsman, H.P. Salmonella Serovar Specific Upregulation of Porcine Defensins 1 and 2 in a Jejunal Epithelial Cell Line. *Vet. Microbiol.* **2009**, *136*, 69–75. [CrossRef]
51. Foster, D.M.; Smith, G.W. Pathophysiology of Diarrhea in Calves. *Vet. Clin. N. Am. Food Anim. Pract.* **2009**, *25*, 13–36. [CrossRef]
52. Hata, T.; Murakami, K.; Nakatani, H.; Yamamoto, Y.; Matsuda, T.; Aoki, N. Isolation of Bovine Milk-Derived Microvesicles Carrying MRNAs and MicroRNAs. *Biochem. Biophys. Res. Commun.* **2010**, *396*, 528–533. [CrossRef]
53. Tsai, K.-W.; Lai, H.-T.; Tsai, T.-C.; Wu, Y.-C.; Yang, Y.-T.; Chen, K.-Y.; Chen, C.-M.; Li, Y.-S.J.; Chen, C.-N. Difference in the Regulation of IL-8 Expression Induced by Uropathogenic *E. Coli* between Two Kinds of Urinary Tract Epithelial Cells. *J. Biomed. Sci.* **2009**, *16*, 91. [CrossRef]
54. Lian, S.; Lin, X.; Zhan, F.; Shen, X.; Liang, Y.; Li, C. Transcriptome Analysis Reveals the Multiple Functions of PBD2 in IPEC-J2 Cells against *E. Coli*. *Int. J. Mol. Sci.* **2022**, *23*, 9754. [CrossRef]
55. Asadpour-Behzadi, A.; Kariminik, A. RIG-1 and MDA5 Are the Important Intracellular Sensors against Bacteria in Septicemia Suffering Patients. *J. Appl. Biomed.* **2018**, *16*, 358–361. [CrossRef]
56. Long, T.M.; Nisa, S.; Donnenberg, M.S.; Hassel, B.A. Enteropathogenic Escherichia Coli Inhibits Type I Interferon- and RNase L-Mediated Host Defense To Disrupt Intestinal Epithelial Cell Barrier Function. *Infect. Immun.* **2014**, *82*, 2802–2814. [CrossRef]
57. Chen, R.; Zhang, K.; Zhang, H.; Gao, C.; Li, C. Analysis of the Antimicrobial Mechanism of Porcine Beta Defensin 2 against *E. Coli* by Electron Microscopy and Differentially Expressed Genes. *Sci. Rep.* **2018**, *8*, 14711. [CrossRef]
58. Dai, C.; Yang, L.; Jin, J.; Wang, H.; Wu, S.; Bao, W. Regulation and Molecular Mechanism of TLR5 on Resistance to Escherichia Coli F18 in Weaned Piglets. *Animals* **2019**, *9*, 735. [CrossRef]
59. Hayashi, F.; Smith, K.D.; Ozinsky, A.; Hawn, T.R.; Yi, E.C.; Goodlett, D.R.; Eng, J.K.; Akira, S. The Innate Immune Response to Bacterial flagellin Is Mediated by Toll-like Receptor 5. *Nature* **2001**, *410*, 5. [CrossRef]
60. Decout, A.; Katz, J.D.; Venkatraman, S.; Ablasser, A. The CGAS–STING Pathway as a Therapeutic Target in Inflammatory Diseases. *Nat. Rev. Immunol.* **2021**, *21*, 548–569. [CrossRef]

61. Zevini, A.; Olagnier, D.; Hiscott, J. Crosstalk between Cytoplasmic RIG-I and STING Sensing Pathways. *Trends Immunol.* **2017**, *38*, 194–205. [CrossRef]
62. Wang, X.; Lin, X.; Wan, Z.; Zuo, J.; Wang, Z.; Xu, Y.; Phouthapane, V.; Han, X.; Zhang, J.; Miao, J. Regulation of YdiV-Induced Biological Characteristics Permits Escherichia Coli Evasion of the Host STING Inflammatory Response. *Vet. Microbiol.* **2021**, *261*, 109207. [CrossRef]
63. Wottawa, F.; Bordoni, D.; Baran, N.; Rosenstiel, P.; Aden, K. The Role of CGAS/STING in Intestinal Immunity. *Eur. J. Immunol.* **2021**, *51*, 785–797. [CrossRef]
64. Palmela, C.; Chevarin, C.; Xu, Z.; Torres, J.; Sevrin, G.; Hirten, R.; Barnich, N.; Ng, S.C.; Colombel, J.-F. Adherent-Invasive Escherichia Coli in Inflammatory Bowel Disease. *Gut* **2018**, *67*, 574–587. [CrossRef]

biomedicines

MDPI

Review

Effects of Physical Cues on Stem Cell-Derived Extracellular Vesicles toward Neuropathy Applications

Danyale Berry [1,2], Justice Ene [3], Aakash Nathani [4], Mandip Singh [4], Yan Li [3,*] and Changchun Zeng [1,2,*]

[1] Department of Industrial and Manufacturing Engineering, FAMU-FSU College of Engineering, Florida Agricultural and Mechanical University, Tallahassee, FL 32310, USA; danyale1.berry@famu.edu

[2] High Performance Materials Institute, FAMU-FSU College of Engineering, Florida State University, Tallahassee, FL 23210, USA

[3] Department of Chemical and Biomedical Engineering, FAMU-FSU College of Engineering, Florida State University, Tallahassee, FL 32310, USA; je17d@fsu.edu

[4] College of Pharmacy and Pharmaceutical Sciences, Florida Agricultural and Mechanical University, Tallahassee, FL 32307, USA; aakash1.nathani@famu.edu (A.N.); mandip.sachdeva@famu.edu (M.S.)

* Correspondence: yli@eng.famu.fsu.edu (Y.L.); zeng@eng.famu.fsu.edu (C.Z.); Tel.: +1-850-410-6320 (Y.L.); Fax: +1-850-410-6150 (Y.L.)

Abstract: The peripheral nervous system undergoes sufficient stress when affected by diabetic conditions, chemotherapeutic drugs, and personal injury. Consequently, peripheral neuropathy arises as the most common complication, leading to debilitating symptoms that significantly alter the quality and way of life. The resulting chronic pain requires a treatment approach that does not simply mask the accompanying symptoms but provides the necessary external environment and neurotrophic factors that will effectively facilitate nerve regeneration. Under normal conditions, the peripheral nervous system self-regenerates very slowly. The rate of progression is further hindered by the development of fibrosis and scar tissue formation, which does not allow sufficient neurite outgrowth to the target site. By incorporating scaffolding supplemented with secretome derived from human mesenchymal stem cells, it is hypothesized that neurotrophic factors and cellular signaling can facilitate the optimal microenvironment for nerve reinnervation. However, conventional methods of secretory vesicle production are low yield, thus requiring improved methods to enhance paracrine secretions. This report highlights the state-of-the-art methods of neuropathy treatment as well as methods to optimize the clinical application of stem cells and derived secretory vesicles for nerve regeneration.

Keywords: peripheral neuropathy; stem cells; extracellular vesicles; electrical stimulation; neurogenesis

1. Introduction

Communication between the central nervous system (CNS) and the peripheral nervous system (PNS) is essential for successful operation of the human body [1,2]. This crosstalk occurs via chemical cues translated as electrical signals [1,2]. During embryonic development, localized neural crest stem cells invaginate to form the brain and the spinal cord, which expand from the neural tube [3]. Later, neural crest stem cells migrate to the dorsal region of the embryo, differentiate into a mesenchymal lineage of PNS derivatives, and give rise to efferent (motor) and afferent (sensory) neurons [3]. Efferent neurons receive signals relayed as motor function, whereas afferent neurons return sensory information translated to chemical signals by the CNS [1,2]. For efficient communication, an intricate network of nerve fibers or axons is required to transmit signals that ensure the self-regulation of bodily systems, the collection of sensory information, and the execution of motor function [1,2]. Axons within the spinal cord branch out and transmit signals from the CNS to the peripheral regions [4]. An inhibitory or excitatory electrical impulse travels through the dendrites to the cell body, then propagates down the axon to the synapse, where information is relayed to the target area [5]. The propagation of the electrical signal is due to Schwann cells (SCs) forming protective segments of myelin sheath separated by nodes of Ranvier to increase conductivity [4,6,7]. Axons within the PNS elongate throughout the trunk and the upper and lower extremities, forming the somatic and autonomic nervous system [1,4,8]. The somatic nervous system encompasses voluntary muscular functions influenced by conscious decisions [1]. The autonomic nervous system governs involuntary function including the regulation of survival instincts and functionality of the circulatory, digestive, urinary, and reproductive systems [1,9]. Short-term and long-term trauma to the PNS can be fatal, causing decreased function of autonomic systems, altered motor function, inaccurate sensory input, and delayed sensory response from the CNS. When peripheral nerves become damaged or diseased, communication with the CNS is disrupted, leading to the most common neurological disease, peripheral neuropathy (PN) [10].

PN is estimated to affect approximately 8.8% of the world population by 2040, primarily affecting older generations [11–14]. Those affected commonly experience muscular atrophy, decreased sensation, mobility, balance, and coordination [13,15]. Other associated symptoms include symmetrical pain, numbness, tingling, or burning sensations at the distal end of the upper and lower extremities [12,16]. As the PN and associated pain continue to escalate, affected people will experience increased risk of further injury due to muscular weakness, altered gait cycle, decreased joint movement and range of motion, and in the worst-case scenario, complete paralysis [13,17,18]. Depending upon the injury mechanism, the recommended treatment approach for superficial injuries encompasses noninvasive therapy. Once the nerve gap surpasses tensionless reconstruction, stem cell-based therapies can provide supportive growth factors to accelerate the natural healing process, potentially replacing conventional invasive therapeutic methods [2]. The intervention of stem cells can assist in maintaining the cellular microenvironment and supplementation of secretory vesicles compacted with regenerative growth factors necessary for reinnervation [19,20]. Thus, understanding the interaction of stem cells with an injured nerve is crucial to successfully manipulate the cellular microenvironment, avoiding unethical complications [21]. Therefore, further investigation into the mechanisms guiding the regenerative influence of stem cells and the increased production of secretory vesicles will effectively manage chronic pain and treat neuropathy [22].

2. Mechanisms of Peripheral Neuropathies

Understanding the diverse etiology behind PN is beneficial to developing appropriate diagnoses and courses of treatment [10]. The accurate identification of the specific condition that attributes to neuropathy is difficult due to a variety of methods used in the diagnosis and classification of origin [15]. Accounting for less than 30%, patients with idiopathic neuropathy are diagnosed without an established mechanism of injury [12,13,23]. Based on diagnosis, neuropathic symptoms are attributed to genetic or developed acquisition, axonal, or demyelinated degeneration and acute or chronic injury progression [12]. According to the method of nerve degeneration, PN can present in several forms such as distal symmetric neuropathy (DSN), sensory neuropathy (SN), and autonomic neuropathy (AN) [10,12].

DSN, also known as length-dependent neuropathy, originates in the most distal portion of the lower extremities and progresses symmetrically to more proximal regions of the body [24]. On the other hand, SN negatively affects proprioception, which reduces thermal and pain sensibility in the upper extremities and more proximal regions, eventually causing complete loss of sensation in the lower and more distal extremities [24]. Finally, AN affects the sympathetic and parasympathetic nervous systems, leading to the neurological dysfunction of one or more organ system [25]. Alongside an in-depth diagnostic workup, the various symptoms of each form of neuropathy can be utilized to identify the underlying cause [10]. To complete a diagnostic evaluation, patient history, neurological examination, assessment of symptom distribution, and further laboratory testing are required to categorize symptoms in preestablished clinical patterns [10]. However, multiple etiologies of neuropathy can be active at once, highlighting the importance of early diagnosis, optimal treatment, and preventative measures to further decrease the occurrence of PN [10]. Within this section, the most prevalent mechanisms of PN are summarized and the specific forms and symptoms of neuropathy are detailed.

2.1. Diabetic Peripheral Neuropathy

Diabetes is prevalent in 6.4% of the worldwide population and is estimated to impact 439 million individuals by 2030 [12,26]. Of all the diabetic patients, 30–50% suffer from diabetic peripheral neuropathy (DPN). Type 1 and type 2 diabetes results from the downregulation of insulin production and absorption, respectively, which disrupts glucose regulation [27]. High levels of glucose in the vasculature affect cellular metabolism and energy production in peripheral nerves, ultimately leading to DPN [14,26,28,29]. Typically, cellular respiration via glucose phosphorylation and glycolysis pathways provides a mechanism of transporting electrons when converting between the oxidative nicotinamide adenine dinucleotide (NAD+) and reductive nicotinamide adenine dinucleotide (NADH) to produce adenosine triphosphate (ATP) in the mitochondria [27,30–32]. However, excess glucose promotes an excess supply of NADH, leading to imbalanced NADH/NAD+ redox signaling [30,32].

This imbalanced environment increases reactive oxygen species (ROS), negatively affecting mitochondrial metabolism and respiration and insulin insufficiency [27,33–36]. Huang et al. investigated the correlation between hyperglycemia and mitochondrial dysfunction concerning neurodegeneration in streptozotocin (STZ)-diabetic rats [34]. As the concentration of glucose increases and insulin uptake decreases, glycolysis discontinues, resulting in ATP depletion, uncontrolled oxidative stress, the downregulation of neurotrophic factors, decreased neurite outgrowth, and the induction of PN [27,30,34,37,38]. As represented in Table 1, DPN is categorized into five major categories based on the type of nerve affected or where that effect occurs.

Table 1. Various types of diabetic neuropathy categorized into five major categories.

Form of DPN	Description	Reference
Focal	Affecting 1 or a singular group of nerves (i.e., carpal tunnel).	[39]
Multifocal Peripheral Neuropathy	Length-dependent motor/ sensory neuropathy.	[24]
Autonomic	Loss of involuntary bodily function.	[40]
Diabetic Amyotrophy (Proximal Neuropathy)	Unilateral or bilateral pain and sensory loss and muscular atrophy in quadriceps, hips, and gluteus maximus.	[24]
Idiopathic Neuropathy	Undetermined etiology of neuropathy.	[41]

Prevalent in more than 80% of patients affected by DPN, length-dependent neuropathy is the most common, typically described as chronic and symmetrically distributed pain, affecting first, more minor, then larger nerves until numb [14,23,24,42,43]. Focal and multifocal diabetic neuropathies such as oculomotor dysfunction and carpal tunnel are atypical, affecting a singular or small bundle of nerves within the cranial, trunk, or limb regions [14,42,44–46]. AN mediates the dysfunction of the urinary, reproductive, gastrointestinal, and cardiac systems, prevalent in less than 65% of both type I and type II diabetics [14,23,47,48]. Finally, diabetic amyotrophy presents as acute anterior burning when touched, pain, and muscular weakness in the quadriceps with spontaneous improvement after months of deterioration [42]. Diabetic neuropathy affects everyone differently, causing neurodegeneration in various forms within the central and peripheral nervous systems [49]. The variation in injury distribution directs treatment toward eliminating the underlying condition and managing developing symptoms [50].

Consequently, the development of chronic diabetic sensory and autonomic neuropathy affects the individual's overall health and finances. DPN requires therapeutic and financial support to adequately manage the emotional, social, and mental health burdens of diabetes and DPN [38,51,52]. Poor adjustment to lifestyle changes necessary to maintain glycemic and psychological control can result in blindness, kidney failure, amputations, and increased risk of anxiety and depression [14,53,54]. To assist, appointments with health care providers and medical specialists, equipment, medication, and living assistance accumulates costly societal and direct expenses [14,55]. In the United Kingdom, DPN has been estimated to cost approximately $£18 billion in direct and £25 billion in indirect societal costs by 2035 [56,57]. Individually, DPN patients spend between $9632 and $24,702 annually, depending upon the form of neuropathy and severity of their condition [14,58].

2.2. Chemotherapy-Induced Peripheral Neuropathy

Cancerous cells are treated with antineoplastic agents that despite optimizing patient survival, introduce life-threatening side effects that can hinder a healthy physical and psychological way of life [59,60]. Depending on the type of chemotherapy, dosage, and duration of treatment, approximately 40% of patients experience chemotherapy-induced peripheral neuropathy (CIPN) [59,60]. CIPN includes progressive length-dependent sensorimotor and autonomic neuropathies caused by prescribed neurotoxic drugs. Chemotherapy is an individualized course of treatment that works to eliminate malignant tumors but also plagues the body with chronic toxicity and compromised immunity [60–62]. It is required that oncologists consider pre-existing conditions and the drug's unpredictable side effects to prevent cancer remission [63,64]. Unfortunately, the utilized drugs are not target-specific [65,66]. Both malignant and healthy cells are inhibited once exposed to the maximum tolerated dose capable of reducing uncontrolled proliferation [67,68]. Although there is a reduction in cancerous agents, the side effect of CIPN becomes more prevalent due to the type, dosage, and administration of the drugs, especially in patients with pre-existing conditions [64,69]. The drugs used to treat various types of cancer include platinum compounds, taxanes, vinca alkaloids, immunomodulators, and proteosome inhibitors, as summarized in Table 2. As a result, patients experience hair loss, bone marrow toxicity, immunosuppression, decreased appetite, and induced nausea and vomiting [65,70,71].

Table 2. Description of the five types of drugs used when treating cancerous agents.

Drug	Treated Condition	CIPN Pathogenesis
Platinum Compounds	Tumors in cranium, digestive, urinary, respiratory, and reproductive systems.	Mitochondrial dysfunction. Increased oxidative stress. Voltage-gated K^+ and Na^+ hyperactivity.
Taxanes	Tumors in breast, ovaries, prostate, lungs, and bladder.	Mitochondrial dysfunction. Increased oxidative stress. Voltage-gated K^+ and Na^+ hyperactivity. Altered functionality of skin-based receptors (Aβ, C, and Aδ nerve fibers).
Vinca Alkaloids	Tumors in kidneys, liver, lungs, breast, and brain. Hematological malignancies, testicular, and non-small cell lung cancer.	Mitochondrial dysfunction. Microtubule function inhibition.
Immunomodulators	Example: thalidomide. MM, glioblastoma, breast, and prostate cancer.	Inhibition of growth factors (VEGF, TNF-α, NF-kB, b-FGF). ROS activation. Induced hypoxia and ischemia.
Proteosome Inhibitors	Example: bortezomib. Progressive, relapsed, or refractory MM.	Mitochondrial dysfunction. Increased oxidative stress. Increased apoptosis via release of Ca^{2+} in endoplasmic reticulum.

Chemotherapeutic agents affect fundamental cellular processes including axonal transport, mitosis, cellular movement, and the management of metabolic and oxidative stress [67,68,72–74]. Cellular communication is possible through the release of neurotransmitters to the presynaptic terminal. Microtubules transport the chemicals along the axon to the presynaptic terminal, which are then secreted as vesicles to receptors in the postsynaptic membrane [1,75,76]. The action potential depolarizes the cellular membrane to activate voltage-gated ion channels that release neurotransmitters via exocytosis [75,77,78]. Neurotransmitter receptors, located in the membrane of the postsynaptic neuron, receive inhibitory or excitatory chemicals via endocytosis to process sensory information and generate muscular contraction [79,80]. Platinum compounds, taxanes, and vinca alkaloids disrupt microtubule function in axonal transport as well as cellular division and homeostatic regulation [74,81–83]. Under oxidative stress, microtubules initiate the release of inflammatory cytokines, directly effecting signaling pathways such as the mitogen-activated protein kinase (MAPK), regulated by stress-activated C-Jun N-terminal kinase (JNK) and p38 MAPK [67,73,81,82,84–86]. MAPK pathways respond to external stimulus that influences cellular function such as proliferation, differentiation, and senescence [85–87]. The activation of JNKs are the result of MAPK phosphorylation, further influencing cellular growth, death, and survival [88]. Lower levels of p38 MAPK are closely related to the autophagy of damaged organelles, playing an active role in cellular survival by tending to homeostatic functions [84]. Chemotherapeutic agents rely on the hyperactivation of p38 MAPK to inhibit cellular growth and activate genotoxic stress-induced apoptosis by disrupting spindle assembly within mitosis [84,85,87]. Neurotoxic agents that promote microtubule dysfunction and the disruption of homeostatic cellular signaling cause CIPN since the chemical cues, proteins, and nutrients required for nerve communication are inhibited [89,90].

2.3. Peripheral Neuropathy via Physical Injury

Physical injury to the nerve instantaneously alters the quality of life of those affected. Trauma to the PNS includes repetitive physical movements, the mechanical deformation of nerves, lacerations, and ischemia [91,92]. Complete recovery from such trauma depends on the severity of the injury. According to the Seddon and Sunderland classification systems, peripheral nerve injuries are divided into five categories [92,93]. To further understand how various degrees of injury are organized, the structural composition of the nerve is shown in Figure 1.

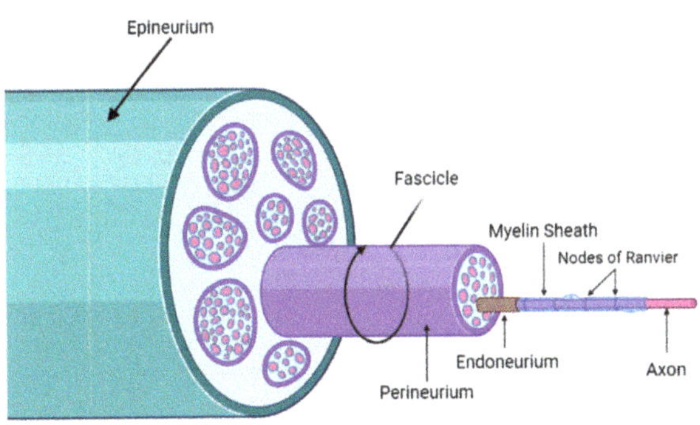

Figure 1. Structural representation of the nerve in PNS.

The epineurium composes the outermost layer of connective tissue, grouping together all fascicles of one peripheral nerve [94]. A bundle of nerve fibers forms a fascicle, surrounded by the perineurium, which protects the nerve by providing it with tensile strength and elasticity [95–98]. Each myelinated nerve fiber is surrounded by the endoneurium, maintaining fluidic pressure between the endoneurial space and the surrounding environment [93,96,99–102]. Beneath the endoneurium, SCs form a nutritional and protective layer of myelin sheath around the axon [101–103]. The axon conducts an action potential from the cell body to the nerve terminal, modulating the release of neurotransmitters [104]. Between each segment of myelin, nodes of Ranvier propagate the transmission of electrical impulses between nerves [101–103]. Once the myelin sheath is damaged, the rate of electrical transmission decreases, often diagnosed as a form of PN [103].

Peripheral nerve injuries are classified into three primary categories by Seddon and further defined by severity by Sunderland, as shown in Figure 2. Seddon's method of classification developed from observed nerve injuries during World War I, focusing on conduction blocks, loss of axon continuity, and complete nerve transection [105,106]. However, Sunderland's focused on the histological structure of each injury [105]. Seddon first defines neuropraxia as the mildest form of nerve injury caused by blockage or compression [93,107]. Neuropraxias are equivalent to Sunderland's description of first-degree injuries [92,98,99]. First-degree injuries primarily block the transmission of electrical impulses without permitting further injury to the axon. Seddon defines axonotmesis, which is the severity of the axon, endoneurium, and perineurium, with little effect on the epineurium [92,99,106,108,109]. Sutherland further describes axonotmesis as second- and third-degree injuries [105,110]. Within second-degree injuries, the axon experiences discontinuity, but the endoneurium and perineurium are still intact [2,98,105,111]. Third-degree injuries damage the axon and endoneurium; however, the perineurium is complete [105,106,110]. This process is attributable to the SC release of cellular signals and the recruitment of macrophages to engulf axonal and myelin debris and begin regeneration [112–115]. Seddon then defines neurotmesis, which is the loss of anatomical continuity within the three layers surrounding the axon [93,109]. In this case, the event of axonal regeneration without intervention is rare [93]. Sunderland describes neurotmesis as fourth- and fifth-degree injuries. Within a fourth-degree injury, the axon, endoneurium, and perineurium are discontinuous, but the epineurium, the outermost layer, is intact [2,110]. Without the guidance of the endoneurium and perineurium, the regenerating axons return unorganized and are constricted by the development of fibrosis and scar tissue blocks. Finally, fifth-degree injuries describe the complete severance of the nerve, requiring medical interventions to treat [92,105,106,108,110].

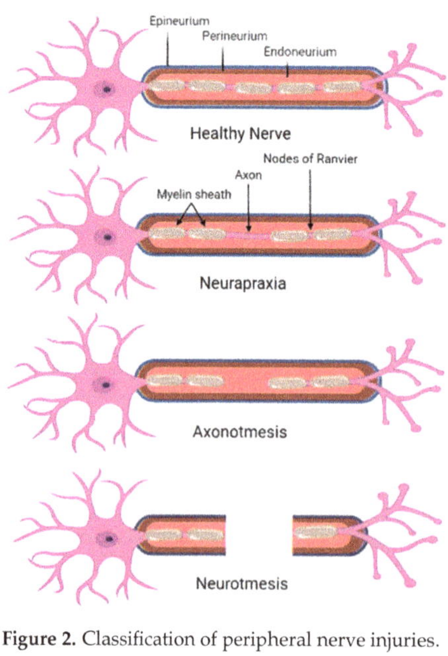

Figure 2. Classification of peripheral nerve injuries.

Beyond third-degree injuries, nerve regeneration becomes increasingly difficult due to impaired axon recovery. Minimal interventions are necessary for complete axon reinnervation with returned functionality to treat first- and second-degree injuries [93,109]. When the injury is substantial enough to damage the perineurium or introduce a nerve gap, surgical and noninvasive treatment methods are practiced to manage symptoms and promote nerve regeneration [108].

2.4. Pathophysiology of Axonal Injury

To maintain neurons distant from the cell body to the synaptic terminal, dynein and kinesin motors actively transport intracellular cargo along axonal microtubules within the cytoskeleton [116,117]. The transport components include secretory membrane vesicles, essential organelles (mitochondria, lysosomes, and lipids), and messenger ribonucleic acid (mRNA) to maintain cellular polarity and migration [118–120]. Following axonotmesis, Wallerian degeneration (WD) occurs at the distal end, causing the axon to self-degenerate in preparation for reinnervation [2,7,121,122]. However, with the discovery of the Wallerian degeneration slow (Wlds) gene mutation in mice, axonal degradation is recognized as an active process [123,124].

Molecular homeostasis of the cellular environment is maintained by the neuroprotective properties of nicotinamide mononucleotide adenylyltransferase (NMNAT) and the NAD+ regulation of gene expression and metabolic and signaling processes [125–127]. NAD+ serves as an essential catalyst for enzymes that regulate energy metabolism, the management of ROS, and overall health of the cell [126,127]. The biosynthesis of NAD+ occurs in three primary pathways with varied precursors requiring several steps for synthesis [128]. The Preiss–Handler pathway converts nicotinic acid (NA) into NAD+ in three steps [126,128,129]. The de novo pathway synthesizes tryptophan (Trp) in 10 steps [126,128,129]. Finally, the salvage pathway can occur in a 2-step process with either nicotinamide (NAM) or nicotinamide riboside (NR) [126,128–130].

The disrupted production of NAD+ is primarily associated with decreased physiological and metabolic functions associated with age and the progression of neurodegenerative diseases, presenting a similar inflammatory response when an axonal injury occurs [131,132]. Demonstrated by metabolic flux analysis, Sasaki et al. concluded that axon fragmentation is induced when sterile alpha and toll/interleukin-1 receptor motif-containing 1 (SARM1) activates an increase in NAD+ synthesis until depletion due to the discontinuation of NMNAT2 [133]. Once NAD+ is consumed by SRAM1 via MAPK signaling, the decreased supply of ATP further expedites WD [134]. However, the overexpression of NMNAT or nicotinamide mononucleotide (NMN) de-amidase halts SARM1 activation, proving neuroprotective abilities following injury [133].

To facilitate the microenvironment for regeneration, subsets of glial cells such as SCs, astrocytes, microglia, and neural progenitor cells promote migration accuracy [135]. Via axo–glial interaction, c-Jun and notch transcription factors within the MAPK kinase extracellular signaling regulation pathway (MEK/ERK) promote the upregulation of transforming growth factor-beta 1 (TGF-β1) and growth factor secretion in repairing SCs (rSCs) [20,136]. As the rSCs develop uninterrupted alignment, the growth of Büngner bands are directionally influenced for successful reinnervation [2,20,137]. This guidance is provided by the influence of macrophages, fibroblasts, and SCs toward self-renewal [2]. Macrophages secrete cytokines of two different phenotypes, pro-inflammatory (M1) or anti-inflammatory (M2), further divided into four subsets (M2a, M2b, M2c, M2d) [138,139]. The fluctuating levels of M1 and M2 macrophages influence the migration, proliferation, and secretion patterns of SCs at the site of injury [138]. Until the fourth day post injury, M1 macrophages engulf fragmented axons and myelin debris during WD [2,138,140,141]. Following the first phase of regeneration, M1 macrophages are polarized to subsets of M2 macrophages to further promote immunoregulation, tissue repair and remodeling, and long-distance axonal growth [138,139]. As treatment progresses, hypoxic conditions promote M2d secretion of vascular endothelial growth factor (VEGF) to extend blood vessels across gaps between nerve segments [138,140,142,143]. The regrown vasculature serves as guidance for bands of Büngner to the target endoneurial tubes [19,138,140,142]. However, the probability of connection without growth misdirection is slim [144]. Uncontrolled branching of growing axons leads to misdirection from the target site [7]. The accumulation of dense scar tissue and fibrosis resulting from fibroblast proliferation flares up inflammation, distracts axonal regeneration, and endoneurial tube reinnervation [2].

3. Approaches to Peripheral Nerve Injury Treatment

The PNS is capable of self-regenerating at a rate of ~1 mm/day [2,7,20,92,98]. Grade 1 and 2 injuries will heal within a few months without assistance [2,7,98]. However, injuries of a high caliber that traumatize the axon and surrounding connective tissue require medical interventions to promote remyelination and active healing [93]. Prior to medical interventions, the primary goal of diagnosis and treatment is to mitigate the underlying mechanism of injury [138,139]. DPN and CIPN progressively alter the external environment encompassing the nerve. To halt neuropathy progression and ensure treatment to the nerve is not reversed, the elimination of toxic medication and nutritional deficiency is the goal. Within personal injuries, the nerve trauma is more instantaneous, leading to a noninvasive therapeutic approach or surgical procedure that will guide regeneration [2].

Noninvasive strategies that promote remyelination include over-the-skin electrical stimulation, steroid hormone therapy, and pharmacological agents. Once a nerve experiences interrupted stimulation to the neuromuscular junction, the release of neurotransmitters for muscular contraction is halted [145]. Therefore, voluntary and involuntary muscular contractions are impaired, increasing neuropathic symptoms [146]. To alleviate pain and improve neuromuscular activity, the PNS is exposed to transcutaneous electrical nerve stimulation (TENS) [147,148]. Electrodes are placed over the skin to stimulate the nerve and induce muscle contraction [145]. The stimulation is modified between high (>80 Hz) or low (<10 Hz) frequency, duration, and intensity depending upon the severity of neuropathic pain (NP) [147,149,150]. As a result, the clinical application of TENS increases blood circulation and axonal transport, decreases inflammation, and reinnervates muscle and nerve fibers [150,151]. Although TENS can alleviate NP, research supporting the influence of TENS in nerve regeneration is limited [152]. In a separate study, TENS has also been observed to reduce the axon count, disorganize cellular arrangement within the tissue, and negatively affect the remaining nerves at the injury site [2]. Externally applied stimuli hinder morphological development in nerve regeneration but positively effect sensory-motor function [152]. Hormonal steroids influence the regulation of physiological functions within the CNS and PNS [153]. These steroids modulate pain sensitivity while providing neuroprotection and the maintenance of SC myelination when PNS nerve injury occurs [153–155]. The utilization of estradiol in neuropathy management treatment directs functional improvement and the regeneration of injured peripheral nerves [156]. In a study by Calabrese et al., animals experiencing pain caused by DPN were treated with testosterone metabolites [157]. DPN induces the expression of toll-like receptor member 4 (TLR4), which increases the production of inflammatory cytokines causing NP [157,158]. Once treated with testosterone metabolites, 3α-diol and dihydrotestosterone (DHT), pro anti-inflammatory cytokines were counteracted, increasing the analgesic properties [157].

The pharmacological treatment of NP is focused on the management and relief of symptoms [159,160]. Commonly, the combination of anti-depressants, anti-convulsant, opioids, and natural products work to reduce the perception of pain resulting from neural hyperexcitation [159,160]. First-line drugs such as tricyclic antidepressants, lidocaine, phenytoin, and capsaicin inhibit the transduction of voltage-gated channels, ligand-gated channels, G protein-coupled receptors (GPCRs), and gamma-aminobutyric acid (GABA) receptors [161]. Natural components including omega-3, curcumin, berberine, lycopene, and naringin possess anti-inflammatory properties by inhibiting the expression of injury-induced chemokines and cytokines [161]. Second- and third-line drugs such as opioids also reduce NP, however, adverse side effects and a high dosage required for effective treatment discourages usage [161]. Once treated with natural or synthetically derived drugs, patients commonly experience a placebo effect or a euphoric relief from pain, without treating the original mechanism [159,160]. Alternatively, topical agents such as tacrolimus (FK506), hyaluronic acid (HA), melatonin, lidocaine, and vitamin B12 actively support the alleviation of NP [147]. Tarcolimus (FK506) counteracts neurotoxicity by increasing the expression of growth-associated protein 43 (GAP-43), known for neuronal plasticity and regeneration [162,163]. HA is naturally found in the extracellular matrix composition, stimulating cluster of differentiation 44 (CD44) expression following a traumatic nerve injury [164,165]. HA can provide a suitable environment for nerve regeneration and recovery when topically administered [165]. Lidocaine targets the mechanism of neurotransmitter release, inhibiting the generation of an action potential required for nerve signal conductance [147]. Finally, vitamin B12 promotes myelination and upregulates gene transcription factors for nerve regeneration and pain management [166]. However, this approach to treatment is passive, lacking specificity to the various types of neuropathies and accompanying symptoms [147,159].

Invasive techniques used to treat severe nerve injuries include nerve graft, allograft, nerve transfer, and conduits. The U.S. Food and Drug Administration (FDA) has approved conduits that are primarily constructed with collagen or hyaluronic acid hydrogels, or synthesized with poly-glycolic acid (PGA), polycaprolactone (PCL), and polyvinyl acetate (PVA), effectively re-establishing functionality (Table 3) [167]. In vitro and rodent-based trials (in vivo) have occurred with a combination of natural and synthetic materials, exploring manufacturing techniques for nerve injury treatment. Standard fabrication methods include dip coating, solvent casting, freeze-drying, micro-patterning, and additive manufacturing [168]. The dip coating, solvent casting, and freeze-drying methods produce conduits with varying sizes and connectivity of pores, decreasing the transfer of nutrients and metabolic waste [168]. With electrospinning and micropatterning, the fiber network resembles the extracellular matrix (ECM) and allows for the strategic alignment of growing axons; however, low reproducibility is a disadvantage [168]. Finally, additive manufacturing is highly reproducible and can control specific morphological features depending on the printing method and material used [168].

Table 3. Beneficial properties of each protein within the ECM.

Protein	Properties	Benefit to Neural Regeneration	Reference
Elastin	Highly elastic, water-soluble, hydrophobic.	Promotes cellular adhesion, proliferation, stem cell differentiation, the release of growth factors, drug delivery.	[169]
Fibrinogen	Produces fibrin network, composed of polypeptide chains.	Facilitate stem cell proliferation, adhesion, and differentiation.	[170]
Laminin	Abundant in native ECM.	Basement membrane. Facilitate cellular attachment, differentiation, and neurite outgrowth.	[171,172]
Silk	Naturally occurring in ECM.	Promotes oxygen and permeability. Biodegradable. Supports SC and neuron growth and attachment.	[173,174]
Collagen	Abundant in native ECM.	Fibroblast proliferation, angiogenesis, regulation of pro- and anti-inflammatory response.	[175,176]
Hyaluronic Acid	Abundant in embryonic tissue and ECM.	Maintains ECM, regulates binding proteins in cellular adhesion, proliferation, pro/anti-inflammatory response depending on molecular weight.	[177]

Protein-based hydrogels and synthetic conduits are engineered with varied concentrations of crosslinking agents to influence the biophysical and biochemical cues that promote cellular proliferation, the secretion of ECM components from seeded SCs, and the organization of regrowing axons [169,178,179]. Adjusting the crosslinking agent allows for the effective treatment of severe injuries of a significant distance and large diameter [169]. Biophysical properties such as the porosity, stiffness, degradation, and biochemical communication between protein binding sites and proliferating cells ensure nutritional support as regenerating axons close the nerve gap [169,179–181].

4. Neurotrophic Support in Neuropathy Treatment

With natural or biomaterials acting alone, conduits lack the mechanical and structural properties necessary to support axon regeneration. However, combining biodegradable polymers with biological proteins produces a biocomposite conduit capable of regulating the biochemical cues and growth factors necessary to support neurite outgrowth without disrupting the surrounding connective tissue [117,178,182]. Growth factors are released from the distal and proximal nerve stumps to generate axoplasmic fluid, forming a neomatrix of fibrin [167,180]. Nerve injuries with significant gaps and are large in diameter have limited neurotrophic support; therefore, additional nutrients are required to see nerve reinnervation to completion [180]. Recent studies support the seeding of stem cells and growth factors within biocomposite conduits to enhance the neomatrix between nerve stumps [108,183,184]. To further increase the probability of axon regeneration, neurotrophic factors such as nerve growth factor (NGF), brain-derived neurotrophic factor (BDNF), glial cell-derived neurotrophic factor (GDNF), and VEGF are released from SCs and localized along the conduit [2,168]. Neurotrophic factors within conduits assist in promoting SC migration, neuronal survival, and axon regeneration [168,173].

4.1. Stem Cell Differentiation

Stem cells are classified into two categories: embryonic (totipotent and pluripotent) and nonembryonic (multipotent, oligopotent, and unipotent), based on where they are derived [185]. Self-renewing pluripotent stem cells express transcription factors for the blastula formation that generate the three germ layers: ectoderm, mesoderm, and endotherm [186–189]. The ectoderm gives rise to the nervous system, the mesoderm gives rise to connective and muscular tissue, and the endoderm gives rise to organ systems throughout the body [190]. Multipotent stem cells, commonly derived from bone marrow, adipose tissue, or dental pulp, experience differentiation into several cell types within one designated germ line [186–188,191]. Once within a specific lineage, differentiation is flexible [185]. Due to increased plasticity, self-renewal, and proliferative properties, totipotent, pluripotent, and multipotent stem cells are most advantageous in tissue engineering [188]. However, there are limitations associated, primarily moral objections when harvesting embryonic stem cells and uncontrolled teratoma formation and immunorejection, once clinically applied [187,188,192].

To harvest, tissue rich in stem cells such as the umbilical cord or placenta, bone marrow, adipose tissue, and peripheral blood is first collected then filtered [188,193]. However, neonatal-derived stem cells from the umbilical cord and placenta are considered unethical, leading to the preferred use of mesenchymal stem cells (MSCs) and induced pluripotent stem cells (iPSCs) harvested from connective tissue within the body [188]. Connective tissue is preferred due to the accessibility, cost effectiveness, and abundance of MSCs, however, the harvesting technique influences the survival and yield of the cells collected [194]. Compared to liposuction, syringe aspiration is the most effective because trauma to the donor site is minimized, and the viability of the cells is maintained [194].

MSCs give rise to different mesenchymal lineages within the mesoderm based on the specific stimuli and signaling required for differentiation [193,195,196]. MSCs are derived from bone marrow and adipose tissue [193,195,197,198]. Cellular components of bone marrow and adipose tissue include sympathetic neurons, SCs, macrophages, regulatory T cells, neutrophils, fibroblasts, pericytes, and endothelial cells [195,197]. The positive markers of CD90, CD73, CD105, and negative markers of CD45, CD34, CD14, CD11b,

CD19, and human leukocyte antigen (HLA-DR) effectively distinguish MSCs from other cellular components in the bone marrow (BM) and adipose tissue [193,194,198–202]. Depending upon the source, whether bone marrow or adipose tissue, the markers present slightly differ [194]. To influence differentiation, MSCs are exposed to specific chemical cocktails that upregulate Wnt signaling for osteogenic, chondrogenic, and cardiogenic differentiation [196,197]. Wnt signaling is highly influential in stem cell division, proliferation, migration, and fate determination to increase neurite outgrowth [5,203]. The differentiation of MSCs to a true neuronal lineage is arguable since neurons and connective tissue reside in a different lineage [190]. To encourage an altered lineage, the activation of Wnt signaling promotes the expression of neuronal and glial cell markers in MSCs after exposure to signals that will influence transdifferentiation [196,198]. The induction medium is supplemented with fibroblast growth factor (FGF), Sonic Hedgehog protein (SHH), retinoic acid (RA), and BDNF over 18 days [198]. Reverse transcription polymerase chain reaction (RT-PCR) is used to confirm the gene expression of neural phenotypes [198]. Immunocytochemistry visually confirmed the morphological changes of neurite extension typically exhibited by neural stem cells [198]. Within this study conducted by Urrutia et al., RT-PCR and immunocytochemistry identified the expression of neuroepithelial stem cell protein (NESTIN), β-tubulin III, synaptophysin, neurofilament light polypeptide (NEFL), neurofilament medium polypeptide (NEFM), dopaminergic neuron marker (NURR1), calcium-binding protein B (S100B), and neurotrophin-3 (NT-3) [198]. Comparing the multiple sources human MSCs were isolated from, neuronal markers were considerably more expressed in adipose-derived mesenchymal stem cells (ASCs) than in BM-MSCs [198].

Identical to embryonic stem cells (ESCs), iPSCs are developed from reprogrammed somatic cells or human fibroblasts by introducing growth factors [193]. In 2007, Takahashi et al. reconditioned human fibroblasts to human iPSCs by utilizing a transcription factor cocktail including octamer transcription factor 3 and 4 (OCT-3/4), sex-determining region Y-box 2 (SOX2), c-Myc gene, and Kruppel-like factor 4 (KLF4), engineered initially by Yamanaka for mice fibroblasts [204–206]. This discovery eliminates the need to transfer the nucleus from somatic cells [206]. However, using c-Myc leads to the death of embryonic stem cells [206]. Alternatively, Yu et al. demonstrated the successful reprogramming of human MSCs to iPSCs using OCT4, SOX2, NANOG gene, and Lin28 gene [206]. The addition of NANOG and LIN28 proved to increase the survival rate and recovery of reprogrammed cells [206]. To verify similarities between iPSCs and ESCs, RT-PCR and Western blot analysis identified comparable gene expressions and undifferentiated cell-surface markers such as OCT3/4, SOX2, NANOG, FGF4, reduced expression 1 (REX1), and growth and differentiation factor 3 (GDF3) [205,207]. Immunocytochemistry also showed consistent morphology and proliferation between the embryonic and induced pluripotent cell lines [205,207]. IPSCs can differentiate into mature neural progenitor cells and astrocytes once introduced to a neural induction medium for 21 days [208]. Kang et al. mapped the morphological, genetic expression, and electrophysiological profile changes endured during iPSCs to neuron differentiation [208]. The morphology of differentiating iPSCs detailed increased dendrites and the lengthening of axons following growth cone development throughout 15 days [208]. Immunostaining confirmed the positive gene expression of mature neurons including NESTIN, paired box 6 (PAX6), SOX2, class III beta-tubulin (Tuj1), glial fibrillary acidic protein (GFAP), synapsin 1, and tyrosine hydroxylase (TH) [208]. The genes identified also influence the upregulation of signaling pathways that regulate stem cell proliferation such as MAPK, ligand–receptor interaction, and Wnt pathways [208]. The electrophysiological profile characterization confirmed the synapse's successful formation by recording excitatory postsynaptic currents [208]. Once the cellular membrane is depolarized, the calcium (Ca^{2+}) current, decreased membrane resistance, and increased membrane capacitance are recorded, confirming signal conductance for effective neural communication [208].

Based on the specific conditions the MSCs are transplanted to, complete neural differentiation is not achieved, however, the phenotypic properties of glial cells are adopted [209].

Once injected, MSCs promote angiogenesis, anti-inflammation, and neuroprotection during the regeneration process through secretome expression by which cells exchange communicative signals [209]. Clinically, compared to MSC injections, the intravenous application of paracrine secretions has gained popularity due to the ability to modulate injury symptoms and facilitate functional recovery [209]. As a cell-free therapeutic method, secretory treatment voids the instability experienced with MSC differentiation and the safety risks associated with stem cell transplantation [210,211].

4.2. The Application of Stem Cells in Neuropathy Treatment

Stem cell treatment of PN-induced chronic pain provides assistive interaction with the damaged cells by inhibiting apoptosis and enhancing cellular survival during regeneration [181,212]. The primary mechanism of pain is attributed to the activation of the Janus kinase 2/signal transducer and activator of transcription 3 (JAK2/STAT3) pathway, p38-MAPK pathway, and Notch signaling once peripheral damage occurs [213]. In response to injury, nerve hyperexcitation from an immune-mediated response and continuous infiltration of proinflammatory cytokines contribute to demyelination and neuronal death [181,212,213]. By releasing anti-inflammatory, angiogenic, and nutritional neurotrophic factors such as BDNF, NT-3, FGF, and VEGF, stem cells strongly regulate the body's natural immunoresponse when peripheral nerve damage occurs [181]. Transplantation of BM-MSCs has been proven to upregulate the expression of anti-inflammatory M2 macrophages, downregulate inflammatory M1 macrophages, and influence the MAPK signaling pathway toward the native SC response to injury [181].

Preclinical trials have primarily focused on the successful delivery and retention of stem cells in neurodegenerative diseases such as Parkinson's disease, Huntington's disease, and ischemic stroke [214]. Traditionally, MSCs have been introduced systemically via intracerebral, intravenous, arterial, and nasal infusion to activate neurogenesis in diseases affecting the CNS [212,213]. Stem cells can cross the blood–brain barrier (BBB), allowing effective migration toward damaged brain tissue [215]. The intracerebral application of MSCs in ischemic stroke has proven to reduce inflammation, inhibit further destruction of the BBB, and promote neurogenesis [215]. However, the limitations of this method compromise the success of treatment due to cell clusters trapped in the respiratory and circulatory system [212,215]. Alternatively, the intravenous and intraarterial application is safer but less effective as many cells do not cross the BBB and develop into blood clots or occlusions that lead to further damage [215]. Intranasal administration allows for the successful migration of stem cells via the olfactory system with MSC detection in brain tissue [215]. Proving their success in neurodegenerative diseases affecting the CNS provides gateway access to pain modulation and neuropathy treatment within the PNS [213].

MSC transplantation to the PNS improves neuropathic symptoms by inhibiting destructive mechanisms while maintaining nerve function and axonal regeneration [213]. Various studies, outlined in Table 4, support MSC mediation of oxidative stress, ROS formation, neural inflammation, and apoptosis through the secretion of neurotrophic factors [213].

Table 4. Studies that utilized MSCs in neuropathic treatment.

MSC Source	Neuropathy Treated	Title of Study	Reference
hUC-MSC	DPN	Human umbilical cord-derived mesenchymal stem cells prevent the progression of early diabetic nephropathy through inhibiting inflammation and fibrosis.	[216]
BM-MSC	DPN	The bone marrow-derived mesenchymal stem cells (BMSCs) alleviate diabetic peripheral neuropathy induced by STZ via activating GSK-3β/β-catenin signaling pathway.	[217]

Table 4. *Cont.*

MSC Source	Neuropathy Treated	Title of Study	Reference
ASC	DPN	Treatment with adipose tissue-derived mesenchymal stem cells exerts anti-diabetic effects, improves long-term complications, and attenuates inflammation in type 2 diabetic rats.	[218]
hMSC	CIPN	Nasal administration of mesenchymal stem cells prevents accelerated age-related tauopathy after chemotherapy in mice.	[219]
BM-MSC	CIPN	Bone marrow-derived mesenchymal stem cells alleviate paclitaxel-induced mechanical allodynia in rats.	[220]
MSC	CIPN	Nasal administration of mesenchymal stem cells reverses chemotherapy-induced peripheral neuropathy in mice.	[221]
ASC	CIPN	Adipose-derived stem cells decrease pain in rat model of oxaliplatin-induced neuropathy: Role of VEGF-A modulation.	[222]
hASC and hUC-MSC	Neuropathic symptoms via partial sciatic nerve ligation	Intravenous administration of human mesenchymal stem cells derived from adipose tissue and umbilical cord improves NP via suppression of neuronal damage and anti-inflammatory actions in rats.	[223]
ASC	Peripheral nerve injury repair for NP relief	Role of adipose tissue grafting and adipose-derived stem cells in peripheral nerve surgery.	[194]

Yu et al. investigated the effect of multiple intravenous infusions of ASC on systemic inflammation and the long-term complications brought on by type 2 diabetes [218]. This study aimed to demonstrate the long-term therapeutic potential of ASCs in pain management and interruption of injury progression [218]. Diabetic rats were treated with ASC infusions once a week for 24 weeks. Blood glucose levels gradually decreased to normal levels throughout treatment after each MSC infusion [218]. Insulin sensitivity increased due to the restoration of islet b cells, which is necessary for a proper pancreatic negative response to glucose [218]. MSC treatment also alleviated inflammation due to an increased expression of M2 macrophage phenotypes, effectively combating the development of fibrosis, which negatively affects other essential bodily systems [218]. Similarly, Xiang et al. concluded that treating MSCs in diabetic rats reduced the expression of proinflammatory interleukin-1b (IL-1b), IL-6, and tumor necrosis factor (TNF-α) and reduced the M1 macrophage secretion of TGF-β within the kidneys [216]. Xiang et al. also observed the secretion of anti-inflammatory and anti-fibrotic factors that effectively improved renal function and inhibited the harmful progression of DPN [216]. Within CIPN, the administration of MSCs reversed the pain in mice exposed to chemotherapeutic medications known to negatively affect mitochondrial function and increase oxidative stress [220,221]. After 24 days of MSC treatment, mitochondrial respiration was restored, attributed to the increased MSC and M2 macrophage expression of IL-10 signaling [221]. The limitations of the systemic administration of MSCs are still an issue, requiring an abundant amount of MSCs in the hope that they stay viable, successfully differentiate, and accurately treat the desired target site [220,224].

As previously stated, the intravenous transplantation of MSCs for nerve regeneration increases the risk of complications that limit treatment capabilities. MSCs undoubtedly promote healing, however, the retention of neural differentiation and capability of effective treatment is not guaranteed [225]. The decreased survival rate requiring multiple injection and the risk of vascular obstruction contributing to stroke encourages research into a more optimal therapeutic approach [225]. Alternatively, the secretome produced from MSCs has been explored due to the production of extracellular vesicles [225]. Extracellular vesicles

(EVs) are secreted organelles from the parent cell, compacted with cargo that promotes regenerative function, induces angiogenesis, and regulates cellular communication [224]. EVs range in size and function including apoptotic bodies (>1000 nm), microvesicles (100–1000 nm), and exosomes (50–150 nm) [226,227]. The variety in size requires differential centrifugation to isolate a pure sample [224,228]. The cargo of EVs is potent with proteins, lipids, mRNA, and microRNA (miRNA), which promotes an enhanced regenerative potential such as the type of cell they are derived from (Figure 3). EVs derived from a specific lineage of stem cells replicate mechanisms of intracellular communication and signaling mediation as the parent cell to encourage regenerative properties [227,228]. For example, EVs derived from differentiated neural MSCs have been shown to stimulate angiogenesis, neurite outgrowth, and regeneration and inhibit inflammation, oxidative stress, and apoptosis [224,229].

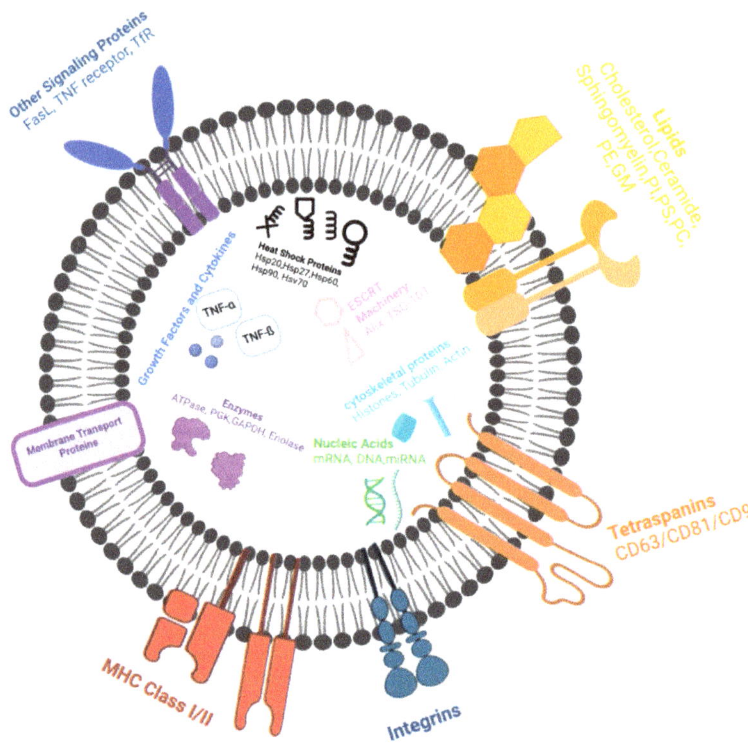

Figure 3. Components of EV cargo. Exosomes are composed of a multitude of proteins, molecules, growth factors, cytokines, lipids, and nucleic acids that influence the exosome structure, cargo organization, secretion, and signaling in multiple biological processes.

4.3. Potential of MSCs Secretome in Nerve Regeneration

Naturally, exosomes within the PNS regulate synaptic activity via neurotransmitters, modulate intracellular and cell-to-cell communication, and facilitate the exchange of biological information to maintain homeostatic conditions [228,230,231]. The primary mode of communication is through the transportation and selective delivery of mRNA, miRNA, and proteins from the donor to the recipient cell. The EV transfer of mRNA facilitates the paracrine exchange of genetic information [224]. MiRNAs are crucial in stimulating gene expression and facilitating cellular proliferation, differentiation, migration, and apoptosis [224]. The delivery of proteins is essential for managing tissue regeneration and providing a mechanism for the EV surface to interact with cellular receptors for targeted delivery [224]. The primary methods of EV uptake include phagocytosis, receptor-mediated endocytosis, and direct fusion with the cellular membrane [227,232]. However, efficient EV consumption depends on the biophysical and mechanical properties that allow the proper interaction for tissue absorption [227]. The size, elasticity, stiffness, and Young's modulus of EVs differs per source of the parent cell [227]. Modification of the EV surface increases migration through the ECM and enhances the attraction of specific surface proteins to cellular receptors for more effective delivery [227].

4.3.1. EV Biogenesis and Transport

The biogenesis of EVs is attributed to the endosomal sorting complex required for transport (ESCRT) mechanism complex, which guides endosomes through the early and late stages of development before exocytosis (Figure 4) [233]. Subunits of ESCRT promote cargo organization and internalization during intraluminal vesicle (ILV) formation, dictated by the expression of seven primary proteins: tumor susceptibility gene 101 (TSG101), Alix, chromatin modified protein 4C (CHMP4C), vascular protein sorting-associated (VPS) protein 4B, vacuolar protein sorting-associated protein (VTA1), hepatocyte growth factor-regulated tyrosine kinase substrate (Hrs), and signal transducing adaptor molecule (STAM1) [233–235]. Once organized within late-endosome development, the Golgi apparatus then supplies ILVs with major histocompatibility complex (MHC) class I and II molecules, growth factor receptors, and RNAs, encompassed by multivesicular bodies (MVBs) [233,236]. The MVBs are then transported to the cellular membrane, guided by cytoskeleton, microtubules, and Ras-associated binding guanosine triphosphates (Rab GTPases), then secreted as exosomes via exocytosis [233,234]. Rab GTPases are crucial during the transport of MVBs to the cellular membrane, specifically Rab27a and Rab27b, during MVB docking and intracellular trafficking [233]. The mechanism by which the cells receive cargo includes ligand–receptor interaction, binding to target receptors on the cellular membrane, membrane fusion, and complete exosome internalization via endocytosis [227,232,233,236]. EVs contain surface markers on the phospholipid bilayer membrane that are attracted to specific sites for targeted delivery [224,226,227,229].

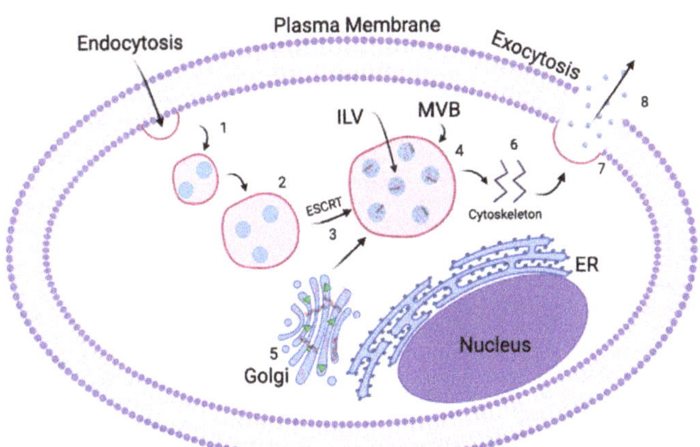

Figure 4. Biogenesis of exosomes. (1) Internalized cargo from the cellular membrane via endocytosis is sorted into (2) early endosomes. (3) ESCRT, tetraspanins, and lipids guide early endosomes through late endosome/MVB maturation, (4) which is concentrated with ILVs. (5) The Golgi apparatus then supplements ILVs with nucleic acids, RNAs, proteins, and MHC II molecules. (6) MVBs are then transported to the plasma membrane via the cytoskeletal and microtubule network. (7) During the transportation process, Rab GTPases guide the docking and fusion of MVB with the plasma membrane. (8) ILVs are secreted as exosomes via exocytosis.

Within neuropathy treatment, incorporating EVs enhances the repair environment with neurotrophic factors such as GDNF (SC recruitment), insulin-like growth factor 1 (IGF-1), TNF-α, and TGF to promote the regeneration of damaged tissue and improve functional recovery [180,237]. The primary source of EVs is derived from BM-MSC and ASCs due to easy access, nonimmunogenic response when transplanted, and the phenotypic alteration of immune-mediated cells responding to injury [237–239]. Due to the therapeutic capabilities of BM-MSCs and ASCs, derived exosomes from each respective stem cell are favorable in drug delivery and the treatment of neuropathy, neurodegenerative diseases, and cancer [237].

4.3.2. Targeted Transplantation of EVs in Neuropathy Treatment

Within neuropathic treatment, the transplantation of exosomes derived from MSCs directly targeted to the injury site will activate signaling pathways that promote angiogenesis, immune response regulation, and the management of the extracellular environment [240,241]. The mentioned effects, which are also highlighted in Table 5, are attributed to the cargo within exosomes. Once EVs are applied to damaged cells, the cargo uptake leads to the downregulation of key factors that negatively affect the quality and health of the cells within the injury site. For example, Song et al. isolated EVs from healthy cortical neurons containing miR-NA-181-3p, which have been shown to suppress neuroinflammation via targeting the CXCL1 gene in astrocytes [242]. Alternatively, EV cargo isolation from damaged PC12 cells containing miRNA-21-5p, known to cause chronic neuroinflammation, upregulated the expression of proinflammatory factors following EV uptake in BV2 cells [243]. The RNA within EV cargo is critical to their therapeutic effect. MiRNA-133b, a regulator of tyrosine hydroxylase production and dopamine transporter, is the best understood MSC-EV mediated treatment regarding cerebral injury [244]. Researchers have transferred MSC-EVs to injured neurons, successfully promoting neural plasticity and neurite outgrowth due to its role in post-transcriptional gene regulation and neuroprotective upregulation [244,245]. However, a more directed approach to treatment will accelerate the healing capabilities associated with EVs. The uptake of EVs continues to be a challenging obstacle to overcome. When injected intravenously, EVs primarily accumulate in organs of the reticuloendothelial system such as the liver or spleen [246]. A further understanding of site-specific EV uptake is needed, specifically toward neuropathy treatment.

Table 5. Studies that utilized exosomes in neuropathy treatment.

Exosome Source	Neuropathy Treated	Title of Study	Reference
hMSC	DPN	Treatment of diabetic peripheral neuropathy with engineered mesenchymal stromal cell-derived exosomes enriched with microRNA-146a provide amplified therapeutic efficacy.	[237]
hBM-MSC	DPN	Exosomes derived from atorvastatin-pretreated MSC accelerate diabetic wound repair by enhancing angiogenesis via AKT/eNOS pathway.	[240]
hBM-MSC	DPN	Melatonin-stimulated MSC-derived exosomes improve diabetic wound healing through regulating macrophage M1 and M2 polarization by targeting the PTEN/AKT pathway.	[241]
SC-EV	DPN	Exosomes derived from Schwann cells ameliorate peripheral neuropathy in type 2 diabetic mice.	[247]
CEC-sEV	CIPN	Small extracellular vesicles ameliorate peripheral neuropathy and enhance chemotherapy of oxaliplatin on ovarian cancer.	[238]
hBM-MSC-EVs	CIPN	Bone marrow mesenchymal stem cells and their derived exosomes resole doxorubicin-induced chemobrain: Critical role of their miRNA cargo.	[248]

Table 5. *Cont.*

Exosome Source	Neuropathy Treated	Title of Study	Reference
hUC-MSC	Microglial activation of NP	Huc-MSCs-derived exosomes attenuate NP by inhibiting activation of the TLR2/MyD88/NF-kB signaling pathway in the spinal microglia by targeting Rasad2.	[249]
MSC	Microglial activation of NP	Mesenchymal stem cell-derived extracellular vesicles carrying miR-99b-3p restrain microglial activation and NP by stimulating autophagy.	[250]
BM-MSC	NP via sciatic nerve chronic constriction injury	Exosomes carried miR-181c-5p alleviates NP in CCI rat models.	[251]
MSC	NP via spinal neuroinflammation	Extracellular vesicles derived from mesenchymal stem cells alleviate neuroinflammation and mechanical allodynia in interstitial cystitis rats by inhibiting NLRP3 inflammasome activation.	[252]
hUC-MSC	Alleviate inflammatory pain	Huc-MSCs-derived exosomes attenuate inflammatory pain by regulating microglia pyroptosis and autophagy via the miR-146a-5p/TRAF6 axis.	[253]

Once applied, the uptake of EVs may occur via five different mechanisms including clathrin-dependent and independent endocytosis, caveolin-mediated invagination, lipid raft-mediated endocytosis, phagocytosis, and macropinocytosis [233]. Clathrin-mediated endocytosis occurs by forming a clathrin-coated vesicle due to deformation in the plasma membrane cytoskeleton [233,254]. The inward budding vesicle is separated from the membrane by dynamin-2 and then further developed through the endocytic pathway [233,254]. Similarly, caveolae-mediated invagination creates a membrane specifically concentrated with glycoproteins and cholesterol, recognized as caveolae [233,254]. Lipid-raft mediated endocytosis is an invagination process that is enriched in cholesterol, sphingolipids, and glycosylphosphatidylinositol (GPI)-anchored proteins, promoting the formation of early endosome [233]. Phagocytosis internalizes EVs into a large vacuole through the rearrangement of the membrane cytoskeleton, identified by the phagocytic marker, lysosomal-associated membrane protein 1 (LAMP-1) [233,254,255]. Alternatively, macropinocytosis promotes the rearrangement of the cytoskeleton into lamellipodia to engulf nonspecific EVs into lysosomes [233,255]. Each method of internalization can co-exist and co-occur [233]. To specifically direct EVs toward damaged nerves for neuropathic treatment, utilizing EVs derived from the parent cell known to be directly involved in nerve injury treatment may influence the targeting capabilities [256]. Common EV markers identified for neuronal regeneration, EV biogenesis, and uptake by neuronal cells include CD81, CD9, and CD63 [257,258]. Further research on the surface protein and chemical dependence is needed to understand which mechanisms govern EV uptake toward neuropathy treatment.

SCs play an influential role in the maintenance of the PNS. The plasticity of SCs allows the transdifferentiation from mature myelinating SCs to immature SCs, then rSCs that initiate the neuroinflammatory response causing NP [259]. Following the dissipation of injured nerve fragments, rSCs supply neurotrophic factors for axonal regeneration, alter the phenotype of immune-responsive M1 macrophages to anti-inflammatory M2 macrophages, and guide Büngner bands to the target site [239]. Due to their crucial role in nerve regeneration, recent studies have explored the application of rSC-derived exosomes in neural regeneration and neuropathic treatment [239]. Further investigation strives to identify the miRNA composition with rSC-derived exosomes directly influencing axonal growth [260]. El-Derany et al. treated CIPN with exosomes derived from BM-MSCs, successfully identifying exosomal miRNAs (miR-21-5p, miR-125b-5p, miR-199a-3p, miR-24-3p, and let-7a-5p) secreted to the damaged nerves [248]. López-Leal et al. demonstrated increased neurite outgrowth once rSC exosomes transferred miRNA21 to damaged tissue, directly activating the expression of c-Jun, SOX2, and the modified regulation of regenerative molecules via the phosphatidylinositol 3-kinase (P13K)/protein kinase B (AKT) signaling pathway [239,261,262]. C-Jun expression activates the repair mechanism of SCs, and SOX2 activates the immune response while inhibiting myelinating factors of rSCs [261]. The PI3K/AKT pathway is active in cellular proliferation, cellular survival, cell cycle progression, cellular plasticity, glucose metabolism, and protein synthesis [262]. Targeting the PI3K/AKT pathway has been explored as a viable option to regulate diabetics and diseases affecting the nervous system [262]. For example, Li et al. successfully alleviated NP induced by chemotherapeutic agents through the supplementation of resveratrol via the PI3K/AKT signaling pathway [263]. As a result, mitochondrial dysfunction improved due to the reduction in oxidative stress and successfully alleviated NP symptoms [263]. Concerning SC function, the PI3K/AKT pathway, which regulates the tuberous sclerosis complex (TSC), activates the mechanistic target of rapamycin complex 1 (mTORC1), playing an important role in the myelination of axons and mRNA protein translation for cellular metabolism, growth, and proliferation [264–268]. Along with the Erk1/2 signaling pathway, this pathway is also influential in SC development and transdifferentiation in response to pathological conditions [267,268].

Of the three types of SCs, the expression of rSCs and derived exosomes is most beneficial in the axonal regeneration and management of NP [261]. However, the utilization of rSC exosomes is limited regarding the number of EVs produced, the loading efficiency of desired cargo, and retention once applied clinically [224,239]. The process of EV isolation has not been optimized to generate large enough quantities to support complete regeneration [224,237]. Additionally, nonfunctional components within EV cargo hinder effective treatment, requiring an abundance of EVs at the injury site [224,239]. Finally, the retention of rSC phenotype expression is unstable [239,269]. Once the injury gap length and time required for reinnervation become extensive, the secretion of neurotrophic factors fades as the cell-to-axon biochemical cascade no longer encourages a regenerative microenvironment [269,270].

4.4. Methods to Increase EV Production

The clinical application of EVs requires mass production and an optimal isolation protocol to ensure that sustainable quantities are obtained [211]. Traditional two-dimensional (2D) cultures produce a low yield of EVs and batch-to-batch variability between cellular passages [211]. A 2D culture does not actively represent the native environment in which cell-to-cell and cell-to-matrix interactions naturally occur within the ECM [271]. To mimic accurate cellular behavior, three-dimensional (3D) culture conditions allow cells to form aggregates for the increased production of EVs [272]. Furthermore, 3D aggregates enhanced by dynamic cellular agitation have been proven to allow for the large-scale production of EVs with an enhanced expression of therapeutic cargo [211,272–274]. Through shear stress, the expression of ESCRT-independent/dependent biogenesis markers significantly increased alongside EV production within the PBS Vertical-Wheel Bioreactor compared to the 2D culture [273]. As a result, the EVs isolated from the 3D culture expressed upregulated therapeutic miRNA secretion consistent with angiogenesis, wound healing, and neuroprotection [273]. Jeske et al. compared the effect of shear stress within the PBS Vertical-Wheel Bioreactor to 2D static culture, investigating the secretion and cargo profile of hMSC-derived EVs [273]. Western blot analysis presented an upregulation in exosomal markers HRS, syntenin-1, CD81, and CD63 in the bioreactor groups compared to the 2D group [273]. Finally, the miRNA cargo within the 3D bioreactor groups, compared to the 2D groups, showed an upregulation in EVs that would effectively promote wound healing such as miR-10, 19a, 19b, 21, 30b, 92a, 126, and 132 [273]. Therefore, culture expansion and increased EV production rely on improving culture conditions, enhancing the external environment, and stimulating signaling pathways that influence cellular secretions [211,271]. Alternatively to the PBS Vertical-Wheel Bioreactor, the spinner flask and rotating wall bioreactors mildly support scaling up for clinical application; however, various limitations discourage utilization. For example, a horizontal impeller is used to agitate the media in spinner flask bioreactors. However, this application of shear stress results in turbulent flows and nonhomogeneous shear zones within the reactor, generating aggregates of different quality [275,276].

Alongside scaling up EV production, the ability to store generated EVs effectively while ensuring a nonsignificant drop in quality is also a limiting factor in the clinical utilization of EVs. EVs are typically stored in PBS or media at 4 °C or −80 °C, as suggested by the International Society for Extracellular Vesicles [277]. However, in 2018, these suggestions were redacted due to the impact of EV preservation and long-term storage on the stability, concentration, and overall function [278]. These storage methods have been shown to significantly decrease EV yield within seven days of storage [279]. The buffer selection, temperature, and storage techniques greatly influence the EV shelf life to optimize current storage techniques.

Regarding a storage buffer, Kawai-Harada et al. developed an EV storage buffer consisting of trehalose and BSA-supplemented PBS-HEPES buffer [279]. This buffer showed better cargo protection than the standard storage techniques without sacrificing any loss in targeting ability, size, or EV morphology [279]. While a promising alternative to standard storage methods, the study on the effects of the EV storage buffer is limited to 7 days. A clinically applicable method would need long-term storage of months to years. This EV storage buffer has yet to be tested on EVs derived from stem cells, as Kawai-Harada et al. utilized HEK293T cell-derived EVs, and it is unlikely that the necessary cargo for neuropathic treatment is stored within these EVs. Therefore, the effects the storage buffer could have on stem cell-derived EV cargo quality are unknown. Another study by Görgens et al. addressed EV storage conditions for up to two years, concluding that buffers composed of trehalose and human albumin showed significant improvement in EV preservation for samples stored at −80 °C [280]. While MSC-derived EVs were studied within this research, the data are inconclusive compared to those of the HEK293T cells utilized. Particle concentration saw a significant improvement after storage, regardless of temperature. Cellular uptake and cargo quantification were not investigated with these EVs. Another limitation, regardless of the storage solution, is that multiple freeze–thaw cycles have been shown to induce membrane disruption and re-micellization, with effects being significant after as few as two cycles [281,282]. Other avenues such as lyophilization and temperature dependency have also been explored with varying levels of success and conflicting results [281,283,284]. These alternative methods share the same limitation of short-term analysis, with no studies testing for the effects on EVs over extended periods. For EVs to be clinically ready, the enormous hurdles of successful scale and proper long-term storage protocols must be addressed to ensure the quality and repeatability of EVs between stocks.

The influence of the external environment on cellular gene expression directly alters the protein synthesis and behavior of the cell [285]. Specifically regarding ESCRT-dependent and -independent biogenesis markers, the upregulation of HRS, TSG101, Alix, sphingomyelin phosphodiesterase 2 (SMPD2), SMPD3, melanocyte including transcription factor (MITF), STAM1, and GTPases Rab27a and Rab27b expression effectively increases the exosome yield [234,273]. ESCRT-dependent exosome biogenesis markers, HRS, TSG101, and Alix, promote endosomal budding, selective cargo sorting, and MBV formation toward exosome release [235]. The ESCRT-independent biogenesis markers include the vital role of lipids and tetraspanins such as CD9, CD63, CD37, CD81, CD82, and CD53 during cargo sorting and exosome budding [235]. Ceramide is a lipid that is essential in the formation of ILVs, generated by the enzyme neutral sphingomyelinase 2 (nSMase2) [234,235]. As one of the primary mechanisms of exosome formation, upregulating nSMase2 expression alongside increased metabolic activity effectively promotes ceramide function within the ESCRT-independent pathway [234]. Once formed, GTPases Rab27a and Rab27b promote the transport and binding of MVBs for release [233,235]. The influence of external stimulus toward increased EV production has been accurately identified in the upregulation of essential exosome biogenesis markers. Wang et al. demonstrated the upregulation of MSC-derived exosomes without increasing the cellular volume [234]. The introduction of norepinephrine, fenoterol, N-methyldopamine, and forskolin to the MSC culture increased exosome production 3-fold [234]. The additional molecules effectively enhanced the nSMase2 promotion of ceramide expression as well as Rab27a and Rab27b, correlating the increased production of exosomes to an abundance of cargo [234,235]. Similarly, the microcarrier-based expansion of hMSCs within 3D PBS Vertical-Wheel Bioreactors compared to base 2D cultures effectively increased the exosome yield 2.5-fold, an upregulation of EV biogenesis markers, and the enhanced expression of neuroprotective microRNA [273]. Aside from environmental cues, direct stimulation of the signaling pathways that control the endolysosomal pathway charged with EV production may produce the largest yield [271].

Electrical Stimulation Promoting Transdifferentiation and EV Production

Electrical stimulation (ES) is a form of neuromodulation commonly used to stimulate damaged nerve fibers that induce chronic pain in spinal cord injuries and peripheral neuropathy [286]. The neuronal response to ES is induced neuroplasticity, which alters the synaptic release of neurotransmitters, cellular behavior, and overall response to injury [286]. Similarly, the cellular response to an electrical field promotes cellular signaling to initiate hMSC transdifferentiation toward a neural lineage and increases exosome production for therapeutic applications, evident in Table 6 [287,288]. Neural-like differentiation, neurite outgrowth, and increased exosome production are attributed to low-level ES combined with growth factors and mechanical cues from the external microenvironment [212,288,289].

ES catalyzes the role of neurotransmitters and receptors in cellular signaling, subsequently increasing the production of EVs [288]. Limited understanding of the relationship between ES and cellular signaling further promotes the investigation of ES on the natural SC response to peripheral nerve injury [290]. Enhanced neural excitation directly alters voltage-gated ion kinetics across the cellular membrane and the synaptic release of neurotransmitters that influence pain modulation and cellular functionality [286]. Hu et al. electrically stimulated dorsal root ganglion (DRG) cells with 100 mV/mm, which effectively increased cellular proliferation as well as the production of glutamate [291]. Glutamate is an excitatory neurotransmitter that mediates the peripheral nerve communication, cellular signaling, and SC secretion of exosomes [290]. Once ES is applied, excess glutamate binds with ionotropic glutamate receptors, causing an influx in Ca^{2+} [290,291]. As a result, Hu et al. highlighted the direct correlation between an upregulation in Ca^{2+} ion concentration and the increased secretion of EVs [288,291]. Similarly, Zhang et al. exposed cardiac-MSCs (C-MSCs) to low-level ES from 2 to 72 h. There was a significant increase in the nSMase2 protein levels, crucial to EV biogenesis and release [292]. Compared to C-MSCs (control), C-MSCs (ES) produced a 38% increase in EV particles/mL concentration and diameter [292]. Alternatively, with high voltage and exposure time, the hyperactive rate of nerve action potential proved to be damaging to the cell [291]. A complete understanding of ES on the cell has yet to be fully understood; however, ES has been confirmed to alter cellular energy metabolism, morphology, phenotype, and Ca^{2+} expression [291,292]. The optimization of ES parameters is necessary to ensure cellular proliferation and the secretion of glutamate and EVs without causing cellular damage or the ability to produce quality EVs. Fukuta et al. isolated EVs from electrically stimulated B16F1 and 3T3 Swiss Albino cultures that effectively increased the particle quantity without compromising the exosome quality [288]. Compared to cultures unexposed to ES, Western blot analysis reflected an insignificant difference in the expression of EV markers CD9, HSP70, and CD81 [288]. The low-level ES permits a Ca^{2+} influx to activate exosome biogenesis and Rho GTPase involvement in the mechanism of cellular exocytosis [288].

The effect of ES can be further enhanced by materials known to possess the ideal biophysical and conductive properties for enhanced EV secretion and MSC neural differentiation. For example, graphene is commonly used in scaffold manufacturing, implant devices, and substrates for cellular differentiation [256,293,294]. Despite graphene's benefits, complex material production places its viability into question. Guo et al. utilized a reduced graphene oxide (rGO) microfiber scaffold to enhance electrical stimulation toward neural differentiation. Further modifications incorporated poly(3,4-ethylenedioxythiophene) (PEDOT), a biocompatible conductive polymer, within the rGO microfibers due to negatively charged carboxylic acid groups. This composite material is bioactive due to rGO and is highly conductive due to the PEDOT, with no significant effect on mechanical properties [212]. Compared to rGO microfibers, rGO–PEDOT hybrid microfibers maintained 99% cellular viability, and increased MSC adhesion and proliferation over five days of ES exposure. Finally, immunostaining and quantitative PCR (qPCR) results expressed Tuj1 and GFAP markers toward neural differentiation [212]. This is attributed to the enhanced electrical–cellular interface and the mechanical and topographical features that influence MSC morphology and gene expression [212].

ES has been shown to enhance the MSC microenvironment for differentiation. To mimic these physiological conditions in a closed system, Naskar et al. fabricated lab-on-a-chip microfluidic devices. They utilized polymethylmethacrylate (PMMA) as the material because it is noncytotoxic, biocompatible, and autoclavable for sterilization [287]. Conduction within the closed microenvironment is possible with pressure sensitive adhesive (PSA) tape and two stationary electrodes. This design allowed for a uniform electric field to stimulate the entire cell population simultaneously. ES was shown to strengthen the differentiation of C2C12 cells to neural-like cells due to the electrophysiological analysis of Ca^{2+} depolarization.

Electroconductive substrates have also been developed and implemented for localized ES during cell proliferation and differentiation. Many conductive polymers were investigated due to their potential as substrates for biological and medical applications, one of the most promising polymers being polyaniline (PANI). It was previously shown to be an excellent matrix that supports cardiac myoblast and nerve cell proliferation and differentiation [295–297]. Thrivikramn et al. attempted to understand the behavior of hMSCs grown on PANI films with tunable conductivity combined with ES. Results showed that the intermittent delivery of low-level ES (100 mV/cm) at 24-h intervals created distinct morphological changes, enhanced cytoskeletal elongation, and the expression of early neural markers such as NESTIN and beta-tubulin III, providing further evidence of the benefit of ES on both neural differentiation and cell proliferation [289].

Table 6. Electrical stimulation to promote transdifferentiation or increased exosome production for peripheral nerve injury treatment.

Title of Study	Cell Culture	ES	ES Duration	ES Method	Reference
Intermittent electrical stimuli for guidance of human mesenchymal stem cell lineage commitment towards neural-like cells on electroconductive substrates.	MSCs	DC; 1 mV–2 V	10 min/day, 3 days	Parallel stainless-steel electrodes PANI film	[289]
Neurogenesis-on-Chip: Electric field modulated transdifferentiation of human mesenchymal stem cell and mouse muscle precursor cell coculture.	hMSCs Murine myoblast	DC ~8 ± 0.06 mV/mm	20 h/day for 9 days	Microfluidic device; graphene oxide (GO) microfiber	[287]
Effectiveness of electrical stimulation on nerve regeneration after crush injury: Comparison between invasive and non-invasive stimulation.	Sciatic nerve crush injury	25 Hz, 1–3 mA, 0.1 ms pulse width	30 min/day 5 times/week for 6 weeks	Implanted wireless cuff electrodes	[298]
Low level electricity increases the secretion of extracellular vesicles from cultured cells.	Murine melanoma cell line, B16F1	0.34 mA/cm^2	60 min Immediate EV isolation	Two Ag–AgCl electrodes with 2.5 cm^2 surface areas	[288]

Table 6. *Cont.*

Title of Study	Cell Culture	ES	ES Duration	ES Method	Reference
The frequency-dependent effect of electrical fields on the mobility of intracellular vesicles in astrocytes.	Rat astrocytes	5 mV/mm; 2 Hz	5 min of constant voltage; 0.1 nms pulse 600 total pulses	Stimulus isolator A365 with 1 KΩ resistor	[299]
Electrical stimulation increases the secretion of cardioprotective extracellular vesicles from cardiac mesenchymal stem cells.	Cardiac MSC	1.5 V/1.8 cm	2–72 h; 1.5 V/1.8 cm voltage, 0.5 Hz frequency, pulse width at 5 ms	Cultured-cell pacer system (IonOptix)	[292]

The molecular mechanism of cellular differentiation and increased EV production following ES exposure is inconclusive [299]. However, various studies have concluded on the increased mobility of secreted vesicles that transport vesicular cargo, neurotransmitters, neuromodulators, hormones, and peptides [299]. Ang et al. concluded that the effect of ES may not directly alter the EV, but the external factors that depict cytoskeleton and motor protein functionality surrounding the vesicles [299]. ES generates an action potential that increases the expression of Ca^{2+}, neural marker proteins, cellular signaling pathways, and exosomal paracrine communication, effectively promoting enhanced cargo produced by MSC-derived EVs [287,300].

Naskar et al. applied a direct current (DC) of low-level ES of ~8 ± 0.06 mV/mm for 20 h/day for nine days to a hMSC and murine myoblast coculture within a microfluidic device [287]. The microfluidic device mimicked native biochemical cues and the directional orientation of the ECM to promote neural differentiation [287]. As a result, the appropriate microenvironment and ES profile successfully promoted the hMSC expression of NESTIN, Tuj1, and MAP2 and intracellular calcium-signaling, signifying neuronal synaptic activity [287]. The condition media also facilitated exosome mRNA protein translation from differentiated neural hMSCs to the myoblasts, exhibiting neural-like phenotypes and morphology [287]. DC stimulation at a low frequency has repeatedly demonstrated successful neural differentiation, increased exosome production, and enhanced axon regeneration [298]. Enhancement of the external environment further amplifies the method by which ES promotes nerve regeneration [212,289,300]. Biocompatible, electroconductive materials such as carbon, graphene, and PANI, enhanced with electrodes, are strategically engineered to mimic the ECM and induce cellular signals congruent with neural differentiation. However, the long-term integration of various biocompatible materials with the host tissue for additional manipulation of the external cellular environment requires further investigation. The studies incorporating biocompatible and electroconductive materials were conducted in vitro in controlled environments. However, Leng et al. successfully utilized carbon nanotube bucky paper in vivo to transplant human retinal pigment epithelium cells within the subretinal space of rats [301]. This study explicitly emphasized that minimal material manipulation is suitable for short-term host interaction. However, functionalization of the material surface is required to extend material capabilities beyond the retina [301].

Depending on the cell type and expected outcome, the parameters for electrical stimulation can range in frequency, direction, magnitude, and current. Therefore, optimization is challenging. However, the primary comparison between low- and high-level frequency and an alternating current (AC), DC, and pulsed current contributes toward an optimized protocol per cell type. An AC flows bidirectionally, causing the charge's magnitude to periodically reverse [300]. A DC produces a consistent and directional charge, effectively guiding the cellular migration toward the anode or cathode [300].

Similarly, a PC, which can be a direct or alternating current, produces a unidirectional or bidirectional current, allowing a dynamic range of electrical frequency, strength, and duration [300,302]. Cellular directional migration during ES stimulation, otherwise known as electrotaxis or galvanotaxis, is influenced by the polarity of the activated intracellular signaling pathways and Golgi apparatus [300,302,303]. However, this phenomenon is cell-type dependent, with MSCs and iPSCs directed toward the anode and neural stem cell (NSC) migration toward the cathode [302–304]. To investigate cellular viability concerning ES duration and current, ASCs stimulated with direct and pulsed currents within a custom agar-salt electrotaxis chamber were exposed to 1200 μA for 3, 6, and 9 h [302]. There was a direct correlation between increased DC exposure and decreased cellular viability. However, the exact duration of pulsed current ES revealed minimal cell death while actively maintaining directional migration toward the anode through Golgi polarization [302].

Regarding frequency, the cellular response to low-level ES includes increased EV production, the upregulation of neural phenotype markers, and extended neurite outgrowth [288,289,300]. This is ultimately beneficial for neuropathic and nerve injury treatment. Alternatively, the high-level frequency that approaches the voltage capacity of the cellular membrane, especially for an extended duration, contributes toward decreased cellular proliferation, viability, and membrane integrity [300,302]. The method and parameters by which the ES was applied differed for each experiment. Each ES chamber was custom-built, thus decreasing the ability to reproduce results quickly. Although the ES parameters were different, favorable results were consistently produced when applying low-frequency levels.

5. Discussion

Damage to the PNS results from physical injury or demyelinating mechanisms that severely alter the microenvironment encompassing the nerves. The current state-of-the-art treatment methods for neuropathic injury do not effectively treat nerve degeneration but instead mask the associated chronic pain. Treating physical damage by nerve graft remains the golden standard; however, donor site morbidity diminishes its success. The transition to artificial nerve grafts utilizing biocompatible and biodegradable materials is a favorable alternative. However, the probability of complete nerve regeneration becomes less than likely as the nerve gap surpasses three centimeters, thus extending the time required for complete regeneration.

The three stages of SC differentiation mediate the pathophysiology of injury response. Once fragmented cellular debris is cleared, rSCs and distal and proximal nerve stumps supplement neurotrophic factors that initiate a cascade of biochemical cues that facilitate the remyelination of damaged nerves and accurately guide regrowing axons to the target site [180]. The signaling pathways most influential in nerve regeneration include PI3K/AKT/mTORC1, MAPK, Notch, Wnt, and JAK2/STAT3. Each pathway influences the cellular response to external stress, determining the cellular fate and the natural immunoresponse to injury. Working together, nerve regeneration is possible; however, large peripheral nerves with significant nerve gaps require additional neurotrophic support [180]. Gapped nerves require more time for neurite outgrowth, decreasing the survivability of rSCs. To overcome this limitation, supplying the nerve conduit with additional factors will maintain the regenerative microenvironment surrounding regrowing nerves. The application of MSCs expressing neural phenotypes and rSCs within the biocomposite conduit will actively modulate the surrounding area. Additionally, rSC-derived exosomes, compacted with cytokines, anti-inflammatory factors, and miRNA, will supply an optimal combination of neurotrophic factors necessary to accelerate the regeneration process.

To further promote the regenerative properties provided by the coculture of neural-like MSC, rSCs, and rSC-derived exosomes, modifications to the external environment enhance the production of rSC exosomes, increasing the probability of clinical applications. Low levels of direct electrical stimulation activate the Rho GTPase and PKC signaling pathways to increase EV production [288]. Within a lab setting, the in vitro application of electrical stimulation requires a device to supply voltage and conductive electrodes. However, the previously described schematic could be more realistic and convenient to the patient within clinical applications. Guo et al. developed a self-generating device powered by triboelectric charging [212]. Incorporating conductive, biocompatible, and biodegradable materials such as carbon nanotubes, enhanced by a triboelectric effect, is an effective method of maintaining a regenerative environment.

6. Conclusions

The PNS is more susceptible to damage than the CNS, which is protected by the skull and spinal column. Due to the associated symptoms, individuals affected by peripheral nerve injuries have trouble navigating through everyday life, preventing effective communication between the CNS and PNS. These symptoms are influenced by mechanisms such as the compression or severance of nerves, classified as Grade I–Grade IV injuries. Once a nerve is severed, the muscular function and sensory information that the nerve innervates are disconnected. The treatment options for various nerve injuries successfully restore function; however, the associated disadvantages discourage long-term use. Fortunately, peripheral nerves can slowly self-regenerate, encouraging the utilization of biocomposite conduits to guide and facilitate axon reinnervation. In conjunction with a biocompatible material, seeding neural-like MSCs, rSCs, and rSC-derived exosomes will further encourage the presence of growth factors necessary for axon growth, myelination, and nerve reinnervation. Difficulties arise when attempting this treatment method. Effective treatment requires accurate mapping of the mechanisms that guide cellular differentiation and release neurotrophic support.

Before exosomal therapeutics can become an effective clinical option, limitations such as upscale, site specificity, storage, and quality assurance must be addressed. Upscaling cellular expansion for EV production has been shown to affect cell quality and, in turn, the cargo and concentration loaded within exosomes. A practical and repeatable upscaling technique that ensures minimal difference in cell and exosome quality from static to large-scale dynamic cultures has yet to be devised. After upscale, long-term storage must also be addressed. It is pivotal to store EVs for long periods in an economically feasible way to ensure clinical viability. Research is inconclusive, and many different methods such as lyophilization, storage buffer, and storage temperature still need to be studied. Despite having some site specificity due to the markers on their surface, EVs often accumulate in unintended sites like the liver or spleen. Current research focuses on increasing site specificity via exosomal surface modifications and cargo. The results are promising, but considering the effects of culture conditions on EV formation, they should be tackled along with engineered modifications to produce more site-specific exosomes. More research on engineered EV surface modifications, storage, particle reconstitution, clearance within the body, and long-term outcomes are all avenues of research that are of interest in cell-free therapy. Furthermore, a method of EV isolation to maximize exosome production as well as the optimal combination of materials necessary to enhance the regenerative microenvironment must be universally established. With EVs becoming more and more prevalent in research, it is critical to note that many safety barriers must be addressed. Regarding MSCs, there are conflicting data regarding safety. While the research suggests human MSC EVs are nontoxic, these studies are in vitro cultures with small dosages relative to those needed in clinical work [305]. Despite being nontoxic, there is conflicting evidence regarding oncogenesis derived from MSC EVs. While EVs cannot grow tumors, they can inhibit or upregulate tumor growth and metastasis [306–308]. In a 2021 study by Tan et al., they proposed that these conflicting data could be due to the heterogeneity of the MSC source, EV isolation methodology, or tumor model utilized [309]. Nonetheless, more must be known about EVs regarding oncogenesis and other safety concerns prior to clinical applications.

Author Contributions: Writing—original draft preparation, D.B.; Writing—review and editing, J.E., A.N., M.S., Y.L. and C.Z.; Project administration, Y.L. and C.Z.; Funding acquisition, Y.L. and C.Z. All authors have read and agreed to the published version of the manuscript.

Funding: D.B. was supported in part by FAMU Title III funding. This work is partially supported by the National Science Foundation (CBET-1917618). Research reported in this publication was also partially supported by the National Institutes of Health (USA) under Award Number R01NS125016.

Acknowledgments: Figures 1–4 were created with BioRender.com. The content is solely the responsibility of the authors and does not necessarily represent the official views of the National Institutes of Health. Support is also appreciated from R16 grant from NIH (1 R16GM149462-01).

Conflicts of Interest: The authors declare no conflicts of interest.

Abbreviations

AC	Alternating current
hASC	Human adipose derived MSC
AKT	Protein kinase B
ATP	Adenosine triphosphate
Aβ	Alpha beta
Aδ	Alpha delta
BBB	Blood–brain barrier
BDNF	Brain-derived neurotrophic factor
b-FGF	Fibroblast growth factor
hBM-MSC	Human bone marrow derived MSC
Ca^{2+}	Calcium
CD44	Cluster of differentiation 44
CHMP4C	Chromatin modified protein 4C
CIPN	Chemotherapy-induced peripheral neuropathy
CNS	Central nervous system
CT	Computerized tomography
DC	Direct current
DHT	Dihydrotestosterone
DPN	Diabetic peripheral neuropathy
DSN	Distal symmetric neuropathy
ECM	Extracellular matrix
ER	Endoplasmic reticulum
ESCs	Embryonic stem cells
ESCRT	Endosomal sorting complex required for transport
EVs	Extracellular vesicles
FasL	Fas ligand
FBS	Fetal bovine serum
FDA	U.S. Food and Drug Administration
FK506	Tacrolimus
GABA	Gamma-aminobutyric acid
GAP-43	Growth-associated protein 43
GDF3	Growth and differentiation factor 3
GDNF	Glial cell-derived neurotrophic factor
GFAP	Glial fibrillary acidic protein
GluN1	Glycine-binding subunits
GM	Gangliosides
GPCR	G protein-coupled receptor
GPI	Glycosylphosphatidylinositol
GTPase	Guanosine triphosphate
HA	Hyaluronic acid
hASC	Human ASC
hBM-MSC	Human BM-MSC
Hrs	Hepatocyte growth factor-regulated tyrosine kinase substrate
HF	High frequency
HLA-DR	Human leukocyte antigen
HPL	Human platelet lysate
Hsc	Heat shock cognate
Hsp	Heat shock protein
hUC	Human umbilical cord
Hz	Hertz
IGF-1	Insulin-like growth factor 1
IL	Interleukin
NAD^+	Oxidative nicotinamide adenine dinucleotide
NADH	Reductive nicotinamide adenine dinucleotide
NAM	Nicotinamide
NEFL	Neurofilament light polypeptide
NEFM	Neurofilament medium polypeptide
NESTIN	Neuroepithelial stem cell protein
NK-kB	Nuclear factor-kappa beta
NGF	Nerve growth factor
nm	Nanometers
NMDA	N-methyl-D-aspartate
NMN	Nicotinamide mononucleotide
NMNAT	Nicotinamide mononucleotide adenylyltransferase
NP	Neuropathic pain
NR	Nicotinamide riboside
nSMase2	Neutral sphingomyelinase 2
NT-3	Neurotrophin-3
NURR1	Dopaminergic neuron marker
OCT-3/4	Octamer transcription factor 3 and 4
P0	Protein zero
PI3K	Phosphatidylinositol 3-kinase
PAX6	Paired box 6
PC	Phosphatidylcholine
PCL	Polycaprolactone
PE	Phosphatidylethanolamine
PGA	Poly-glycolic acid
PI	Phosphatidylinositol
PLA	Polylactic acid
PLGA	Poly-dl-lactic-co-glycolic acid
PMP22	Peripheral myelin protein-22
PN	Peripheral neuropathy
PNS	Peripheral nervous system
PS	Phosphatidylserine
PSA	Pressure sensitive adhesive tape
PVA	Polyvinyl acetate
qPCR	Quantitative polymerase chain reaction
RA	Retinoic acid
Rab GTPases	Ras-associated binding guanosine triphosphates
REX1	Reduced expression 1
ROS	Reactive oxygen species
rSCs	Repair Schwann cells
RT-PCR	Reverse transcription polymerase chain reaction
S100B	Calcium-binding protein B
SARM1	Sterile alpha and toll/interleukin-1 receptor motif-containing 1
SC	Schwann cell
SHH	Sonic Hedgehog protein
SMPD2	Sphingomyelin phosphodiesterase 2
SOX2	Sex determining region Y-box 2
STAM1	Signal transducing adaptor molecule
STZ	Streptozotocin
TENS	Transcutaneous electrical nerve stimulation

ILV	Intraluminal vesicles	TfR	Transferrin receptor
iPSCs	Induced pluripotent stem cells	TGF-β1	Transforming growth factor-beta 1
JNK	C-Jun N-terminal kinase	TH	Tyrosine hydroxylase
K^+	Potassium	TLR4	Toll-like receptor member 4
KLF4	Kruppel-like factor 4	TNF-α	Tumor necrosis factor
kPa	Kilopascal		
LAMP1	Lysosomal-associated membrane protein 1	Trp	Tryptophan
LF	Low frequency	TRAIL	TNF related apoptosis-inducing ligand
mA	Milliamps	TSG	Tumor susceptibility gene
MAL	Myelin and lymphocyte protein	Tuj1	Class III beta-tubulin
MAPK	Mitogen-activated protein kinase	hUM-MSC	Human umbilical cord derived MSC
MEK/ERK	Kinase extracellular signaling regulation pathway	VEGF	Vascular endothelial growth factor
MHC	Major histocompatibility complex	VPS	Vascular protein sorting-associated protein
miRNA	MicroRNA	VTA1	Vacuolar protein sorting-associated protein
MITF	Melanocyte including transcription factor	WD	Wallerian degeneration
MM	Multiple myeloma	WHO	World Health Organization
MRI	Magnetic resonance imaging	Wlds	Wallerian degeneration slow
mRNA	Messenger RNA	μs	Microseconds
MSCs	Mesenchymal stromal cells	μm	Micrometers
MVB	Multivesicular bodies	2D	Two-dimensional
NA	Nicotinic acid	3D	Three-dimensional
Na^+	Sodium		

References

1. Jakob, M.O.; Kofoed-Branzk, M.; Deshpande, D.; Murugan, S.; Klose, C.S.N. An Integrated View on Neuronal Subsets in the Peripheral Nervous System and Their Role in Immunoregulation. *Front. Immunol.* **2021**, *12*, 679055. [CrossRef]
2. Hussain, G.; Wang, J.; Rasul, A.; Anwar, H.; Qasim, M.; Zafar, S.; Aziz, N.; Razzaq, A.; Hussain, R.; de Aguilar, J.-L.G.; et al. Current Status of Therapeutic Approaches against Peripheral Nerve Injuries: A Detailed Story from Injury to Recovery. *Int. J. Biol. Sci.* **2020**, *16*, 116–134. [CrossRef]
3. Butler, S.J.; Bronner, M.E. From classical to current: Analyzing peripheral nervous system and spinal cord lineage and fate. *Dev. Biol.* **2015**, *398*, 135–146. [CrossRef]
4. Jortner, B.S. Preparation and Analysis of the Peripheral Nervous System. *Toxicol. Pathol.* **2010**, *39*, 66–72. [CrossRef] [PubMed]
5. He, C.-W.; Liao, C.-P.; Pan, C.-L. Wnt signalling in the development of axon, dendrites and synapses. *Open Biol.* **2018**, *8*, 180116. [CrossRef] [PubMed]
6. Fallon, M.; Tadi, P. Histology, Schwann Cells. In *BTI—StatPearls*; StatPearls Publishing: Treasure Island, FL, USA, 2022.
7. Houschyar, K.S.; Momeni, A.; Pyles, M.N.; Cha, J.Y.; Maan, Z.N.; Duscher, D.; Jew, O.S.; Siemers, F.; van Schoonhoven, J. The Role of Current Techniques and Concepts in Peripheral Nerve Repair. *Plast. Surg. Int.* **2016**, *2016*, 4175293. [CrossRef] [PubMed]
8. Catala, M.; Kubis, N. Chapter 3—Gross anatomy and development of the peripheral nervous system. In *Handbook of Clinical Neurology*; Said, G., Krarup, C., Eds.; Elsevier: Amsterdam, The Netherlands, 2013; pp. 29–41.
9. Gordan, R.; Gwathmey, J.K.; Xie, L.-H. Autonomic and endocrine control of cardiovascular function. *World J. Cardiol.* **2015**, *7*, 204–214. [CrossRef]
10. Lehmann, H.C.; Wunderlich, G.; Fink, G.R.; Sommer, C. Diagnosis of peripheral neuropathy. *Neurol. Res. Pract.* **2020**, *2*, 20. [CrossRef]
11. Hanewinckel, R.; Drenthen, J.; van Oijen, M.; Hofman, A.; van Doorn, P.A.; Ikram, M.A. Prevalence of polyneuropathy in the general middle-aged and elderly population. *Neurology* **2016**, *87*, 1892–1898. [CrossRef]
12. Hanewinckel, R.; van Oijen, M.; Ikram, M.A.; van Doorn, P.A. The epidemiology and risk factors of chronic polyneuropathy. *Eur. J. Epidemiol.* **2016**, *31*, 5–20. [CrossRef]
13. Kneis, S.; Wehrle, A.; Müller, J.; Maurer, C.; Ihorst, G.; Gollhofer, A.; Bertz, H. It's never too late—Balance and endurance training improves functional performance, quality of life, and alleviates neuropathic symptoms in cancer survivors suffering from chemotherapy-induced peripheral neuropathy: Results of a randomized controlled trial. *BMC Cancer* **2019**, *19*, 414. [CrossRef]
14. Zakin, E.; Abrams, R.; Simpson, D.M. Diabetic Neuropathy. *Semin. Neurol.* **2019**, *39*, 560–569. [CrossRef]
15. Nesbit, S.A.; Sharma, R.; Waldfogel, J.M.; Zhang, A.; Bennett, W.L.; Yeh, H.-C.; Chelladurai, Y.; Feldman, D.; Robinson, K.A.; Dy, S.M. Non-pharmacologic treatments for symptoms of diabetic peripheral neuropathy: A systematic review. *Curr. Med Res. Opin.* **2019**, *35*, 15–25. [CrossRef]
16. Khdour, M.R. Treatment of diabetic peripheral neuropathy: A review. *J. Pharm. Pharmacol.* **2020**, *72*, 863–872. [CrossRef]
17. Reeves, N.D.; Orlando, G.; Brown, S.J. Sensory-Motor Mechanisms Increasing Falls Risk in Diabetic Peripheral Neuropathy. *Medicina* **2021**, *57*, 457. [CrossRef]
18. Staszel, J.P.; Miknevich, M. Not Always as It Seems: A Case of Ascending Paralysis. *Am. J. Phys. Med. Rehabil.* **2020**, *99*, e32–e34. [CrossRef]
19. Gordon, T. Peripheral Nerve Regeneration and Muscle Reinnervation. *Int. J. Mol. Sci.* **2020**, *21*, 8652. [CrossRef]
20. Stassart, R.M.; Woodhoo, A. Axo-glial interaction in the injured PNS. *Dev. Neurobiol.* **2021**, *81*, 490–506. [CrossRef] [PubMed]

21. Gao, P.; Jiang, D.; Liu, W.; Li, H.; Li, Z. Urine-derived Stem Cells, A New Source of Seed Cells for Tissue Engineering. *Curr. Stem Cell Res. Ther.* **2016**, *11*, 547–553. [CrossRef] [PubMed]
22. Huang, Z.; Powell, R.; Phillips, J.B.; Haastert-Talini, K. Perspective on Schwann Cells Derived from Induced Pluripotent Stem Cells in Peripheral Nerve Tissue Engineering. *Cells* **2020**, *9*, 2497. [CrossRef] [PubMed]
23. Freeman, R.; Gewandter, J.S.; Faber, C.G.; Gibbons, C.; Haroutounian, S.; Lauria, G.; Levine, T.; Malik, R.A.; Singleton, J.R.; Smith, A.G.; et al. Idiopathic distal sensory polyneuropathy. *Neurology* **2020**, *95*, 1005–1014. [CrossRef] [PubMed]
24. Said, G. Diabetic neuropathy—A review. *Nat. Clin. Pract. Neurol.* **2007**, *3*, 331–340. [CrossRef] [PubMed]
25. Vinik, A.I.; Maser, R.E.; Mitchell, B.D.; Freeman, R. Diabetic Autonomic Neuropathy. *Diabetes Care* **2003**, *26*, 1553–1579. [CrossRef] [PubMed]
26. Nolan, C.J.; Damm, P.; Prentki, M. Type 2 diabetes across generations: From pathophysiology to prevention and management. *Lancet* **2011**, *378*, 169–181. [CrossRef] [PubMed]
27. Mizukami, H.; Osonoi, S. Pathogenesis and Molecular Treatment Strategies of Diabetic Neuropathy Collateral Glucose-Utilizing Pathways in Diabetic Polyneuropathy. *Int. J. Mol. Sci.* **2020**, *22*, 94. [CrossRef] [PubMed]
28. Raza, C.; Riaz, H.A.; Anjum, R.; Shakeel, N.U.A. Repair strategies for injured peripheral nerve: Review. *Life Sci.* **2020**, *243*, 117308. [CrossRef] [PubMed]
29. Hogg, P.J.; McLachlan, E.M. Blood vessels and nerves: Together or not? *Lancet* **2002**, *360*, 1714. [CrossRef] [PubMed]
30. Wu, J.; Jin, Z.; Zheng, H.; Yan, L.-J. Sources and implications of NADH/NAD(+) redox imbalance in diabetes and its complications. *Diabetes Metab. Syndr. Obes.* **2016**, *9*, 145–153.
31. Casem, M.L. Chapter 11—Cell Metabolism. In *Case Studies in Cell Biology*; Casem, M.L., Ed.; Academic Press: Boston, MA, USA, 2016; pp. 263–281.
32. Bouché, C.; Serdy, S.; Kahn, C.R.; Goldfine, A.B. The Cellular Fate of Glucose and Its Relevance in Type 2 Diabetes. *Endocr. Rev.* **2004**, *25*, 807–830. [CrossRef]
33. Kopp, W.A.-O. How Western Diet and Lifestyle Drive The Pandemic of Obesity and Civilization Diseases. *Diabetes Metab. Syndr. Obes. Targets Ther.* **2019**, *12*, 2221–2236. [CrossRef]
34. Huang, T.-J.; Price, S.A.; Chilton, L.; Calcutt, N.A.; Tomlinson, D.R.; Verkhratsky, A.; Fernyhough, P. Insulin Prevents Depolarization of the Mitochondrial Inner Membrane in Sensory Neurons of Type 1 Diabetic Rats in the Presence of Sustained Hyperglycemia. *Diabetes* **2003**, *52*, 2129–2136. [CrossRef] [PubMed]
35. Russell, J.W.; Golovoy, D.; Vincent, A.M.; Mahendru, P.; Olzmann, J.A.; Mentzer, A.; Feldman, E.L. High glucose-induced oxidative stress and mitochondrial dysfunction in neurons. *FASEB J.* **2002**, *16*, 1738–1748. [CrossRef]
36. Samakidou, G.; Eleftheriadou, I.; Tentolouris, A.; Papanas, N.; Tentolouris, N. Rare diabetic neuropathies: It is not only distal symmetrical polyneuropathy. *Diabetes Res. Clin. Pract.* **2021**, *177*, 108932. [CrossRef] [PubMed]
37. Yagihashi, S.; Mizukami, H.; Sugimoto, K. Mechanism of diabetic neuropathy: Where are we now and where to go? *J. Diabetes Investig.* **2011**, *2*, 18–32. [CrossRef] [PubMed]
38. Burgess, J.; Frank, B.; Marshall, A.; Khalil, R.S.; Ponirakis, G.; Petropoulos, I.N.; Cuthbertson, D.J.; Malik, R.A.; Alam, U. Early Detection of Diabetic Peripheral Neuropathy: A Focus on Small Nerve Fibres. *Diagnostics* **2021**, *11*, 165. [CrossRef] [PubMed]
39. Mandeville, R.; Wali, A.; Park, C.; Groessl, E.; Walker, F.O.; Cartwright, M.S. Cost-effectiveness of neuromuscular ultrasound in focal neuropathies. *Neurology* **2019**, *92*, e2674–e2678. [CrossRef]
40. Bansal, V.; Kalita, J.; Misra, U.K. Diabetic neuropathy. *Postgrad. Med. J.* **2006**, *82*, 95. [CrossRef]
41. Sharma, D.; Jaggi, A.S.; Bali, A. Clinical evidence and mechanisms of growth factors in idiopathic and diabetes-induced carpal tunnel syndrome. *Eur. J. Pharmacol.* **2018**, *837*, 156–163. [CrossRef]
42. Said, G. Focal and multifocal diabetic neuropathies. *Arq. De Neuro-Psiquiatr.* **2007**, *65*, 1272–1278. [CrossRef]
43. Watson, J.C.; Dyck, P.J.B. Peripheral Neuropathy: A Practical Approach to Diagnosis and Symptom Management. *Mayo Clin. Proc.* **2015**, *90*, 940–951. [CrossRef]
44. Singh, J.; Aslam, A.; Rajbhandari, S. Diagnosis and Treatment of a Typical Painful Neuropathy Due to "Insulin Neuritis" in Patients with Diabetes. *Open Access J. Neurol. Neurosurg.* **2018**, *9*, 555759. [CrossRef]
45. Kim, S.H.; Baek, C.-O.; Lee, K.A.; Jin, H.Y.; Baek, H.S.; Park, T.S. Neuropathic truncal pain in patients with type 2 diabetes mellitus relieved by topical cream and nerve block. *Korean J. Intern. Med.* **2014**, *29*, 120–122. [CrossRef] [PubMed]
46. Hameed, S.; Cascella, M. Multifocal Motor Neuropathy. In *BTI—StatPearls*; StatPearls Publishing: Treasure Island, FL, USA, 2022.
47. Spallone, V.A.-O.X. Update on the Impact, Diagnosis and Management of Cardiovascular Autonomic Neuropathy in Diabetes: What Is Defined, What Is New, and What Is Unmet. *Diabetes Metab. J.* **2019**, *43*, 3–30. [CrossRef] [PubMed]
48. Spallone, V.; Ziegler, D.; Freeman, R.; Bernardi, L.; Frontoni, S.; Pop-Busui, R.; Stevens, M.; Kempler, P.; Hilsted, J.; Tesfaye, S.; et al. Cardiovascular autonomic neuropathy in diabetes: Clinical impact, assessment, diagnosis, and management. *Diabetes/Metab. Res. Rev.* **2011**, *27*, 639–653. [CrossRef] [PubMed]
49. Ferris, J.K.; Inglis, J.T.; Madden, K.M.; Boyd, L.A. Brain and Body: A Review of Central Nervous System Contributions to Movement Impairments in Diabetes. *Diabetes* **2019**, *69*, 3–11. [CrossRef]
50. Azhary, H.; Farooq, M.U.; Bhanushali, M.; Majid, A.; Kassab, M.Y. Peripheral neuropathy: Differential diagnosis and management. *Am. Fam. Physician* **2010**, *81*, 887–892.
51. Zis, P.; Sarrigiannis, P.G.; Rao, D.G.; Hadjivassiliou, M. Gluten neuropathy: Prevalence of neuropathic pain and the role of gluten-free diet. *J. Neurol.* **2018**, *265*, 2231–2236. [CrossRef]

52. Robinson, D.J.; Coons, M.; Haensel, H.; Vallis, M.; Yale, J.F. Diabetes and Mental Health. *Can. J. Diabetes* **2018**, *42*, S130–S141. [CrossRef]
53. Garrett, C.; Doherty, A. Diabetes and mental health. *Clin. Med.* **2014**, *14*, 669. [CrossRef]
54. Kiyani, M.; Yang, Z.; Charalambous, L.T.; Adil, S.M.; Lee, H.J.; Yang, S.; Pagadala, P.; Parente, B.; Spratt, S.E.; Lad, S.P. Painful diabetic peripheral neuropathy: Health care costs and complications from 2010 to 2015. *Neurol. Clin. Pract.* **2020**, *10*, 47–57. [CrossRef]
55. O'Connor, A.B. Neuropathic Pain. *Pharm. Econ.* **2009**, *27*, 95–112. [CrossRef]
56. Hex, N.; Bartlett, C.; Wright, D.; Taylor, M.; Varley, D. Estimating the current and future costs of Type 1 and Type 2 diabetes in the UK, including direct health costs and indirect societal and productivity costs. *Diabet. Med.* **2012**, *29*, 855–862. [CrossRef]
57. Chapman, D.; Foxcroft, R.; Dale-Harris, L.; Ronte, H.; Bidgoli, F.; Bellary, S. Insights for Care: The Healthcare Utilisation and Cost Impact of Managing Type 2 Diabetes-Associated Microvascular Complications. *Diabetes Ther.* **2019**, *10*, 575–585. [CrossRef]
58. Sadosky, A.; Schaefer, C.; Mann, R.; Bergstrom, F.; Baik, R.; Parsons, B.; Nalamachu, S.; Nieshoff, E.; Stacey, B.R.; Anschel, A.; et al. Burden of illness associated with painful diabetic peripheral neuropathy among adults seeking treatment in the US: Results from a retrospective chart review and cross-sectional survey. *Diabetes Metab. Syndr. Obes.* **2013**, *6*, 79–92. [CrossRef]
59. Seretny, M.; Currie, G.L.; Sena, E.S.; Ramnarine, S.; Grant, R.; MacLeod, M.R.; Colvin, L.A.; Fallon, M. Incidence, prevalence, and predictors of chemotherapy-induced peripheral neuropathy: A systematic review and meta-analysis. *Pain* **2014**, *155*, 2461–2470. [CrossRef] [PubMed]
60. Selvy, M.; Kerckhove, N.; Pereira, B.; Barreau, F.; Nguyen, D.; Busserolles, J.; Giraudet, F.; Cabrespine, A.; Chaleteix, C.; Soubrier, M.; et al. Prevalence of Chemotherapy-Induced Peripheral Neuropathy in Multiple Myeloma Patients and its Impact on Quality of Life: A Single Center Cross-Sectional Study. *Front. Pharmacol.* **2021**, *12*, 637593. [CrossRef] [PubMed]
61. Pike, C.T.; Birnbaum, H.G.; Muehlenbein, C.E.; Pohl, G.M.; Natale, R.B. Healthcare costs and workloss burden of patients with chemotherapy-associated peripheral neuropathy in breast, ovarian, head and neck, and nonsmall cell lung cancer. *Chemother. Res. Pract.* **2012**, *2012*, 913848. [CrossRef] [PubMed]
62. Schirrmacher, V. From chemotherapy to biological therapy: A review of novel concepts to reduce the side effects of systemic cancer treatment (Review). *Int. J. Oncol.* **2019**, *54*, 407–419. [CrossRef] [PubMed]
63. Pucci, C.; Martinelli, C.; Ciofani, G. Innovative approaches for cancer treatment: Current perspectives and new challenges. *Ecancermedicalscience* **2019**, *13*, 961. [CrossRef] [PubMed]
64. Staff, N.P.; Grisold, A.; Grisold, W.; Windebank, A.J. Chemotherapy-induced peripheral neuropathy: A current review. *Ann. Neurol.* **2017**, *81*, 772–781. [CrossRef] [PubMed]
65. Almohammadi, A.; Alqarni, A.; Alraddadi, R.; Alzahrani, F. Assessment of Patients' Knowledge in Managing Side Effects of Chemotherapy: Case of King Abdul-Aziz University Hospital. *J. Cancer Educ.* **2019**, *35*, 334–338. [CrossRef]
66. Oun, R.; Moussa, Y.E.; Wheate, N.J. The side effects of platinum-based chemotherapy drugs: A review for chemists. *Dalton Trans.* **2018**, *47*, 6645–6653. [CrossRef]
67. Behranvand, N.; Nasri, F.; Emameh, R.Z.; Khani, P.; Hosseini, A.; Garssen, J.; Falak, R. Chemotherapy: A double-edged sword in cancer treatment. *Cancer Immunol. Immunother.* **2022**, *71*, 507–526. [CrossRef]
68. Chortkoff, B.; Stenehjem, D. 38—Chemotherapy, Immunosuppression, and Anesthesia. In *Pharmacology and Physiology for Anesthesia*, 2nd ed.; Hemmings, H.C., Egan, T.D., Eds.; Elsevier: Philadelphia, PA, USA, 2019; pp. 753–768.
69. Fallon, M.T. Neuropathic pain in cancer. *Br. J. Anaesth.* **2013**, *111*, 105–111. [CrossRef] [PubMed]
70. Gupta, K.; Walton, R.; Kataria, S.P. Chemotherapy-Induced Nausea and Vomiting: Pathogenesis, Recommendations, and New Trends. *Cancer Treat. Res. Commun.* **2021**, *26*, 100278. [CrossRef] [PubMed]
71. Nurgalieva, Z.; Liu, C.-C.; Du, X.L. Chemotherapy use and risk of bone marrow suppression in a large population-based cohort of older women with breast and ovarian cancer. *Med. Oncol.* **2011**, *28*, 716–725. [CrossRef] [PubMed]
72. Nicolini, G.; Monfrini, M.; Scuteri, A. Axonal Transport Impairment in Chemotherapy-Induced Peripheral Neuropathy. *Toxics* **2015**, *3*, 322–341. [CrossRef] [PubMed]
73. Parker, A.L.; Kavallaris, M.; McCarroll, J.A. Microtubules and Their Role in Cellular Stress in Cancer. *Front. Oncol.* **2014**, *4*, 153. [CrossRef] [PubMed]
74. De Iuliis, F.; Taglieri, L.; Salerno, G.; Lanza, R.; Scarpa, S. Taxane induced neuropathy in patients affected by breast cancer: Literature review. *Crit. Rev. Oncol.* **2015**, *96*, 34–45. [CrossRef]
75. Rizo, J. Mechanism of neurotransmitter release coming into focus. *Protein Sci.* **2018**, *27*, 1364–1391. [CrossRef]
76. Costanzi, S.; Machado, J.-H.; Mitchell, M. Nerve Agents: What They Are, How They Work, How to Counter Them. *ACS Chem. Neurosci.* **2018**, *9*, 873–885. [CrossRef]
77. Südhof, T.C. Calcium Control of Neurotransmitter Release. *Cold Spring Harb. Perspect. Biol.* **2012**, *4*, a011353. [CrossRef]
78. Lipscombe, D.; Toro, C.P. Chapter 13—Biophysics of Voltage-Gated Ion Channels. In *From Molecules to Networks*, 3rd ed.; Byrne, J.H., Heidelberger, R., Waxham, M.N., Eds.; Academic Press: Boston, MA, USA, 2014; pp. 377–407.
79. Hyman, S.E. Neurotransmitters. *Curr. Biol.* **2005**, *15*, R154–R158. [CrossRef]
80. Lines, J.; Martin, E.D.; Kofuji, P.; Aguilar, J.; Araque, A. Astrocytes modulate sensory-evoked neuronal network activity. *Nat. Commun.* **2020**, *11*, 3689. [CrossRef]
81. Hammond, E.A.; Pitz, M.; Shay, B. Neuropathic Pain in Taxane-Induced Peripheral Neuropathy: Evidence for Exercise in Treatment. *Neurorehabilit. Neural Repair* **2019**, *33*, 792–799. [CrossRef] [PubMed]

82. Malacrida, A.; Meregalli, C.; Rodriguez-Menendez, V.; Nicolini, G. Chemotherapy-Induced Peripheral Neuropathy and Changes in Cytoskeleton. *Int. J. Mol. Sci.* **2019**, *20*, 2287. [CrossRef] [PubMed]
83. Hagiwara, H.; Sunada, Y. Mechanism of taxane neurotoxicity. *Breast Cancer* **2004**, *11*, 82–85. [CrossRef] [PubMed]
84. Cuadrado, A.; Nebreda, A.R. Mechanisms and functions of p38 MAPK signalling. *Biochem. J.* **2010**, *429*, 403–417. [CrossRef] [PubMed]
85. Sui, X.; Kong, N.; Ye, L.; Han, W.; Zhou, J.; Zhang, Q.; He, C.; Pan, H. p38 and JNK MAPK pathways control the balance of apoptosis and autophagy in response to chemotherapeutic agents. *Cancer Lett.* **2014**, *344*, 174–179. [CrossRef]
86. Chen, J.; Ye, C.; Wan, C.; Li, G.; Peng, L.; Peng, Y.; Fang, R. The Roles of c-Jun N-Terminal Kinase (JNK) in Infectious Diseases. *Int. J. Mol. Sci.* **2021**, *22*, 9640. [CrossRef] [PubMed]
87. Zhang, W.; Liu, H.T. MAPK signal pathways in the regulation of cell proliferation in mammalian cells. *Cell Res.* **2002**, *12*, 9–18. [CrossRef]
88. Bubici, C.; Papa, S. JNK signalling in cancer: In need of new, smarter therapeutic targets. *Br. J. Pharmacol.* **2013**, *171*, 24–37. [CrossRef] [PubMed]
89. Fukuda, Y.; Li, Y.; Segal, R.A. A Mechanistic Understanding of Axon Degeneration in Chemotherapy-Induced Peripheral Neuropathy. *Front. Neurosci.* **2017**, *11*, 481. [CrossRef]
90. Tian, N.; Hanson, K.A.; Canty, A.J.; Vickers, J.C.; King, A.E. Microtubule-dependent processes precede pathological calcium influx in excitotoxin-induced axon degeneration. *J. Neurochem.* **2020**, *152*, 542–555. [CrossRef]
91. Feinberg, J.H.; Nadler, S.F.; Krivickas, L.S. Peripheral nerve injuries in the athlete. *Sports Med.* **1997**, *24*, 385–408. [CrossRef] [PubMed]
92. Tosti, R.; Rossy, W.; Sanchez, A.; Lee, S.G. Burners, Stingers, and Other Brachial Plexus Injuries in the Contact Athlete. *Oper. Tech. Sports Med.* **2016**, *24*, 273–277. [CrossRef]
93. Campbell, W.W. Evaluation and management of peripheral nerve injury. *Clin. Neurophysiol.* **2008**, *119*, 1951–1965. [CrossRef] [PubMed]
94. Wang, M.L.; Rivlin, M.; Graham, J.G.; Beredjiklian, P.K. Peripheral nerve injury, scarring, and recovery. *Connect. Tissue Res.* **2019**, *60*, 3–9. [CrossRef]
95. Barral, J.-P.; Croibier, A. Chapter 1—Some preliminary thoughts. In *Manual Therapy for the Cranial Nerves*; Barral, J.-P., Croibier, A., Eds.; Churchill Livingstone: Edinburgh, UK, 2009; pp. 1–5.
96. Liu, Q.; Wang, X.; Yi, S. Pathophysiological Changes of Physical Barriers of Peripheral Nerves After Injury. *Front. Neurosci.* **2018**, *12*, 597. [CrossRef]
97. Reina, M.A.; Boezaart, A.P.; Tubbs, R.S.; Zasimovich, Y.; Fernández-Domínguez, M.; Fernández, P.; Sala-Blanch, X. Another (Internal) Epineurium: Beyond the Anatomical Barriers of Nerves. *Clin. Anat.* **2020**, *33*, 199–206. [CrossRef]
98. Grinsell, D.; Keating, C.P. Peripheral Nerve Reconstruction after Injury: A Review of Clinical and Experimental Therapies. *BioMed Res. Int.* **2014**, *2014*, 698256. [CrossRef]
99. Chaney, B.; Nadi, M. *Axonotmesis*; StatPearls Publishing: Treasure Island, FL, USA, 2022.
100. Stadelmann, C.; Timmler, S.; Barrantes-Freer, A.; Simons, M. Myelin in the Central Nervous System: Structure, Function, and Pathology. *Physiol. Rev.* **2019**, *99*, 1381–1431. [CrossRef]
101. Rasband, M.N.; Peles, E. Mechanisms of node of Ranvier assembly. *Nat. Rev. Neurosci.* **2021**, *22*, 7–20. [CrossRef]
102. Arancibia-Carcamo, I.L.; Attwell, D. The node of Ranvier in CNS pathology. *Acta Neuropathol.* **2014**, *128*, 161–175. [CrossRef] [PubMed]
103. Kaji, R. Physiology of conduction block in multifocal motor neuropathy and other demyelinating neuropathies. *Muscle Nerve* **2003**, *27*, 285–296. [CrossRef] [PubMed]
104. Debanne, D.; Campanac, E.; Bialowas, A.; Carlier, E.; Alcaraz, G. Axon Physiology. *Physiol. Rev.* **2011**, *91*, 555–602. [CrossRef]
105. Sunderland, S.S. The anatomy and physiology of nerve injury. *Muscle Nerve* **1990**, *13*, 771–784. [CrossRef] [PubMed]
106. Seddon, H.J. THREE TYPES OF NERVE INJURY. *Brain* **1943**, *66*, 237–288. [CrossRef]
107. Seddon, H.J. A Classification of Nerve Injuries. *Br. Med. J.* **1942**, *2*, 237–239. [CrossRef] [PubMed]
108. Vijayavenkataraman, S. Nerve guide conduits for peripheral nerve injury repair: A review on design, materials and fabrication methods. *Acta Biomater.* **2020**, *106*, 54–69. [CrossRef]
109. Andrei, M.; Ioana, M.R.; Mircea, E.D. Underlying histopathology of peripheral nerve injury and the classical nerve repair techniques. *Romanian Neurosurg.* **2019**, *33*, 17–22. [CrossRef]
110. Lee, D.-H. Clinical Efficacy of Electroneurography in Acute Facial Paralysis. *J. Audiol. Otol.* **2016**, *20*, 8–12. [CrossRef]
111. Gorgey, A.S.; Chandrasekaran, S.; Davis, J.; Bersch, I.; Goldberg, G. Electrical stimulation and denervated muscles after spinal cord injury. *Neural Regen. Res.* **2020**, *15*, 1397–1407. [CrossRef]
112. Gaudet, A.D.; Popovich, P.G.; Ramer, M.S. Wallerian degeneration: Gaining perspective on inflammatory events after peripheral nerve injury. *J. Neuroinflamm.* **2011**, *8*, 110. [CrossRef]
113. Bhandari, P.S. Management of peripheral nerve injury. *J. Clin. Orthop. Trauma* **2019**, *10*, 862–866. [CrossRef]
114. Burnett, M.G.; Zager, E.L. Pathophysiology of peripheral nerve injury: A brief review. *Neurosurg. Focus* **2004**, *16*, E1. [CrossRef] [PubMed]
115. Zhang, K.; Jiang, M.; Fang, Y. The Drama of Wallerian Degeneration: The Cast, Crew, and Script. *Annu. Rev. Genet.* **2021**, *55*, 93–113. [CrossRef] [PubMed]

116. Siddiqui, N.; Straube, A. Intracellular cargo transport by kinesin-3 motors. *Biochemistry* **2017**, *82*, 803–815. [CrossRef] [PubMed]
117. Pillai, M.M.; Sathishkumar, G.; Houshyar, S.; Senthilkumar, R.; Quigley, A.F.; Shanthakumari, S.; Padhye, R.; Bhattacharyya, A. Nanocomposite-Coated Silk-Based Artificial Conduits: The Influence of Structures on Regeneration of the Peripheral Nerve. *ACS Appl. Bio Mater.* **2020**, *3*, 4454–4464. [CrossRef]
118. Garcin, C.; Straube, A. Microtubules in cell migration. *Essays Biochem.* **2019**, *63*, 509–520.
119. Bandyopadhyay, D.; Cyphersmith, A.; Zapata, J.A.; Kim, Y.J.; Payne, C.K. Lysosome Transport as a Function of Lysosome Diameter. *PLoS ONE* **2014**, *9*, e86847. [CrossRef]
120. Guedes-Dias, P.; Holzbaur, E.L.F. Axonal transport: Driving synaptic function. *Science* **2019**, *366*, eaaw9997. [CrossRef]
121. Peters, O.M.; Weiss, A.; Metterville, J.; Song, L.; Logan, R.; Smith, G.A.; Schwarzschild, M.A.; Mueller, C.; Brown, R.H.; Freeman, M. Genetic diversity of axon degenerative mechanisms in models of Parkinson's disease. *Neurobiol. Dis.* **2021**, *155*, 105368. [CrossRef]
122. Coleman, M.P.; Freeman, M.R. Wallerian Degeneration, WldS, and Nmnat. *Annu. Rev. Neurosci.* **2010**, *33*, 245–267. [CrossRef]
123. Freeman, M.R. Signaling mechanisms regulating Wallerian degeneration. *Curr. Opin. Neurobiol.* **2014**, *27*, 224–231. [CrossRef]
124. Liu, H.-W.; Smith, C.B.; Schmidt, M.S.; Cambronne, X.A.; Cohen, M.S.; Migaud, M.E.; Brenner, C.; Goodman, R.H. Pharmacological bypass of NAD+ salvage pathway protects neurons from chemotherapy-induced degeneration. *Proc. Natl. Acad. Sci. USA* **2018**, *115*, 10654–10659. [CrossRef] [PubMed]
125. Brazill, J.M.; Li, C.; Zhu, Y.; Zhai, R.G. NMNAT: It's an NAD^+ synthase... It's a chaperone... It's a neuroprotector. *Curr. Opin. Genet. Dev.* **2017**, *44*, 156–162. [CrossRef] [PubMed]
126. Covarrubias, A.J.; Perrone, R.; Grozio, A.; Verdin, E. NAD+ metabolism and its roles in cellular processes during ageing. *Nat. Rev. Mol. Cell Biol.* **2020**, *22*, 119–141. [CrossRef] [PubMed]
127. She, J.; Sheng, R.; Qin, Z.-H. Pharmacology and Potential Implications of Nicotinamide Adenine Dinucleotide Precursors. *Aging Dis.* **2021**, *12*, 1879–1897. [CrossRef] [PubMed]
128. Giroud-Gerbetant, J.; Joffraud, M.; Giner, M.P.; Cercillieux, A.; Bartova, S.; Makarov, M.V.; Zapata-Pérez, R.; Sánchez-García, J.L.; Houtkooper, R.H.; Migaud, M.E.; et al. A reduced form of nicotinamide riboside defines a new path for NAD+ biosynthesis and acts as an orally bioavailable NAD+ precursor. *Mol. Metab.* **2019**, *30*, 192–202. [CrossRef] [PubMed]
129. Williams, P.A.; Harder, J.M.; Cardozo, B.H.; Foxworth, N.E.; John, S.W.M. Nicotinamide treatment robustly protects from inherited mouse glaucoma. *Commun. Integr. Biol.* **2018**, *11*, e1356956. [CrossRef]
130. Kennedy, B.E.; Sharif, T.; Martell, E.; Dai, C.; Kim, Y.; Lee, P.W.; Gujar, S.A. NAD+ salvage pathway in cancer metabolism and therapy. *Pharmacol. Res.* **2016**, *114*, 274–283. [CrossRef]
131. Johnson, S.; Imai, S.I. NAD (+) biosynthesis, aging, and disease. *F1000Research* **2018**, *7*, 132. [CrossRef]
132. Bignon, Y.; Rinaldi, A.; Nadour, Z.; Poindessous, V.; Nemazanyy, I.; Lenoir, O.; Fohlen, B.; Weill-Raynal, P.; Hertig, A.; Karras, A.; et al. Cell stress response impairs de novo NAD+ biosynthesis in the kidney. *J. Clin. Investig.* **2022**, *7*, e153019. [CrossRef]
133. Sasaki, Y.; Nakagawa, T.; Mao, X.; DiAntonio, A.; Milbrandt, J. NMNAT1 inhibits axon degeneration via blockade of SARM1-mediated NAD+ depletion. *eLife* **2016**, *5*, e19749. [CrossRef] [PubMed]
134. Walker, L.J.; Summers, D.W.; Sasaki, Y.; Brace, E.; Milbrandt, J.; DiAntonio, A. MAPK signaling promotes axonal degeneration by speeding the turnover of the axonal maintenance factor NMNAT2. *eLife* **2017**, *6*, e22540. [CrossRef] [PubMed]
135. Rigby, M.J.; Gomez, T.M.; Puglielli, L. Glial Cell-Axonal Growth Cone Interactions in Neurodevelopment and Regeneration. *Front. Neurosci.* **2020**, *14*, 203. [CrossRef]
136. Ullah, R.; Yin, Q.; Snell, A.H.; Wan, L. RAF-MEK-ERK pathway in cancer evolution and treatment. *Semin. Cancer Biol.* **2022**, *85*, 123–154. [CrossRef] [PubMed]
137. Jessen, K.R.; Mirsky, R.; Lloyd, A.C. Schwann Cells: Development and Role in Nerve Repair. *Cold Spring Harb. Perspect. Biol.* **2015**, *7*, a020487. [CrossRef] [PubMed]
138. Rios, R.; Jablonka-Shariff, A.; Broberg, C.; Snyder-Warwick, A.K. Macrophage roles in peripheral nervous system injury and pathology: Allies in neuromuscular junction recovery. *Mol. Cell. Neurosci.* **2021**, *111*, 103590. [CrossRef]
139. Zhang, J.; Li, Y.; Duan, Z.; Kang, J.; Chen, K.; Li, G.; Weng, C.; Zhang, D.; Zhang, L.; Wang, J.; et al. The effects of the M2a macrophage-induced axonal regeneration of neurons by arginase 1. *Biosci. Rep.* **2020**, *40*, BSR20193031. [CrossRef] [PubMed]
140. Chen, P.; Piao, X.; Bonaldo, P. Role of macrophages in Wallerian degeneration and axonal regeneration after peripheral nerve injury. *Acta Neuropathol.* **2015**, *130*, 605–618. [CrossRef] [PubMed]
141. Hirata, K.; Kawabuchi, M. Myelin phagocytosis by macrophages and nonmacrophages during Wallerian degeneration. *Microsc. Res. Tech.* **2002**, *57*, 541–547. [CrossRef] [PubMed]
142. Cattin, A.-L.; Burden, J.J.; Van Emmenis, L.; Mackenzie, F.E.; Hoving, J.J.; Calavia, N.G.; Guo, Y.; McLaughlin, M.; Rosenberg, L.H.; Quereda, V.; et al. Macrophage-Induced Blood Vessels Guide Schwann Cell-Mediated Regeneration of Peripheral Nerves. *Cell* **2015**, *162*, 1127–1139. [CrossRef] [PubMed]
143. Lai, Y.; Wahyuningtyas, R.; Aui, S.; Chang, K. Autocrine VEGF signalling on M2 macrophages regulates PD-L1 expression for immunomodulation of T cells. *J. Cell. Mol. Med.* **2019**, *23*, 1257–1267. [CrossRef]
144. de Ruiter, G.C.; Spinner, R.J.; Verhaagen, J.; Malessy, M.J. Misdirection and guidance of regenerating axons after experimental nerve injury and repair. *J. Neurosurg.* **2014**, *120*, 493–501. [CrossRef]
145. Juel, V.C. Evaluation of Neuromuscular Junction Disorders in the Electromyography Laboratory. *Neurol. Clin.* **2012**, *30*, 621–639. [CrossRef]

146. Jimsheleishvili, S.; Marwaha, K.; Sherman, A.L. Physiology, Neuromuscular Transmission. In *BTI—StatPearls*; StatPearls Publishing: Treasure Island, FL, USA, 2021.
147. Sommer, C.; Cruccu, G. Topical Treatment of Peripheral Neuropathic Pain: Applying the Evidence. *J. Pain Symptom Manag.* **2016**, *53*, 614–629. [CrossRef]
148. Dreibati, B.; Lavet, C.; Pinti, A.; Poumarat, G. Influence of electrical stimulation frequency on skeletal muscle force and fatigue. *Ann. Phys. Rehabil. Med.* **2010**, *53*, 266–277. [CrossRef]
149. Gibson, W.; Wand, B.M.; O'Connell, N.E. Transcutaneous electrical nerve stimulation (TENS) for neuropathic pain in adults. *Cochrane Database Syst. Rev.* **2017**, *9*, CD011976. [PubMed]
150. Kulikova, N.; Khalilovich, A.-Z.M.; Konchugova, T.; Rachin, A.; Chkheidze, T.; Kulchitskaya, D.; Anatoliy, F.; Sanina, N.P.; Ivanova, E. Analgesic effects of high-frequency and low-frequency TENS currents in patients with distal neuropathy. *Eur. J. Transl. Myol.* **2022**, *32*, 10687. [CrossRef] [PubMed]
151. Al-Zamil, M.; Minenko, I.A.; Kulikova, N.G.; Alade, M.; Petrova, M.M.; Pronina, E.A.; Romanova, I.V.; Narodova, E.A.; Nasyrova, R.F.; Shnayder, N.A. Clinical Experience of High Frequency and Low Frequency TENS in Treatment of Diabetic Neuropathic Pain in Russia. *Healthcare* **2022**, *10*, 250. [CrossRef]
152. Baptista, A.F.; Gomes, J.R.; Oliveira, J.T.; Santos, S.M.; Vannier-Santos, M.A.; Martinez, A.M. High- and low-frequency transcutaneous electrical nerve stimulation delay sciatic nerve regeneration after crush lesion in the mouse. *J. Peripher. Nerv. Syst.* **2008**, *13*, 71–80. [CrossRef]
153. Melcangi, R.C.; Magnaghi, V.; Martini, L. Steroid metabolism and effects in central and peripheral glial cells. *J. Neurobiol.* **1999**, *40*, 471–483. [CrossRef]
154. Coronel, M.F.; Labombarda, F.; González, S.L. Neuroactive steroids, nociception and neuropathic pain: A flashback to go forward. *Steroids* **2016**, *110*, 77–87. [CrossRef]
155. Rupprecht, R. Neuroactive steroids: Mechanisms of action and neuropsychopharmacological properties. *Psychoneuroendocrinology* **2003**, *28*, 139–168. [CrossRef] [PubMed]
156. Pieretti, S.; Di Giannuario, A.; Di Giovannandrea, R.; Marzoli, F.; Piccaro, G.; Minosi, P.; Aloisi, A.M. Gender differences in pain and its relief. *Ann. Dell'istituto Super. Di Sanita* **2016**, *52*, 184–189.
157. Calabrese, D.; Giatti, S.; Romano, S.; Porretta-Serapiglia, C.; Bianchi, R.; Milanese, M.; Bonanno, G.; Caruso, D.; Viviani, B.; Gardoni, F.; et al. Diabetic neuropathic pain: A role for testosterone metabolites. *J. Endocrinol.* **2014**, *221*, 1–13. [CrossRef]
158. Piao, Y.; Gwon, D.H.; Kang, D.-W.; Hwang, T.W.; Shin, N.; Kwon, H.H.; Shin, H.J.; Yin, Y.; Kim, J.-J.; Hong, J.; et al. TLR4-mediated autophagic impairment contributes to neuropathic pain in chronic constriction injury mice. *Mol. Brain* **2018**, *11*, 11. [CrossRef]
159. Finnerup, N.B.; Sindrup, S.H.; Jensen, T.S. The evidence for pharmacological treatment of neuropathic pain. *Pain* **2010**, *150*, 573–581. [CrossRef]
160. Yang, K.; Wang, Y.; Li, Y.-W.; Chen, Y.-G.; Xing, N.; Lin, H.-B.; Zhou, P.; Yu, X.-P. Progress in the treatment of diabetic peripheral neuropathy. *Biomed. Pharmacother.* **2022**, *148*, 112717. [CrossRef] [PubMed]
161. Lim, E.Y.; Kim, Y.T. Food-Derived Natural Compounds for Pain Relief in Neuropathic Pain. *BioMed Res. Int.* **2016**, *2016*, 7917528. [CrossRef] [PubMed]
162. Keswani, S.C.; Chander, B.; Hasan, C.; Griffin, J.W.; McArthur, J.C.; Hoke, A. FK506 is neuroprotective in a model of antiretroviral toxic neuropathy. *Ann. Neurol.* **2003**, *53*, 57–64. [CrossRef] [PubMed]
163. Zuber, M.; Donnerer, J. Effect of FK506 on Neurotransmitter Content and Expression of GAP-43 in Neurotoxin-Lesioned Peripheral Sensory and Sympathetic Neurons. *Pharmacology* **2002**, *66*, 44–50. [CrossRef]
164. Su, Y.-C.; Shen, Y.-P.; Li, T.-Y.; Ho, T.-Y.; Chen, L.-C.; Wu, Y.-T. The Efficacy of Hyaluronic Acid for Carpal Tunnel Syndrome: A Randomized Double-Blind Clinical Trial. *Pain Med.* **2021**, *22*, 2676–2685. [CrossRef] [PubMed]
165. Jou, I.; Wu, T.; Hsu, C.; Yang, C.; Huang, J.; Tu, Y.; Lee, J.; Su, F.; Kuo, Y. High molecular weight form of hyaluronic acid reduces neuroinflammatory response in injured sciatic nerve via the intracellular domain of CD44. *J. Biomed. Mater. Res. Part B Appl. Biomater.* **2021**, *109*, 673–680. [CrossRef] [PubMed]
166. Julian, T.; Syeed, R.; Glascow, N.; Angelopoulou, E.; Zis, P. B12 as a Treatment for Peripheral Neuropathic Pain: A Systematic Review. *Nutrients* **2020**, *12*, 2221. [CrossRef]
167. Kehoe, S.; Zhang, X.F.; Boyd, D. FDA approved guidance conduits and wraps for peripheral nerve injury: A review of materials and efficacy. *Injury* **2012**, *43*, 553–572. [CrossRef]
168. Kang, N.-U.; Lee, S.-J.; Gwak, S.-J. Fabrication Techniques of Nerve Guidance Conduits for Nerve Regeneration. *Yonsei Med. J.* **2022**, *63*, 114–123. [CrossRef]
169. Costa, F.; Silva, R.; Boccaccini, A.R. 7—Fibrous protein-based biomaterials (silk, keratin, elastin, and resilin proteins) for tissue regeneration and repair. In *Peptides and Proteins As Biomaterials for Tissue Regeneration and Repair*; Barbosa, M.A., Martins, M.C.L., Eds.; Woodhead Publishing: Thorston, UK, 2018; pp. 175–204.
170. Nelson, D.W.; Gilbert, R.J. Extracellular Matrix-Mimetic Hydrogels for Treating Neural Tissue Injury: A Focus on Fibrin, Hyaluronic Acid, and Elastin-Like Polypeptide Hydrogels. *Adv. Healthc. Mater.* **2021**, *10*, 2101329. [CrossRef]
171. Chang, W.; Shah, M.B.; Zhou, G.; Walsh, K.; Rudraiah, S.; Kumbar, S.G.; Yu, X. Polymeric nanofibrous nerve conduits coupled with laminin for peripheral nerve regeneration. *Biomed. Mater.* **2020**, *15*, 035003. [CrossRef]

172. Neal, R.A.; Tholpady, S.S.; Foley, P.L.; Swami, N.; Ogle, R.C.; Botchwey, E.A. Alignment and composition of laminin-polycaprolactone nanofiber blends enhance peripheral nerve regeneration. *J. Biomed. Mater. Res. Part A* **2012**, *100A*, 406–423. [CrossRef] [PubMed]
173. Carvalho, C.R.; Chang, W.; Silva-Correia, J.; Reis, R.L.; Oliveira, J.M.; Kohn, J. Engineering Silk Fibroin-Based Nerve Conduit with Neurotrophic Factors for Proximal Protection after Peripheral Nerve Injury. *Adv. Health Mater.* **2021**, *10*, e2000753. [CrossRef] [PubMed]
174. Magaz, A.; Faroni, A.; Gough, J.E.; Reid, A.J.; Li, X.; Blaker, J.J. Bioactive Silk-Based Nerve Guidance Conduits for Augmenting Peripheral Nerve Repair. *Adv. Health Mater.* **2018**, *7*, e1800308. [CrossRef] [PubMed]
175. Mathew-Steiner, S.S.; Roy, S.; Sen, C.K. Collagen in Wound Healing. *Bioengineering* **2021**, *8*, 63. [CrossRef] [PubMed]
176. Sensharma, P.; Madhumathi, G.; Jayant, R.D.; Jaiswal, A.K. Biomaterials and cells for neural tissue engineering: Current choices. *Mater. Sci. Eng. C* **2017**, *77*, 1302–1315. [CrossRef]
177. Abatangelo, G.; Vindigni, V.; Avruscio, G.; Pandis, L.; Brun, P. Hyaluronic Acid: Redefining Its Role. *Cells* **2020**, *9*, 1743. [CrossRef]
178. Nune, M.; Bhat, M.; Nagarajan, A. Design of ECM Functionalized Polycaprolactone Aligned Nanofibers for Peripheral Nerve Tissue Engineering. *J. Med. Biol. Eng.* **2022**, *42*, 147–156. [CrossRef]
179. Soucy, J.; Sani, E.S.; Portillo-Lara, R.; Diaz, D.; Dias, F.; Weiss, A.S.; Koppes, A.; Koppes, R.A.; Annabi, N. Photocrosslinkable Gelatin/Tropoelastin Hydrogel Adhesives for Peripheral Nerve Repair. *Tissue Eng. Part A* **2018**, *24*, 1393–1405. [CrossRef]
180. Rebowe, R.; Rogers, A.; Yang, X.; Kundu, S.C.; Smith, T.L.; Li, Z. Nerve Repair with Nerve Conduits: Problems, Solutions, and Future Directions. *J. Hand Microsurg.* **2018**, *10*, 61–65. [CrossRef] [PubMed]
181. Liu, M.; Li, K.; Wang, Y.; Zhao, G.; Jiang, J. Stem Cells in the Treatment of Neuropathic Pain: Research Progress of Mechanism. *Stem Cells Int.* **2020**, *2020*, 8861251. [CrossRef] [PubMed]
182. Ye, H.; Chen, J.; Li, Y.-Q.; Yang, J.; Hsu, C.-C.; Cao, T.-T. A hyaluronic acid granular hydrogel nerve guidance conduit promotes regeneration and functional recovery of injured sciatic nerves in rats. *Neural Regen. Res.* **2023**, *18*, 657–663. [CrossRef] [PubMed]
183. Pabari, A.; Lloyd-Hughes, H.; Seifalian, A.M.; Mosahebi, A. Nerve conduits for peripheral nerve surgery. *Plast. Reconstr. Surg.* **2014**, *133*, 1420–1430. [CrossRef] [PubMed]
184. Kubiak, C.A.; Grochmal, J.; Kung, T.A.; Cederna, P.S.; Midha, R.; Kemp, S.W.P. Stem-cell–based therapies to enhance peripheral nerve regeneration. *Muscle Nerve* **2020**, *61*, 449–459. [CrossRef] [PubMed]
185. Zakrzewski, W.; Dobrzyński, M.; Szymonowicz, M.; Rybak, Z. Stem cells: Past, present, and future. *Stem Cell Res. Ther.* **2019**, *10*, 68. [CrossRef]
186. Sobhani, A.; Khanlarkhani, N.; Baazm, M.; Mohammadzadeh, F.; Najafi, A.; Mehdinejadiani, S.; Sargolzaei Aval, F. Multipotent Stem Cell and Current Application. *Acta Medica Iran.* **2017**, *55*, 6–23.
187. Tatullo, M.; Gargiulo, I.C.; Dipalma, G.; Ballini, A.; Inchingolo, A.M.; Paduanelli, G.; Nguyen, C.đ.K.; Inchingolo, A.D.; Makeeva, I.; Scacco, S.; et al. 17—Stem cells and regenerative medicine. In *Translational Systems Medicine and Oral Disease*; Sonis, S.T., Villa, A., Eds.; Academic Press: Cambridge, MA, USA, 2020; pp. 387–407.
188. Poliwoda, S.; Noor, N.; Downs, E.; Schaaf, A.; Cantwell, A.; Ganti, L.; Kaye, A.D.; Mosel, L.I.; Carroll, C.B.; Viswanath, O.; et al. Stem cells: A comprehensive review of origins and emerging clinical roles in medical practice. *Orthop. Rev.* **2022**, *14*, 37498. [CrossRef]
189. Lu, V.; Roy, I.J.; Teitell, M.A. Nutrients in the fate of pluripotent stem cells. *Cell Metab.* **2021**, *33*, 2108–2121. [CrossRef]
190. Kiecker, C.; Bates, T.; Bell, E. Molecular specification of germ layers in vertebrate embryos. *Cell. Mol. Life Sci.* **2016**, *73*, 923–947. [CrossRef]
191. Guasti, L.; New, S.E.; Hadjidemetriou, I.; Palmiero, M.; Ferretti, P. Plasticity of human adipose-derived stem cells—Relevance to tissue repair. *Int. J. Dev. Biol.* **2018**, *62*, 431–439. [CrossRef]
192. Guo, N.-N.; Liu, L.-P.; Zheng, Y.-W.; Li, Y.-M. Inducing human induced pluripotent stem cell differentiation through embryoid bodies: A practical and stable approach. *World J. Stem Cells* **2020**, *12*, 25–34. [CrossRef]
193. Priester, C.; MacDonald, A.; Dhar, M.; Bow, A. Examining the Characteristics and Applications of Mesenchymal, Induced Pluripotent, and Embryonic Stem Cells for Tissue Engineering Approaches across the Germ Layers. *Pharmaceuticals* **2020**, *13*, 344. [CrossRef] [PubMed]
194. Shin, A.; Saffari, T.; Saffari, S.; Vyas, K.; Mardini, S. Role of adipose tissue grafting and adipose-derived stem cells in peripheral nerve surgery. *Neural Regen. Res.* **2022**, *17*, 2179–2184. [CrossRef] [PubMed]
195. Méndez-Ferrer, S.; Scadden, D.T.; Sánchez-Aguilera, A. Bone marrow stem cells: Current and emerging concepts. *Ann. New York Acad. Sci.* **2015**, *1335*, 32–44. [CrossRef] [PubMed]
196. Visweswaran, M.; Pohl, S.; Arfuso, F.; Newsholme, P.; Dilley, R.; Pervaiz, S.; Dharmarajan, A. Multi-lineage differentiation of mesenchymal stem cells—To Wnt, or not Wnt. *Int. J. Biochem. Cell Biol.* **2015**, *68*, 139–147. [CrossRef]
197. Bunnell, B.A.; Flaat, M.; Gagliardi, C.; Patel, B.; Ripoll, C. Adipose-derived stem cells: Isolation, expansion and differentiation. *Methods* **2008**, *45*, 115–120. [CrossRef] [PubMed]
198. Urrutia, D.N.; Caviedes, P.; Mardones, R.; Minguell, J.J.; Vega-Letter, A.M.; Jofre, C.M. Comparative study of the neural differentiation capacity of mesenchymal stromal cells from different tissue sources: An approach for their use in neural regeneration therapies. *PLoS ONE* **2019**, *14*, e0213032. [CrossRef] [PubMed]
199. Gao, Y.; Jiao, Y.; Nie, W.; Lian, B.; Wang, B. In vitro proliferation and differentiation potential of bone marrow-derived mesenchymal stem cells from ovariectomized rats. *Tissue Cell* **2014**, *46*, 450–456. [CrossRef]

200. Jang, S.; Cho, H.-H.; Cho, Y.-B.; Park, J.-S.; Jeong, H.-S. Functional neural differentiation of human adipose tissue-derived stem cells using bFGF and forskolin. *BMC Cell Biol.* **2010**, *11*, 25. [CrossRef]
201. Mildmay-White, A.; Khan, W. Cell Surface Markers on Adipose-Derived Stem Cells: A Systematic Review. *Curr. Stem Cell Res. Ther.* **2017**, *12*, 484–492. [CrossRef]
202. Palumbo, P.; Lombardi, F.; Siragusa, G.; Cifone, M.G.; Cinque, B.; Giuliani, M. Methods of Isolation, Characterization and Expansion of Human Adipose-Derived Stem Cells (ASCs): An Overview. *Int. J. Mol. Sci.* **2018**, *19*, 1897. [CrossRef]
203. Hayat, R.; Manzoor, M.; Hussain, A. Wnt signaling pathway: A comprehensive review. *Cell Biol. Int.* **2022**, *46*, 863–877. [CrossRef] [PubMed]
204. Yamanaka, S. Strategies and New Developments in the Generation of Patient-Specific Pluripotent Stem Cells. *Cell Stem Cell* **2007**, *1*, 39–49. [CrossRef] [PubMed]
205. Takahashi, K.; Tanabe, K.; Ohnuki, M.; Narita, M.; Ichisaka, T.; Tomoda, K.; Yamanaka, S. Induction of Pluripotent Stem Cells from Adult Human Fibroblasts by Defined Factors. *Cell* **2007**, *131*, 861–872. [CrossRef] [PubMed]
206. Yu, J.; Vodyanik, M.A.; Smuga-Otto, K.; Antosiewicz-Bourget, J.; Frane, J.L.; Tian, S.; Nie, J.; Jonsdottir, G.A.; Ruotti, V.; Stewart, R.; et al. Induced pluripotent stem cell lines derived from human somatic cells. *Science* **2007**, *318*, 1917–1920. [CrossRef] [PubMed]
207. Wilmut, I. The First Direct Reprogramming of Adult Human Fibroblasts. *Cell Stem Cell* **2007**, *1*, 593–594. [CrossRef] [PubMed]
208. Kang, S.; Chen, X.; Gong, S.; Yu, P.; Yau, S.; Su, Z.; Zhou, L.; Yu, J.; Pan, G.; Shi, L. Characteristic analyses of a neural differentiation model from iPSC-derived neuron according to morphology, physiology, and global gene expression pattern. *Sci. Rep.* **2017**, *7*, 12233. [CrossRef]
209. Pajer, K.; Bellák, T.; Nógrádi, A. Stem Cell Secretome for Spinal Cord Repair: Is It More than Just a Random Baseline Set of Factors? *Cells* **2021**, *10*, 3214. [CrossRef]
210. Ocansey, D.K.W.; Xu, X.; Zhang, L.; Mao, F. Mesenchymal stem cell-derived exosome: The likely game-changer in stem cell research. *Biocell* **2022**, *46*, 1169–1172. [CrossRef]
211. Gowen, A.; Shahjin, F.; Chand, S.; Odegaard, K.E.; Yelamanchili, S.V. Mesenchymal Stem Cell-Derived Extracellular Vesicles: Challenges in Clinical Applications. *Front. Cell Dev. Biol.* **2020**, *8*, 149. [CrossRef]
212. Guo, W.; Zhang, X.; Yu, X.; Wang, S.; Qiu, J.; Tang, W.; Li, L.; Liu, H.; Wang, Z.L. Self-Powered Electrical Stimulation for Enhancing Neural Differentiation of Mesenchymal Stem Cells on Graphene-Poly(3,4-ethylenedioxythiophene) Hybrid Microfibers. *ACS Nano* **2016**, *10*, 5086–5095. [CrossRef]
213. Al-Massri, K.F.; Ahmed, L.A.; El-Abhar, H.S. Mesenchymal stem cells in chemotherapy-induced peripheral neuropathy: A new challenging approach that requires further investigations. *J. Tissue Eng. Regen. Med.* **2020**, *14*, 108–122. [CrossRef]
214. Gama, K.B.; Santos, D.S.; Evangelista, A.F.; Silva, D.N.; De Alcântara, A.C.; Dos Santos, R.R.; Soares, M.B.P.; Villarreal, C.F. Conditioned Medium of Bone Marrow-Derived Mesenchymal Stromal Cells as a Therapeutic Approach to Neuropathic Pain: A Preclinical Evaluation. *Stem Cells Int.* **2018**, *2018*, 8179013. [CrossRef]
215. Gao, L.; Xu, W.; Li, T.; Chen, J.; Shao, A.; Yan, F.; Chen, G. Stem Cell Therapy: A Promising Therapeutic Method for Intracerebral Hemorrhage. *Cell Transplant.* **2018**, *27*, 1809–1824. [CrossRef] [PubMed]
216. Xiang, E.; Han, B.; Zhang, Q.; Rao, W.; Wang, Z.; Chang, C.; Zhang, Y.; Tu, C.; Li, C.; Wu, D. Human umbilical cord-derived mesenchymal stem cells prevent the progression of early diabetic nephropathy through inhibiting inflammation and fibrosis. *Stem Cell Res. Ther.* **2020**, *11*, 336. [CrossRef] [PubMed]
217. He, D.; Xu, Y.; Xiong, X.; Yin, C.; Lei, S.; Cheng, X. The bone marrow-derived mesenchymal stem cells (BMSCs) alleviate diabetic peripheral neuropathy induced by STZ via activating GSK-3β/β-catenin signaling pathway. *Environ. Toxicol. Pharmacol.* **2020**, *79*, 103432. [CrossRef] [PubMed]
218. Yu, S.; Cheng, Y.; Zhang, L.; Yin, Y.; Xue, J.; Li, B.; Gong, Z.; Gao, J.; Mu, Y. Treatment with adipose tissue-derived mesenchymal stem cells exerts anti-diabetic effects, improves long-term complications, and attenuates inflammation in type 2 diabetic rats. *Stem Cell Res. Ther.* **2019**, *10*, 333. [CrossRef]
219. Zamorano, M.; Alexander, J.F.; Catania, D.; Dharmaraj, S.; Kavelaars, A.; Heijnen, C.J. Nasal administration of mesenchymal stem cells prevents accelerated age-related tauopathy after chemotherapy in mice. *Immun. Ageing* **2023**, *20*, 5. [CrossRef]
220. Sezer, G.; Yay, A.H.; Sarica, Z.S.; Gonen, Z.B.; Onder, G.O.; Alan, A.; Yilmaz, S.; Saraymen, B.; Bahar, D. Bone marrow-derived mesenchymal stem cells alleviate paclitaxel-induced mechanical allodynia in rats. *J. Biochem. Mol. Toxicol.* **2022**, *36*, e23207. [CrossRef]
221. Boukelmoune, N.; Laumet, G.; Tang, Y.; Ma, J.; Mahant, I.; Singh, S.K.; Nijboer, C.; Benders, M.; Kavelaars, A.; Heijnen, C.J. Nasal administration of mesenchymal stem cells reverses chemotherapy-induced peripheral neuropathy in mice. *Brain Behav. Immun.* **2021**, *93*, 43–54. [CrossRef]
222. Mannelli, L.D.C.; Tenci, B.; Micheli, L.; Vona, A.; Corti, F.; Zanardelli, M.; Lapucci, A.; Clemente, A.M.; Failli, P.; Ghelardini, C. Adipose-derived stem cells decrease pain in a rat model of oxaliplatin-induced neuropathy: Role of VEGF-A modulation. *Neuropharmacology* **2017**, *131*, 166–175. [CrossRef] [PubMed]
223. Miyano, K.; Ikehata, M.; Ohshima, K.; Yoshida, Y.; Nose, Y.; Yoshihara, S.-I.; Oki, K.; Shiraishi, S.; Uzu, M.; Nonaka, M.; et al. Intravenous administration of human mesenchymal stem cells derived from adipose tissue and umbilical cord improves neuropathic pain via suppression of neuronal damage and anti-inflammatory actions in rats. *PLoS ONE* **2022**, *17*, e0262892. [CrossRef] [PubMed]

224. Nagelkerke, A.; Ojansivu, M.; van der Koog, L.; Whittaker, T.E.; Cunnane, E.M.; Silva, A.M.; Dekker, N.; Stevens, M.M. Extracellular vesicles for tissue repair and regeneration: Evidence, challenges and opportunities. *Adv. Drug Deliv. Rev.* **2021**, *175*, 113775. [CrossRef] [PubMed]
225. Lukomska, B.; Stanaszek, L.; Zuba-Surma, E.; Legosz, P.; Sarzynska, S.; Drela, K. Challenges and Controversies in Human Mesenchymal Stem Cell Therapy. *Stem Cells Int.* **2019**, *2019*, 9628536. [CrossRef]
226. Antes, T.J.; Middleton, R.C.; Luther, K.M.; Ijichi, T.; Peck, K.A.; Liu, W.J.; Valle, J.; Echavez, A.K.; Marbán, E. Targeting extracellular vesicles to injured tissue using membrane cloaking and surface display. *J. Nanobiotechnol.* **2018**, *16*, 61. [CrossRef]
227. Fu, P.; Zhang, J.; Li, H.; Mak, M.; Xu, W.; Tao, Z. Extracellular vesicles as delivery systems at nano-/micro-scale. *Adv. Drug Deliv. Rev.* **2021**, *179*, 113910. [CrossRef] [PubMed]
228. Pegtel, D.M.; Peferoen, L.; Amor, S. Extracellular vesicles as modulators of cell-to-cell communication in the healthy and diseased brain. *Philos. Trans. R. Soc. B Biol. Sci.* **2014**, *369*, 20130516. [CrossRef]
229. Toribio, V.; Morales, S.; López-Martín, S.; Cardeñes, B.; Cabañas, C.; Yáñez-Mó, M. Development of a quantitative method to measure EV uptake. *Sci. Rep.* **2019**, *9*, 10522. [CrossRef]
230. Takeda, Y.S.; Xu, Q. Neuronal Differentiation of Human Mesenchymal Stem Cells Using Exosomes Derived from Differentiating Neuronal Cells. *PLoS ONE* **2015**, *10*, e0135111. [CrossRef]
231. Hercher, D.; Nguyen, M.Q.; Dworak, H. Extracellular vesicles and their role in peripheral nerve regeneration. *Exp. Neurol.* **2022**, *350*, 113968. [CrossRef]
232. Raposo, G.; Stahl, P.D. Extracellular vesicles: A new communication paradigm? *Nat. Rev. Mol. Cell Biol.* **2019**, *20*, 509–510. [CrossRef] [PubMed]
233. Gurung, S.; Perocheau, D.; Touramanidou, L.; Baruteau, J. The exosome journey: From biogenesis to uptake and intracellular signalling. *Cell Commun. Signal.* **2021**, *19*, 47. [CrossRef] [PubMed]
234. Wang, J.; Bonacquisti, E.E.; Brown, A.D.; Nguyen, J. Boosting the Biogenesis and Secretion of Mesenchymal Stem Cell-Derived Exosomes. *Cells* **2020**, *9*, 660. [CrossRef]
235. Xie, S.; Zhang, Q.; Jiang, L. Current Knowledge on Exosome Biogenesis, Cargo-Sorting Mechanism and Therapeutic Implications. *Membranes* **2022**, *12*, 498. [CrossRef] [PubMed]
236. Urbanelli, L.; Magini, A.; Buratta, S.; Brozzi, A.; Sagini, K.; Polchi, A.; Tancini, B.; Emiliani, C. Signaling Pathways in Exosomes Biogenesis, Secretion and Fate. *Genes* **2013**, *4*, 152–170. [CrossRef]
237. Fan, B.; Chopp, M.; Zhang, Z.G.; Liu, X.S. Treatment of diabetic peripheral neuropathy with engineered mesenchymal stromal cell-derived exosomes enriched with microRNA-146a provide amplified therapeutic efficacy. *Exp. Neurol.* **2021**, *341*, 113694. [CrossRef]
238. Zhang, Y.; Li, C.; Qin, Y.; Cepparulo, P.; Millman, M.; Chopp, M.; Kemper, A.; Szalad, A.; Lu, X.; Wang, L.; et al. Small extracellular vesicles ameliorate peripheral neuropathy and enhance chemotherapy of oxaliplatin on ovarian cancer. *J. Extracell. Vesicles* **2021**, *10*, e12073. [CrossRef]
239. Wong, F.C.; Ye, L.; Demir, I.E.; Kahlert, C. Schwann cell-derived exosomes: Janus-faced mediators of regeneration and disease. *Glia* **2021**, *70*, 20–34. [CrossRef]
240. Yu, M.; Liu, W.; Li, J.; Lu, J.; Lu, H.; Jia, W.; Liu, F. Exosomes derived from atorvastatin-pretreated MSC accelerate diabetic wound repair by enhancing angiogenesis via AKT/eNOS pathway. *Stem Cell Res. Ther.* **2020**, *11*, 350. [CrossRef]
241. Liu, W.; Yu, M.; Xie, D.; Wang, L.; Ye, C.; Zhu, Q.; Liu, F.; Yang, L. Melatonin-stimulated MSC-derived exosomes improve diabetic wound healing through regulating macrophage M1 and M2 polarization by targeting the PTEN/AKT pathway. *Stem Cell Res. Ther.* **2020**, *11*, 259. [CrossRef]
242. Song, H.; Zhang, X.; Chen, R.; Miao, J.; Wang, L.; Cui, L.; Ji, H.; Liu, Y. Cortical Neuron-Derived Exosomal MicroRNA-181c-3p Inhibits Neuroinflammation by Downregulating CXCL1 in Astrocytes of a Rat Model with Ischemic Brain Injury. *Neuroimmunomodulation* **2019**, *26*, 217–233. [CrossRef] [PubMed]
243. Yin, Z.; Han, Z.; Hu, T.; Zhang, S.; Ge, X.; Huang, S.; Wang, L.; Yu, J.; Li, W.; Wang, Y.; et al. Neuron-derived exosomes with high miR-21-5p expression promoted polarization of M1 microglia in culture. *Brain, Behav. Immun.* **2020**, *83*, 270–282. [CrossRef] [PubMed]
244. Katsuda, T.; Ochiya, T. Molecular signatures of mesenchymal stem cell-derived extracellular vesicle-mediated tissue repair. *Stem Cell Res. Ther.* **2015**, *6*, 212. [CrossRef] [PubMed]
245. Yang, Q.; Zhao, Q.; Yin, Y. miR-133b is a potential diagnostic biomarker for Alzheimer's disease and has a neuroprotective role. *Exp. Ther. Med.* **2019**, *18*, 2711–2718. [CrossRef] [PubMed]
246. Wiklander, O.P.B.; Nordin, J.Z.; O'Loughlin, A.; Gustafsson, Y.; Corso, G.; Mäger, I.; Vader, P.; Lee, Y.; Sork, H.; Seow, Y.; et al. Extracellular vesicle in vivo biodistribution is determined by cell source, route of administration and targeting. *J. Extracell. Vesicles* **2015**, *4*, 26316. [CrossRef] [PubMed]
247. Wang, L.; Chopp, M.; Szalad, A.; Lu, X.; Zhang, Y.; Wang, X.; Cepparulo, P.; Lu, M.; Li, C.; Zhang, Z.G. Exosomes Derived From Schwann Cells Ameliorate Peripheral Neuropathy in Type 2 Diabetic Mice. *Diabetes* **2020**, *69*, 749–759. [CrossRef] [PubMed]
248. El-Derany, M.O.; Noureldein, M.H. Bone marrow mesenchymal stem cells and their derived exosomes resolve doxorubicin-induced chemobrain: Critical role of their miRNA cargo. *Stem Cell Res. Ther.* **2021**, *12*, 322. [CrossRef]

249. Gao, X.; Gao, L.-F.; Zhang, Y.-N.; Kong, X.-Q.; Jia, S.; Meng, C.-Y. Huc-MSCs-derived exosomes attenuate neuropathic pain by inhibiting activation of the TLR2/MyD88/NF-κB signaling pathway in the spinal microglia by targeting Rsad2. *Int. Immunopharmacol.* **2023**, *114*, 109505. [CrossRef]
250. Gao, X.; Gao, L.-F.; Kong, X.-Q.; Zhang, Y.-N.; Jia, S.; Meng, C.-Y. Mesenchymal stem cell-derived extracellular vesicles carrying miR-99b-3p restrain microglial activation and neuropathic pain by stimulating autophagy. *Int. Immunopharmacol.* **2023**, *115*, 109695. [CrossRef]
251. Zhang, Y.; Ye, G.; Zhao, J.; Chen, Y.; Kong, L.; Sheng, C.; Yuan, L. Exosomes carried miR-181c-5p alleviates neuropathic pain in CCI rat models. *An. da Acad. Bras. de Cienc.* **2022**, *94*, e20210564. [CrossRef]
252. Zhang, C.; Huang, Y.; Ouyang, F.; Su, M.; Li, W.; Chen, J.; Xiao, H.; Zhou, X.; Liu, B. Extracellular vesicles derived from mesenchymal stem cells alleviate neuroinflammation and mechanical allodynia in interstitial cystitis rats by inhibiting NLRP3 inflammasome activation. *J. Neuroinflammation* **2022**, *19*, 80. [CrossRef]
253. Hua, T.; Yang, M.; Song, H.; Kong, E.; Deng, M.; Li, Y.; Li, J.; Liu, Z.; Fu, H.; Wang, Y.; et al. Huc-MSCs-derived exosomes attenuate inflammatory pain by regulating microglia pyroptosis and autophagy via the miR-146a-5p/TRAF6 axis. *J. Nanobiotechnology* **2022**, *20*, 324. [CrossRef]
254. Anakor, E.; Le Gall, L.; Dumonceaux, J.; Duddy, W.J.; Duguez, S. Exosomes in Ageing and Motor Neurone Disease: Biogenesis, Uptake Mechanisms, Modifications in Disease and Uses in the Development of Biomarkers and Therapeutics. *Cells* **2021**, *10*, 2930. [CrossRef] [PubMed]
255. French, K.C.; Antonyak, M.A.; Cerione, R.A. Extracellular vesicle docking at the cellular port: Extracellular vesicle binding and uptake. *Semin. Cell Dev. Biol.* **2017**, *67*, 48–55. [CrossRef] [PubMed]
256. Zhang, Y.; Liu, Y.; Liu, H.; Tang, W.H. Exosomes: Biogenesis, biologic function and clinical potential. *Cell Biosci.* **2019**, *9*, 19. [CrossRef] [PubMed]
257. Vader, P.; Mol, E.A.; Pasterkamp, G.; Schiffelers, R.M. Extracellular vesicles for drug delivery. *Adv. Drug Deliv. Rev.* **2016**, *106*, 148–156. [CrossRef] [PubMed]
258. He, J.; Ren, W.; Wang, W.; Han, W.; Jiang, L.; Zhang, D.; Guo, M. Exosomal targeting and its potential clinical application. *Drug Deliv. Transl. Res.* **2022**, *12*, 2385–2402. [CrossRef] [PubMed]
259. Dong, R.; Liu, Y.; Yang, Y.; Wang, H.; Xu, Y.; Zhang, Z. MSC-Derived Exosomes-Based Therapy for Peripheral Nerve Injury: A Novel Therapeutic Strategy. *BioMed Res. Int.* **2019**, *2019*, 6458237. [CrossRef] [PubMed]
260. De Gregorio, C.; Díaz, P.; López-Leal, R.; Manque, P.; Court, F.A. Purification of Exosomes from Primary Schwann Cells, RNA Extraction, and Next-Generation Sequencing of Exosomal RNAs. In *Schwann Cells: Methods and Protocols*; Monje, P.V., Kim, H.A., Eds.; Springer: New York, NY, USA, 2018; pp. 299–315.
261. López-Leal, R.; Díaz-Viraqué, F.; Catalan, R.J.; Saquel, C.; Enright, A.; Iraola, G.; Court, F.A. Schwann cell reprogramming into repair cells increases exosome-loaded miRNA-21 promoting axonal growth. *J. Cell Sci.* **2020**, *133*, jcs239004. [CrossRef] [PubMed]
262. Long, H.-Z.; Cheng, Y.; Zhou, Z.-W.; Luo, H.-Y.; Wen, D.-D.; Gao, L.-C. PI3K/AKT Signal Pathway: A Target of Natural Products in the Prevention and Treatment of Alzheimer's Disease and Parkinson's Disease. *Front. Pharmacol.* **2021**, *12*, 648636. [CrossRef]
263. Li, X.; Yang, S.; Wang, L.; Liu, P.; Zhao, S.; Li, H.; Jiang, Y.; Guo, Y.; Wang, X. Resveratrol inhibits paclitaxel-induced neuropathic pain by the activation of PI3K/Akt and SIRT1/PGC1α pathway. *J. Pain Res.* **2019**, *12*, 879–890. [CrossRef]
264. Figlia, G.; Norrmén, C.; Pereira, J.A.; Gerber, D.; Suter, U. Dual function of the PI3K-Akt-mTORC1 axis in myelination of the peripheral nervous system. *eLife* **2017**, *6*, e29241. [CrossRef]
265. Sengupta, S.; Peterson, T.R.; Sabatini, D.M. Regulation of the mTOR complex 1 pathway by nutrients, growth factors, and stress. *Mol. Cell* **2010**, *40*, 310–322. [CrossRef]
266. Dibble, C.C.; Cantley, L.C. Regulation of mTORC1 by PI3K signaling. *Trends Cell Biol.* **2015**, *25*, 545–555. [CrossRef]
267. Magnaghi, V.; Castelnovo, L.F.; Bonalume, V.; Melfi, S.; Ballabio, M.; Colleoni, D. Schwann cell development, maturation and regeneration: A focus on classic and emerging intracellular signaling pathways. *Neural Regen. Res.* **2017**, *12*, 1013–1023. [CrossRef]
268. Ishii, A.; Furusho, M.; Bansal, R. Mek/ERK1/2-MAPK and PI3K/Akt/mTOR signaling plays both independent and cooperative roles in Schwann cell differentiation, myelination and dysmyelination. *Glia* **2021**, *69*, 2429–2446. [CrossRef]
269. Jessen, K.R.; Mirsky, R. The Success and Failure of the Schwann Cell Response to Nerve Injury. *Front. Cell. Neurosci.* **2019**, *13*, 33. [CrossRef]
270. Liu, T.; Wang, Y.; Lu, L.; Liu, Y. SPIONs mediated magnetic actuation promotes nerve regeneration by inducing and maintaining repair-supportive phenotypes in Schwann cells. *J. Nanobiotechnol.* **2022**, *20*, 159. [CrossRef]
271. Phan, J.; Kumar, P.; Hao, D.; Gao, K.; Farmer, D.; Wang, A. Engineering mesenchymal stem cells to improve their exosome efficacy and yield for cell-free therapy. *J. Extracell. Vesicles* **2018**, *7*, 1522236. [CrossRef]
272. Yuan, X.; Sun, L.; Jeske, R.; Nkosi, D.; York, S.B.; Liu, Y.; Grant, S.C.; Meckes, D.G.; Li, Y. Engineering extracellular vesicles by three-dimensional dynamic culture of human mesenchymal stem cells. *J. Extracell. Vesicles* **2022**, *11*, e12235. [CrossRef]
273. Jeske, R.; Liu, C.; Duke, L.; Canonicco Castro, M.L.; Muok, L.; Arthur, P.; Singh, M.; Jung, S.; Sun, L.; Li, Y. Upscaling human mesenchymal stromal cell production in a novel vertical-wheel bioreactor enhances extracellular vesicle secretion and cargo profile. *Bioact. Mater.* **2023**, *25*, 732–747. [CrossRef]

274. Gobin, J.; Muradia, G.; Mehic, J.; Westwood, C.; Couvrette, L.; Stalker, A.; Bigelow, S.; Luebbert, C.C.; Bissonnette, F.S.-D.; Johnston, M.J.W.; et al. Hollow-fiber bioreactor production of extracellular vesicles from human bone marrow mesenchymal stromal cells yields nanovesicles that mirrors the immuno-modulatory antigenic signature of the producer cell. *Stem Cell Res. Ther.* **2021**, *12*, 127. [CrossRef]
275. Ghasemian, M.; Layton, C.; Nampe, D.; Nieden, N.I.Z.; Tsutsui, H.; Princevac, M. Hydrodynamic characterization within a spinner flask and a rotary wall vessel for stem cell culture. *Biochem. Eng. J.* **2020**, *157*, 107533. [CrossRef]
276. de Sousa Pinto, D.; Bandeiras, C.; de Almeida Fuzeta, M.; Rodrigues, C.A.V.; Jung, S.; Hashimura, Y.; Tseng, R.J.; Milligan, W.; Lee, B.; Ferreira, F.C.; et al. Scalable Manufacturing of Human Mesenchymal Stromal Cells in the Vertical-Wheel Bioreactor System: An Experimental and Economic Approach. *Biotechnol. J.* **2019**, *14*, e1800716. [CrossRef]
277. Witwer, K.W.; Buzás, E.I.; Bemis, L.T.; Bora, A.; Lässer, C.; Lötvall, J.; Nolte-'t Hoen, E.N.; Piper, M.G.; Sivaraman, S.; Skog, J.; et al. Standardization of sample collection, isolation and analysis methods in extracellular vesicle research. *J. Extracell. Vesicles* **2013**, *2*, 20360. [CrossRef]
278. Théry, C.; Witwer, K.W.; Aikawa, E.; Alcaraz, M.J.; Anderson, J.D.; Andriantsitohaina, R.; Antoniou, A.; Arab, T.; Archer, F.; Atkin-Smith, G.K.; et al. Minimal information for studies of extracellular vesicles 2018 (MISEV2018): A position statement of the International Society for Extracellular Vesicles and update of the MISEV2014 guidelines. *J. Extracell. Vesicles* **2018**, *7*, 1535750. [CrossRef]
279. Kawai-Harada, Y.; El Itawi, H.; Komuro, H.; Harada, M. Evaluation of EV Storage Buffer for Efficient Preservation of Engineered Extracellular Vesicles. *Int. J. Mol. Sci.* **2023**, *24*, 12841. [CrossRef]
280. Görgens, A.; Corso, G.; Hagey, D.W.; Wiklander, R.J.; Gustafsson, M.O.; Felldin, U.; Lee, Y.; Bostancioglu, R.B.; Sork, H.; Liang, X.; et al. Identification of storage conditions stabilizing extracellular vesicles preparations. *J. Extracell. Vesicles* **2022**, *11*, e12238. [CrossRef]
281. Gelibter, S.; Marostica, G.; Mandelli, A.; Siciliani, S.; Podini, P.; Finardi, A.; Furlan, R. The impact of storage on extracellular vesicles: A systematic study. *J. Extracell. Vesicles* **2022**, *11*, e12162. [CrossRef]
282. Luhtala, N.; Aslanian, A.; Yates, J.R., 3rd; Hunter, T. Secreted Glioblastoma Nanovesicles Contain Intracellular Signaling Proteins and Active Ras Incorporated in a Farnesylation-dependent Manner. *J. Biol. Chem.* **2017**, *292*, 611–628. [CrossRef]
283. Charoenviriyakul, C.; Takahashi, Y.; Nishikawa, M.; Takakura, Y. Preservation of exosomes at room temperature using lyophilization. *Int. J. Pharm.* **2018**, *553*, 1–7. [CrossRef]
284. Cheng, Y.; Zeng, Q.; Han, Q.; Xia, W. Effect of pH, temperature and freezing-thawing on quantity changes and cellular uptake of exosomes. *Protein Cell* **2018**, *10*, 295–299. [CrossRef]
285. Buccitelli, C.; Selbach, M. mRNAs, proteins and the emerging principles of gene expression control. *Nat. Rev. Genet.* **2020**, *21*, 630–644. [CrossRef]
286. Knotkova, H.; Hamani, C.; Sivanesan, E.; Le Beuffe, M.F.E.; Moon, J.Y.; Cohen, S.P.; Huntoon, M.A. Neuromodulation for chronic pain. *Lancet* **2021**, *397*, 2111–2124. [CrossRef]
287. Naskar, S.; Kumaran, V.; Markandeya, Y.S.; Mehta, B.; Basu, B. Neurogenesis-on-Chip: Electric field modulated transdifferentiation of human mesenchymal stem cell and mouse muscle precursor cell coculture. *Biomaterials* **2020**, *226*, 119522. [CrossRef]
288. Fukuta, T.; Nishikawa, A.; Kogure, K. Low level electricity increases the secretion of extracellular vesicles from cultured cells. *Biochem. Biophys. Rep.* **2020**, *21*, 100713. [CrossRef]
289. Thrivikraman, G.; Madras, G.; Basu, B. Intermittent electrical stimuli for guidance of human mesenchymal stem cell lineage commitment towards neural-like cells on electroconductive substrates. *Biomaterials* **2014**, *35*, 6219–6235. [CrossRef]
290. Campana, W.M.; Mantuano, E.; Azmoon, P.; Henry, K.; Banki, M.A.; Kim, J.H.; Pizzo, D.P.; Gonias, S.L. Ionotropic glutamate receptors activate cell signaling in response to glutamate in Schwann cells. *FASEB J.* **2016**, *31*, 1744–1755. [CrossRef]
291. Hu, M.; Hong, L.; Liu, C.; Hong, S.; He, S.; Zhou, M.; Huang, G.; Chen, Q. Electrical stimulation enhances neuronal cell activity mediated by Schwann cell derived exosomes. *Sci. Rep.* **2019**, *9*, 4206. [CrossRef]
292. Zhang, H.; Shen, Y.; Kim, I.-M.; Liu, Y.; Cai, J.; Berman, A.E.; Nilsson, K.R.; Weintraub, N.L.; Tang, Y. Electrical Stimulation Increases the Secretion of Cardioprotective Extracellular Vesicles from Cardiac Mesenchymal Stem Cells. *Cells* **2023**, *12*, 875. [CrossRef]
293. Sanchez, V.C.; Jachak, A.; Hurt, R.H.; Kane, A.B. Biological Interactions of Graphene-Family Nanomaterials: An Interdisciplinary Review. *Chem. Res. Toxicol.* **2012**, *25*, 15–34. [CrossRef]
294. Kalbacova, M.; Broz, A.; Kong, J.; Kalbac, M. Graphene substrates promote adherence of human osteoblasts and mesenchymal stromal cells. *Carbon* **2010**, *48*, 4323–4329. [CrossRef]
295. Bidez, P.R.; Li, S.; MacDiarmid, A.G.; Venancio, E.C.; Wei, Y.; Lelkes, P.I. Polyaniline, an electroactive polymer, supports adhesion and proliferation of cardiac myoblasts. *J. Biomater. Sci. Polym. Ed.* **2006**, *17*, 199–212. [CrossRef]
296. Wang, H.-J.; Ji, L.-W.; Li, D.-F.; Wang, J.-Y. Characterization of Nanostructure and Cell Compatibility of Polyaniline Films with Different Dopant Acids. *J. Phys. Chem. B* **2008**, *112*, 2671–2677. [CrossRef]
297. Oren, R.; Sfez, R.; Korbakov, N.; Shabtai, K.; Cohen, A.; Erez, H.; Dormann, A.; Cohen, H.; Shappir, J.; Spira, M.; et al. Electrically conductive 2D-PAN-containing surfaces as a culturing substrate for neurons. *J. Biomater. Sci. Polym. Ed.* **2004**, *15*, 1355–1374. [CrossRef]
298. Ju, C.; Park, E.; Kim, T.; Kim, T.; Kang, M.; Lee, K.-S.; Park, S.-M. Effectiveness of electrical stimulation on nerve regeneration after crush injury: Comparison between invasive and non-invasive stimulation. *PLoS ONE* **2020**, *15*, e0233531. [CrossRef]

299. Wang, Y.; Burghardt, T.P.; Worrell, G.A.; Wang, H.-L. The frequency-dependent effect of electrical fields on the mobility of intracellular vesicles in astrocytes. *Biochem. Biophys. Res. Commun.* **2020**, *534*, 429–435. [CrossRef]
300. Cheng, H.; Huang, Y.; Yue, H.; Fan, Y. Electrical Stimulation Promotes Stem Cell Neural Differentiation in Tissue Engineering. *Stem Cells Int.* **2021**, *2021*, 6697574. [CrossRef]
301. Leng, T.; Fishman, H.A. Carbon nanotube bucky paper as an artificial support membrane for retinal cell transplantation. *Ophthalmic Surg. Lasers Imaging Retin.* **2013**, *44*, 73–76. [CrossRef]
302. Lee, M.H.; Park, Y.J.; Hong, S.H.; Koo, M.-A.; Cho, M.; Park, J.-C. Pulsed Electrical Stimulation Enhances Consistency of Directional Migration of Adipose-Derived Stem Cells. *Cells* **2021**, *10*, 2846. [CrossRef]
303. Banks, T.A.; Luckman, P.S.B.; Frith, J.E.; Cooper-White, J.J. Effects of electric fields on human mesenchymal stem cell behaviour and morphology using a novel multichannel device. *Integr. Biol.* **2015**, *7*, 693–712. [CrossRef]
304. Feng, J.-F.; Liu, J.; Zhang, X.-Z.; Zhang, L.; Jiang, J.-Y.; Nolta, J.; Zhao, M. Guided Migration of Neural Stem Cells Derived from Human Embryonic Stem Cells by an Electric Field. *Stem Cells* **2012**, *30*, 349–355. [CrossRef]
305. Maji, S.; Yan, I.K.; Parasramka, M.; Mohankumar, S.; Matsuda, A.; Patel, T. In vitro toxicology studies of extracellular vesicles. *J. Appl. Toxicol.* **2017**, *37*, 310–318. [CrossRef]
306. Lin, S.; Zhu, B.; Huang, G.; Zeng, Q.; Wang, C. Microvesicles derived from human bone marrow mesenchymal stem cells promote U2OS cell growth under hypoxia: The role of PI3K/AKT and HIF-1α. *Hum. Cell* **2019**, *32*, 64–74. [CrossRef]
307. Lee, J.-K.; Park, S.-R.; Jung, B.-K.; Jeon, Y.-K.; Lee, Y.-S.; Kim, M.-K.; Kim, Y.-G.; Jang, J.-Y.; Kim, C.-W. Exosomes derived from mesenchymal stem cells suppress angiogenesis by down-regulating VEGF expression in breast cancer cells. *PLoS ONE* **2013**, *8*, e84256. [CrossRef]
308. Rodini, C.O.; da Silva, P.B.G.; Assoni, A.F.; Carvalho, V.M.; Okamoto, O.K. Mesenchymal stem cells enhance tumorigenic properties of human glioblastoma through independent cell-cell communication mechanisms. *Oncotarget* **2018**, *9*, 24766–24777. [CrossRef]
309. Tan, T.T.; Lai, R.C.; Padmanabhan, J.; Sim, W.K.; Choo, A.B.H.; Lim, S.K. Assessment of Tumorigenic Potential in Mesenchymal-Stem/Stromal-Cell-Derived Small Extracellular Vesicles (MSC-sEV). *Pharmaceuticals* **2021**, *14*, 345. [CrossRef]

biomedicines

MDPI

Review

Potential for Therapeutic-Loaded Exosomes to Ameliorate the Pathogenic Effects of α-Synuclein in Parkinson's Disease

David J. Rademacher

Department of Microbiology and Immunology and Core Imaging Facility, Stritch School of Medicine, Loyola University Chicago, Maywood, IL 60153, USA; drademacher@luc.edu; Tel.: +1-708-216-3395

Abstract: Pathogenic forms of α-synuclein (α-syn) are transferred to and from neurons, astrocytes, and microglia, which spread α-syn pathology in the olfactory bulb and the gut and then throughout the Parkinson's disease (PD) brain and exacerbate neurodegenerative processes. Here, we review attempts to minimize or ameliorate the pathogenic effects of α-syn or deliver therapeutic cargo into the brain. Exosomes (EXs) have several important advantages as carriers of therapeutic agents including an ability to readily cross the blood–brain barrier, the potential for targeted delivery of therapeutic agents, and immune resistance. Diverse cargo can be loaded via various methods, which are reviewed herein, into EXs and delivered into the brain. Genetic modification of EX-producing cells or EXs and chemical modification of EX have emerged as powerful approaches for the targeted delivery of therapeutic agents to treat PD. Thus, EXs hold great promise for the development of next-generation therapeutics for the treatment of PD.

Keywords: exosomes; extracellular vesicles; Parkinson's disease; pathogenesis; therapeutics; α-synuclein; neurodegeneration; genetic modification; chemical modification

1. Introduction

Extracellular vesicles (EVs) are membrane-enclosed particles released by cells into the extracellular space [1,2]. EVs can be classified as exosomes (EXs), microvesicles, or apoptotic bodies based on their origin and size [1–3]. EXs are enclosed within a single phospholipid bilayer, secreted by all cell types, formed by the inward invagination of the endosomal membrane and fusion of the multivesicular body (MVB), and are typically 30–150 nm in diameter [1,3–5]. Microvesicles are EVs that form from direct outward budding from the cell's plasma membrane and are typically 100 nm to 1 μm in diameter [1–5]. Although the route of microvesicle formation is not fully understood, it is thought to require cytoskeleton components, molecular motors, and fusion machinery [6]. Apoptotic bodies are EVs formed during apoptosis and released into the extracellular space; they range in diameter from 50 nm to 5 μm [3]. Apoptotic bodies form through the separation of the cell's plasma membrane from the cytoskeleton due to increased hydrostatic pressure after the cell contracts [7]. EVs contain thousands of different biologically active molecules, including nucleic acids, proteins, lipids, and metabolites [8–11]. Here, we focus on the most extensively studied EVs, typically designated as EXs, which play key roles in intercellular communication by delivering biologically active cargo to recipient cells, thereby altering the recipient cell's functions [12,13]. Thus, EXs hold great promise for developing next-generation delivery vehicles of therapeutic agents.

2. Role of EXs in the Pathogenesis of Parkinson's Disease

Parkinson's disease (PD) is the second most common neurodegenerative disease in the world after Alzheimer's disease, affecting 1–2% of the population over the age of 65 [14]. There are approximately seven million PD cases in the world; approximately one million of those cases are in the United States [15]. As the population ages, the burden on society attributable to PD is expected to increase substantially. The main pathological changes in PD are a progressive loss of dopamine (DA)-secreting neurons in the substantia nigra, a significant decrease of DA in the striatum, and the appearance of eosinophilic inclusions in the cytoplasm of DA neurons in the substantia nigra, namely Lewy bodies (LBs) [16]. The progressive loss of nigrostriatal neurons leads to the appearance of classical parkinsonian motor symptoms (e.g., bradykinesia, tremor, and rigidity) and numerous non-motor symptoms (e.g., depression, constipation, pain, gastrointestinal dysfunction, and sleep problems) [17,18]. The presence of α-synuclein (α-syn) aggregates in LBs [16], approximately 90% of which are phosphorylated on serine residue 129 [19], and the finding that mutations in the α-syn gene, *SNCA*, cause familial PD [20–23] and accelerate the pathogenic aggregation of α-syn [24,25], strongly suggested a role for α-syn in the pathogenesis of PD.

Prions are infectious agents in which the conformationally altered protein, PrP^{Sc}, recruits and corrupts its counterpart protein, PrP^{C}, generating self-propagating, misfolded species that spread from cell to cell [26]. According to the prion hypothesis of PD [27], like prion proteins, misfolded α-syn is transmitted from diseased cells to healthy cells, thereby spreading α-syn pathology in the PD brain [28,29]. The notion that EXs can be used as a carrier of toxic, misfolded proteins, such as α-syn, is an important tenet of the prion hypothesis of PD and is well supported by evidence. In vitro experiments provided the first evidence that newly synthesized monomeric and aggregated α-syn was released into the extracellular environment [30–32], a finding consistent with the presence of α-syn in human cerebrospinal fluid and blood plasma in both PD and normal human subjects [33,34]. Interestingly, EXs provide an environment conducive to α-syn aggregation [35]. In vitro studies have demonstrated α-syn release in EXs from donor neurons, uptake by recipient neurons, and subsequent cell death of recipient neurons [36–38]. When EXs harvested from the brain tissue of dementia with Lewy bodies patients were injected into the brains of mice, α-syn was taken up by neurons and astrocytes, and intracellular α-syn accumulation was observed [39]. Additional support for the prion hypothesis of PD comes from a study that examined the EXs isolated from the serum of PD patients, which contained a higher content of α-syn phosphorylated at serine residue 129 and oligomeric and monomeric α-syn than controls. In vitro studies demonstrated that the PD EXs, which contained an abundant amount of toxic, misfolded α-syn, were taken up by recipient cells, and acted as a seed or template to induce the aggregation of endogenous α-syn in recipient neurons. Interestingly, in human midbrain DA neuron cell cultures, pathogenic, misfolded α-syn was secreted in EXs via an autophagic secretory pathway [40]. Moreover, PD EX administration to mice resulted in DA neuron degeneration, microglial cell activation, and motor deficits [41]. Notably, neuron-to-neuron, neuron-to-microglia, microglia-to-neuron, neuron-to-astrocyte, and astrocyte-to-neuron transfer of α-syn has been demonstrated (Figure 1) [42–46].

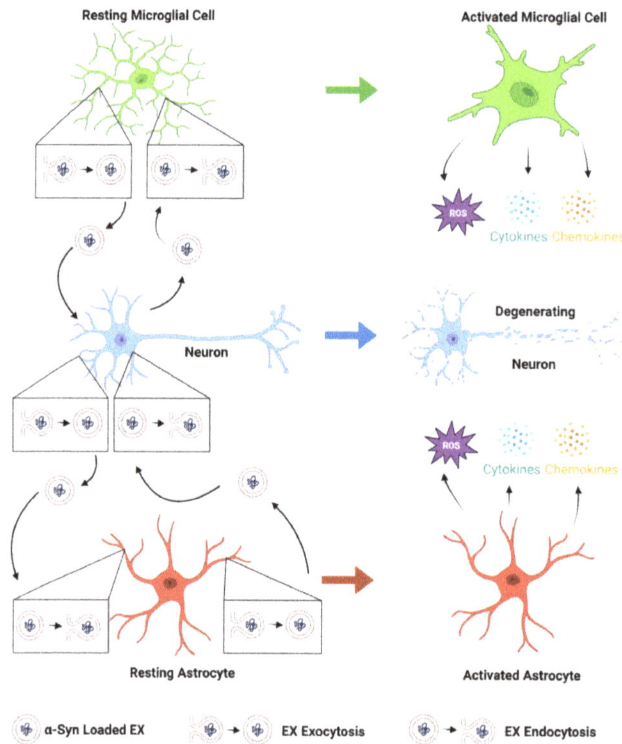

Figure 1. The transfer of α-syn to and from neurons, astrocytes, and microglia. The transfer of α-syn to astrocytes and microglia results in their activation. Activated astrocytes and microglia release ROS, pro-inflammatory cytokines and chemokines, which contribute to the neurodegenerative processes in PD. The figure was created with BioRender.com https://app.biorender.com/ (accessed on 24 March 2023).

3. Role of Microglia in the Pathogenesis of PD

Microglia, the main resident immune cells in the brain, can have beneficial and harmful effects on PD depending, in part, on their activation state. Concerning their harmful effects on PD, microglia have been implicated in the pathogenesis of PD. Positron emission tomography imaging demonstrated microglia activation in the substantia nigra and striatum of PD patients [47]. Increased microglia activation in the midbrain was correlated with a loss of DA-secreting nerve terminals in the striatum [48]. In addition, activated microglia were more frequently observed near LBs containing α-syn and near dying neurons [49].

Concerning their beneficial effects, microglia can enhance neuronal survival by releasing trophic factors, clearing debris, dead cells, and misfolded α-syn aggregates in PD [50–53]. However, α-syn activates microglia (Figure 1) [53,54]. Activation of microglia induces an oxidative stress response, including the release of reactive oxygen species (ROS) and nitric oxide, the production of NADPH oxidase, and the release of pro-inflammatory cytokines and chemokines (Figure 1) [55–57]. Inflammation and oxidative stress can lead to neuron dysfunction and cell death (Figure 1) [58,59], effects that have been linked to the pathogenesis of PD [60], and it is known that microglia release EXs [61]. There is evidence to support the notion that α-syn can be transferred from microglia to neurons via EXs and induce α-syn aggregation in the recipient neurons (Figure 1), an effect that is exacerbated by microglia-derived pro-inflammatory cytokines. In addition, microglial EXs isolated from PD patients induced α-syn aggregation and cell-to-cell transfer of α-syn, DA neuron degeneration in the substantia nigra, and motor deficits in mice [45].

4. Role of Astrocytes in the Pathogenesis of PD

In common with microglia, astrocytes have beneficial and harmful effects on PD. Astrocytes can enhance neuronal survival by releasing trophic factors, antioxidants, and other factors that protect against oxidative stress [62–64]. Although a consensus has not been reached on the degree of astrocyte activation in the PD brain [65,66], α-syn aggregates have been observed in human astrocytes [67], and there is considerable evidence suggesting that α-syn activates astrocytes that, in turn, result in the astrocytic release of pro-inflammatory cytokines, chemokines, and ROS, microglial cell activation, and neuronal cell death (Figure 1) [53,68,69].

5. Pathogenic α-Syn-Containing EXs as Therapeutic Targets

Given the abundance of evidence implicating α-syn-containing EXs in the pathogenesis of PD, a logical therapeutic approach for PD is to minimize or eliminate the pathogenic effects of α-syn-containing EXs. This could be accomplished by decreasing EX biogenesis in parent cells, removing pathogenic EXs from circulation, and inhibiting EX uptake by the recipient cells (Figure 2A–D).

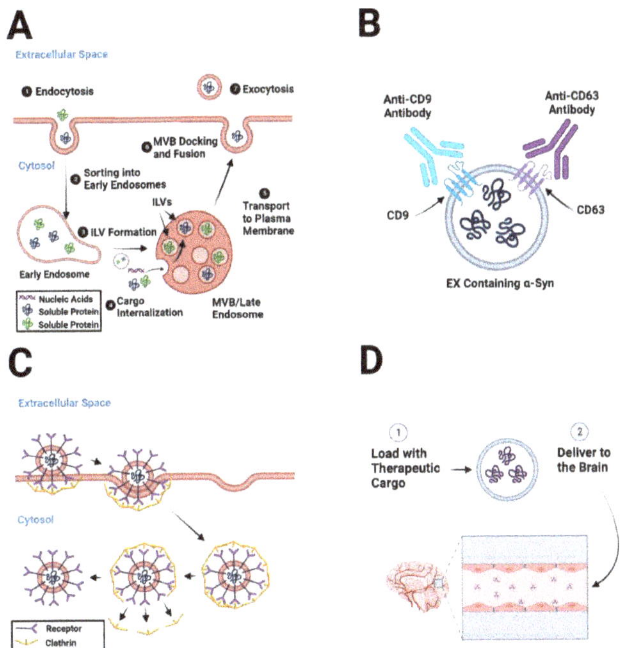

Figure 2. Approaches to minimize or eliminate the pathogenic effects of α-syn-containing EXs in PD. (**A**). The major steps in the biogenesis of α-syn-containing EXs. Therapeutic approaches may target key proteins involved in each of these steps. (**B**). An EX that contains pathogenic, misfolded α-syn and expresses the tetraspanins, CD9 and CD63, is sequestered by antibodies directed against CD9 and CD63 and then cleared from circulation. (**C**). α-Syn-containing EXs are taken up by recipient cells by clathrin-mediated endocytosis. Therapeutic approaches may target proteins involved in EX uptake. Note that there are numerous ways that EXs can be taken up by recipient cells including caveolin-mediated endocytosis, lipid raft-mediated endocytosis, micropinocytosis, phagocytosis, and membrane fusion [70]. (**D**). There are numerous ways to load therapeutic cargos into EXs and deliver them to target cells in the brain, as described in the text. The figure was created with BioRender.com https://app.biorender.com/ (accessed on 24 March 2023).

5.1. Decreasing EX Biogenesis

Several proteins responsible for EX biogenesis have been identified as targets to decrease pathogenic EX formation. EXs are formed by the invagination of the MVB system and their fusion with the plasma membrane [71]. As EX formation requires either endosomal sorting complexes required for transport (EXCRT)-dependent or ESCRT-independent cargo sorting at the MVB and MVB-plasma membrane fusion, related proteins can be regarded as potential therapeutic targets (Figure 2A) [72]. Two extensively studied proteins are the ALG-2-interacting protein X (ALIX) and the Rab protein [73–75]. During EX biogenesis, ALIX proteins are associated with the invagination of the MVB membrane by recruiting ESCRT proteins. Treatment with ALIX small interfering RNA (siRNA) and siRNA directed against the ALIX ligand, syntenin, suppressed ALIX function, resulting in reduced EX biogenesis [73]. Rab27a and Rab27b are notable as they are involved in the process of MVB fusion with the plasma membrane [71,76]. Knockdown or silencing of Rab27a and Rab27b reduced the number of EXs released [77]. In addition, the inhibition of two Rab27 effectors, Slp4 and Slac2b, also reduced the number of EXs released [76]. GW4869 is a potent neutral sphingomyelinase inhibitor that blocks EX production by preventing the formation of intraluminal vesicles (ILVs) (Figure 2A) [78]. Pretreatment of α-syn-activated microglia with GW4869 decreased the release of cathepsin L-containing EXs from microglia, which prevented neuronal death [79]. Similarly, treatment with GW4869 decreased EX release by activated microglia and prevented the death of DA neurons in midbrain slice cultures [80]. Systemic administration of DDL-112, an inhibitor of neutral sphingomyelinase, decreased EX biogenesis, reduced the number of α-syn aggregates in the substantia nigra, and improved motor function in an α-syn mouse model of PD [81].

5.2. Depleting Circulating Pathogenic EXs

After EXs are released from parent cells, they are either taken up by neighboring cells or travel to distant recipient cells to deliver their cargo. One interesting strategy to deplete pathogenic EXs from circulation is to use EX-specific antibodies so that EXs can be removed by the immune system (Figure 2B). The administration of anti-CD9 and anti-CD63 antibodies resulted in phagocytosis of the antibody-bound EXs by macrophages (Figure 2B) [82].

5.3. Inhibiting EX Uptake by Recipient Cells

In an attempt to ameliorate EX-mediated pathogenic cell-to-cell communication, researchers have inhibited EX uptake by recipient cells (Figure 2C) [83,84]. Endocytosis inhibitors have been heavily studied as potential therapeutics, as EXs are primarily taken up by recipient cells via endocytosis [70]. Cytochalasin D inhibits phagocytosis and endocytosis by blocking actin polymerization and inducing depolymerization of actin filaments [83]. Cancer-associated fibroblast-derived EXs were not effectively taken up by cancer cells in the presence of cytochalasin D [83]. Dynasore blocked the uptake of cancer cell-derived EXs due to an endocytosis-inhibiting effect [84]. In addition, the destabilization of lipid rafts in the plasma membrane is another strategy for inhibiting EX uptake (Figure 2C) [85,86].

6. The Therapeutic Effects of Stem Cells Are Mediated by EXs

In recent years, some non-pharmacological methods, such as gene therapy and stem cell therapy, have been considered potential therapeutics for neurodegenerative diseases including PD [87,88]. Mesenchymal stem cells (MSCs) are multipotent progenitor cells that can be isolated from a wide variety of tissues (e.g., bone marrow, adipose tissue, dental tissues, skin, salivary gland, and limb buds) [89]. MSCs are considered therapeutic agents due to their effects on several biological processes, such as immune regulation, oxidative stress, and cytokine secretion [90]. For example, MSCs exert significant antioxidant effects in neurodegenerative diseases [91,92]. While MSC transplantation has been employed in the treatment of several diseases, such as cancer, nerve injury, and neurodegeneration [93–95], several studies have shown that MSC transplantation may cause tumors, embolisms, and abnormal cell differentiation [96], limiting the clinical translation of MSC transplantation as a therapy for PD. Importantly, MSCs exert their biological effects mainly by the secretion of EXs. Thus, the use of EXs derived from MSCs retains the therapeutic potency of MSCs, while preventing the possible damage caused by MSCs [97].

Bone marrow-derived stem cells (BMSCs), in common with other stem cells, can be differentiated into different cells under different physiological conditions. BMSCs can selectively migrate to a site of damage, and interact with neurons and glia, where they stimulate the production of growth factors, such as brain-derived neurotrophic factor (BDNF) and nerve growth factor [98,99]. BMSCs have beneficial effects in models of neurodegenerative diseases [100]. For example, the injection of BMSC-derived EXs into the DA-depleted striatum improved parkinsonian behavior, tyrosine hydroxylase expression, and decreased protein levels of interleukin-6, interleukin-1β, tumor necrosis factor-α, and ROS in the substantia nigra in a rat PD model [101]. It is known that BMSCs mediate their effects through paracrine activities [102]. Importantly, the paracrine activities of BMSCs are mediated through EXs [103].

7. EXs as Therapeutic Delivery Systems in PD

The first-line treatment for PD is the administration of DA and/or by administering agents that increase DA in the brain, specifically, the striatum. Although DA-replacement therapy benefits many PD patients, its therapeutic window is limited due to its decreasing efficacy and increasing side effects, such as dyskinesias [104,105]. Importantly, delivering DA to the brain or agents that increase DA in the brain is difficult due to the blood–brain barrier (BBB). For example, although L-3,4-dihydroxyphenylalanine (L-DOPA) is the most effective treatment for PD symptoms, approximately 1% of the L-DOPA administered systemically reaches the brain [106]. After L-DOPA has reached the brain, it must be converted to DA by DOPA decarboxylase, which is less active in the brains of patients with PD [107]. Moreover, long-term administration of L-DOPA is marred by the emergence of abnormal involuntary movements called L-DOPA-induced dyskinesias [106].

EXs have the potential to serve as carriers of therapeutic agents into the diseased PD brain, in part, due to their ability to readily cross the BBB [108,109], the potential for targeted delivery of exosomal cargo over long distances, and immune resistance [110]. The intravenous administration of DA-encapsulated blood EXs readily crossed the BBB and delivered DA to the brain, including the striatum and substantia nigra. DA-encapsulated EXs increased brain DA content by greater than fifteen-fold and resulted in motor behavioral improvements and increases in DA synthetic enzymes and enzymes against oxidative stress in a 6-hydroxydopamine (6-OHDA) model of PD. Importantly, compared to the intravenous administration of free DA, DA-encapsulated EXs had greater therapeutic efficacy and lower toxicity [111]. Intranasal administration of catalase-loaded EXs was neuroprotective in a 6-OHDA model of PD [112]. The administration of MSC-derived EXs rescued DA neurons in a 6-OHDA model of PD [113]. Stem cell-derived EXs carry beneficial microRNAs (miRNAs) that reduce neuroinflammation in animal models of PD. For example, miR-133b, one of the miRNAs downregulated in PD, can promote neurite outgrowth in both in vitro and in vivo models of PD [114]. In addition, EXs isolated from human neural stem cells (NSCs) exerted a protective effect on PD pathology in a 6-OHDA in vitro and an in vivo mouse model of PD by reducing intracellular ROS and counteracting the activation of apoptotic pathways. NSC-derived EXs carry anti-inflammatory factors and specific miRNAs (i.e., has-miR-182-5p, has-miR-183-5p, has-miR-9, and has-let-7) involved in cell differentiation that contributed to decreased cell loss [115].

8. Strategies to Load EXs with Therapeutic Cargo

After EXs are isolated from tissues, body fluids, or cell culture medium by differential or gradient ultracentrifugation, co-precipitation, size exclusion chromatography, or field flow fractionation [116] then purified to remove unwanted material, they can be loaded with cargo. Notably, EXs are endowed with an aqueous core and a lipid bilayer that allow both hydrophilic and lipophilic cargo to be loaded [117]. In addition to the delivery of small therapeutic compounds, EXs have a natural capacity to transport siRNA, short hairpin RNA (shRNA), miRNA, and proteins [118]. Strategies for loading cargo into EXs include incubation, transfection, and physical treatments.

8.1. Incubation

8.1.1. Incubation of Desired Cargo with EXs

The simplest way to load cargo into EXs is to incubate the desired cargo with EXs or EX-secreting cells to allow the cargo to diffuse into the EXs, following its concentration gradient. Several types of cargo, such as small molecule drugs, nucleic acids, proteins, and peptides have been loaded into EXs using this method [119–121]. Notably, BDNF has been loaded into macrophage-derived EXs and delivered into the brain [120] while the anti-inflammatory and anti-oxidative stress agent, co-enzyme Q10, has been loaded into EXs obtained from adipose-derived stem cells [121]. The strength of the incubation strategy is that it is technically easy and has minimal effects on the structural integrity of the EXs. However, the loading efficiency is low, and the amount of cargo loaded is difficult to control due to the physical and chemical properties of the cargo and EX. For example, hydrophilic drugs tend to reside in the aqueous phase of the interior of EXs, while hydrophobic drugs are more stable in the EX lipid bilayer [122,123]. In addition, pH can influence loading efficiency. When the hydrophilic compound, doxorubicin, was loaded into macrophage-derived EXs, a pH of 8.0 facilitated the diffusion of the compound across the EX lipid bilayer [124].

8.1.2. Incubation of Desired Cargo with EX-Secreting Cells

Drugs and nanomaterials were incubated with EX-secreting cells to generate cargo-loaded EXs. Some small molecule drugs directly pass across the lipid bilayer of parent cells, are packaged into ILVs, and then secreted as EXs. For example, macrophages were incubated with curcumin to generate curcumin-loaded EXs, which were able to cross the BBB and enter the brain [125]. In addition, nanomaterials were incubated with EX-secreting cells to generate cargo-loaded EXs. Although they may induce autophagy and may be destroyed in lysosomes, undegraded nanomaterials are exocytosed within EXs [126]. For example, doxorubicin-loaded silicone nanoparticles were incubated with cancer cells to obtain nanoparticle-loaded EXs for the treatment of lung cancer [126].

8.2. Transfection or Transduction

Transfection or transduction is the most common strategy for stably loading nucleic acids, proteins, and peptides into EXs. Using transfection reagents, specific plasmids are transduced into cells to ectopically express the desired nucleic acids, proteins, or peptides that are later packaged into EXs. For example, MSCs have been transfected with a miR-122-expressing plasmid using a Lipofectamine-based protocol to generate miR-122-enriched EXs [127]. HEK293 cells have been transduced with designed plasmids to generate catalase mRNA-loaded EXs that target the brain to treat PD [128]. HEK293 cells were transfected with lentivirus to generate EXs loaded with translocase of the outer mitochondrial membrane 40 (Tom40). EX-mediated delivery of Tom40 protected cells against hydrogen peroxide-induced oxidative stress [129]. Other types of cells can be transfected with vectors that express proteins and peptides to generate protein- or peptide-loaded EXs [130,131]. In addition, EXs can be directly transfected with nucleic acids by chemical treatment. HEK293 cells have been transfected with siRNA by a heat-shock protocol [132] and cell-derived EXs have been transfected with miR-497 and miR-126 by commercially available kits [133,134]. Although transfection is a common strategy for loading nucleic acids, proteins, or peptides into EXs, the loading efficiency is low [135] and direct chemical transfection of EXs introduces impurities [136].

8.3. Physical Treatments

Physical treatments produce micropores in the EX membrane or membrane recombination that promotes the entry of cargo into EXs to achieve cargo-loaded EXs. Physical treatments include sonication, electroporation, extrusion, the freeze-thaw method, incubation with membrane permeabilizers, and dialysis.

8.3.1. Sonication

Sonication is a physical strategy that applies an extra mechanical shear force to weaken the EX membrane, which promotes the loading of EX cargo [137]. Cancer cell-derived EXs incubated with the anti-cancer drug, gemcitabine, were sonicated. The loading capacity of gemcitabine-loaded EXs was more than four times greater than that of those obtained using the incubation approach [137]. Other researchers have reported that the sonication method results in a higher loading capacity than the incubation approach (e.g., [124]). In addition, nanoparticles and catalase have been loaded into EXs via sonication [112,138]. Note, however, that the sonication method has the potential to produce significant membrane damage. For example, a significant decrease in EX membrane microviscosity was observed after sonication, an effect that was completely reversed after incubating the EXs for 1 h at 37 °C after sonication [139]. Thus, sonication is a simple and effective method for loading cargo into EXs with high loading capacity.

8.3.2. Electroporation

Electroporation is a strategy for loading cargo into EXs through the use of an extra electrical field that produces micropores on the EX membrane to increase permeability. Drugs, nucleic acids, and nanomaterials have all been loaded into EXs using electroporation [139–141]. Although drugs can diffuse, in accordance with their concentration gradient, into EXs via the incubation method, the use of electroporation can significantly increase drug loading efficiency. Researchers have developed modified dendritic cell-derived EXs, which specifically target the brain, by introducing a brain targeting peptide, rabies virus glycoprotein (RVG), on the exterior surface of the EX. An anti-α-syn short hairpin RNA-minicircle (shRNA-MC) construct was loaded into RVG EXs via electroporation. Intravenous administration of shRNA-MC-loaded EXs decreased α-syn aggregation, attenuated the loss of DA-secreting neurons, and improved clinical symptoms in an α-syn preformed fibril model of PD [142].

8.3.3. Extrusion

Extrusion is a physical procedure that utilizes a syringe-based extruder and mechanical force. In this approach, the cargo and EXs are loaded into the extruder equipped with a porous membrane. The extrusion process causes the EXs membrane to collapse and blend with cargo to form cargo-loaded EXs after repeated extrusions under specific parameters [143]. This approach has been taken to load the antioxidant, catalase, into EXs and then deliver the catalase-loaded EXs to the brain as a potential anti-PD therapeutic. The extrusion method resulted in high loading efficiency, sustained release of catalase, and protection of the catalase cargo from degradation by proteases. When administered to mice intranasally, a considerable amount of catalase was detected in the brain and the catalase-loaded EXs had a neuroprotective effect in a 6-OHDA model of PD [112].

8.3.4. Freeze-Thaw Method

The first step of this method is to incubate the isolated EXs with the to-be-loaded cargo for a specific amount of time at room temperature. Next, the EX and cargo solution is rapidly frozen at −80 °C or below, then the solution is thawed at room temperature [112]. For better cargo loading, the aforementioned process is repeated for at least three cycles. Although the freeze-thaw approach is simple and effective to load various cargo (e.g., drugs, proteins, and peptides) into EXs, it has a lower cargo-loading capacity than the sonication and extrusion methods [144] and multiple freeze-thaw cycles could inactivate proteins and induce EX aggregation.

8.3.5. Incubation with Membrane Permeabilizers

Saponin is a surfactant molecule that can form complexes with cholesterol in cell membranes and generate pores, thus leading to an increase in membrane permeabilization [145]. Membrane permeabilizers significantly increase the loading capacity of a variety of cargo into EXs, at least compared to the incubation method [144]. Incubation with saponin resulted in an eleven-fold greater loading of a hydrophilic compound compared to the incubation method [122]. Given the concerns about the hemolytic activity of saponin [145], the concentration of saponin during drug loading should be low, and the EXs should be purified after incubation with saponin.

8.3.6. Dialysis

This method involves placing a mixture of cargo and EXs onto dialysis membranes, which are dialyzed by stirring to obtain cargo-loaded EXs. Compared to the incubation approach, the dialysis procedure has increased the amount of cargo loaded into EXs more than eleven-fold [122]. In addition, the dialysis system can be used to reduce the intra-exosomal pH gradient to generate a pH gradient between the inside and the outside of the exosomal membrane [146]. Although the pH gradient modification increases the loading of miRNA and siRNA into EXs, it may induce the degradation of proteins and peptides [146]. Whereas some studies have reported good cellular uptake of cargo-loaded EXs obtained via the dialysis method [147], others have reported poor cellular uptake [122]. Although the dialysis method appears to be a relatively simple and effective EX-cargo loading technique, researchers should carefully consider the type of loading cargo and whether to use a pH gradient modification.

8.3.7. Comparing Different Loading Methods

The advantages and disadvantages of the different loading approaches are given in Table 1. Note that loading compounds in EXs, regardless of the loading method, may result in greater stability, increased bioavailability, and reduced immunogenicity, as well as preserving the activity of the cargo (as the cargo is protected from degradation) [112,148]. The packaging of the hydrophobic compound, curcumin, in EXs substantially increased its stability in aqueous solutions. The solubility of curcumin-loaded EX was five-fold higher than free curcumin.

Although studies directly comparing exosomal loading by the different loading methods are sparse, the exosomal loading efficiency and cellular uptake of catalase across different loading methods have been assessed. The loading efficiency of catalase into EXs by incubation, the freeze-thaw method, incubation in the presence of saponin, sonication, and extrusion were 4.9%, 14.7%, 18.5%, 22.2%, and 26.1%, respectively. The uptake of catalase-loaded EXs by PC12 cells by incubation, the freeze-thaw method, and sonication were 10%, 15%, and 40%, respectively [112]. Interestingly, regardless of the loading method, the cellular uptake of catalase-loaded EXs was substantially greater than that of poly(lactic-co-glycolic acid) nanoparticles [112], which have been used for the delivery of L-DOPA to the brain to treat PD [149]. The loading efficiencies of the small molecule, porphyrin, into EXs by incubation, electroporation, extrusion, incubation in the presence of saponin, and dialysis were compared. Compared to the loading efficiency of porphyrin into EXs by incubation, the loading efficiency of porphyrin into EXs was increased more than eleven-fold by incubation in the presence of saponin and dialysis but not by electroporation or extrusion [122]. These researchers also observed a four-fold increase in drug uptake by breast cancer cells for EXs loaded by incubation in the presence of saponin and electroporation compared to the uptake of drugs not loaded into EXs [122]. When electroporation and sonication were used to load the highly hydrophobic compound, paclitaxel, into EXs, more than 3 times and more than 19 times, respectively, of paclitaxel was loaded into EXs than when the incubation method was used [139].

Table 1. Advantages and disadvantages, type of cargo that can be loaded, and whether a therapeutic cargo has been used to treat PD for each loading method.

Loading Method	Advantages	Disadvantages	Type of Cargo Loaded	Therapeutic Cargo for PD
Incubation	Simple Minimal effects on EX structure	Low loading capacity Hard to control the amount of cargo loaded	Small drugs, nucleic acids, proteins, peptides	BDNF, co-enzyme Q10, curcumin, DA
Transfection	Easy	Low loading efficiency Possible introduction of impurities	Nucleic acids, proteins, peptides	Catalase mRNA, Tom40
Sonication	Simple High loading capacity	Produces damage to EX membrane	Small drugs, proteins, peptides	None
Electroporation	High loading efficiency	Produces damage to EX membrane Potential to induce EX aggregation	Small drugs, nucleic acids, nanoparticles	shRNA-MC
Extrusion	High loading capacity	Produces damage to EX membrane	Small drugs, proteins, peptides	Catalase
Freeze-Thaw Method	Simple and effective	Potential to inactivate proteins Potential to induce EX aggregation Potential for liposome-EX fusion	Small drugs, proteins, peptides	None
Incubation with Membrane Permeabilizers	Easy High loading capacity	Hemolytic activity of saponin	Small drugs, proteins, peptides	None
Dialysis	Simple High loading capacity	Cellular uptake of dialysis-loaded EX is variable Potential to degrade proteins and peptides	Small drugs, nucleic acids, proteins, peptides	None

9. Strategies to Target EXs to the Brain

9.1. Exploit EX Homing/Tropism

Cells of different origins are known to home in on specific locations in vivo. For example, immune cells preferentially target sites with immunological activity, such as the spleen, to a greater extent than control cells [150]. There is support for the idea that EXs possess intrinsic tropisms based on their cells of origin [151], an attribute that decreases the probability of off-target effects and can be exploited for organ-targeted delivery of EX cargo. For example, EXs secreted from cortical neurons preferentially bind and are endocytosed by neurons [152]. In addition, systemic administration of NSC-derived EXs resulted in preferential brain targeting whereas systemic administration of MSC-derived EXs did not [153]. Notably, brain endothelial cell-derived EXs crossed the BBB and delivered anti-cancer drugs to brain tumors [154].

The currently available methods for EX engineering can be classified into two main approaches: (1) genetic engineering, and (2) chemical modification. Genetic engineering is effective for displaying genetically engineered proteins on the surface of EXs, although it is limited to genetically encodable peptides and proteins. The chemical modification approach can be used to functionalize EXs with a wide range of molecules by using noncovalent or covalent interactions. However, this approach is challenging because of the complexity of the EX membrane and the issues associated with separating unreacted chemicals from the EXs [155].

9.2. Genetic Engineering

One interesting approach to target EXs to the brain has been to genetically modify EX-producing cells by transfecting genes expressing a targeting moiety (e.g., peptides, receptors) with exosomal membrane components, such as tetraspanins, lysosomal membrane-associated protein 2B (LAMP2B), or the C1C2 domain of lactadherin [156,157]. The cells transfected with these vectors generate surface-modified EXs that express the targeting moieties via the natural EX biogenesis process. The EXs produced from genetically engineered cells stably display the introduced target moiety on their surface [158]. For example, cells were transfected with a fusion protein comprised of LAMP2B and RVG, and the cells generated EXs with RVG embedded in the exosomal membrane. These RVG-expressing EXs more readily localized to the brain due to the cell surface expression of receptors for RVG by neurons and glia [159]. Intravenous administration of RVG-expressing EXs resulted in a two-fold greater accumulation of EXs in the brain and a substantial accumulation of EXs in the heart and muscle, which also express receptors for RVG (i.e., nicotinic acetylcholine receptors) [151]. Notably, intravenous administration of a slightly modified RVG peptide, RVG-9R, has been used to transport siRNA to neurons to produce a neuron-specific knockdown [160]. In addition, intravenous administration of RVG-expressing EXs loaded with *GAPDH* siRNA specifically delivered the siRNA to neurons and glial cells in the brain, resulting in an approximately two-fold knockdown of GAPDH mRNA compared to non-treated mice [141]. In an attempt to reduce the expression of mutant huntingtin (mHTT) protein, the root cause of Huntington's disease, mice received tail vein injections of a plasmid containing an RVG, LAMP2B, and mHTT siRNA under the control of a cytomegalovirus promoter. When the plasmid was taken up by hepatocytes, the cytomegalovirus promoter directed the localization of the RVG tag to the EX surface. The RVG-tagged, mHTT siRNA penetrated the BBB, was delivered to the cerebral cortex and striatum, decreased levels of mHTT protein and toxic aggregates in the cerebral cortex and striatum, and ameliorated behavioral deficits in three mouse modes of Huntington's disease [161].

9.3. Chemical Modification

The surface of EXs can be directly engineered via chemical modifications for inducing targetability of therapeutic EXs. One approach is to use covalent attachments of targeting moieties, such as click chemistry, and the other approach uses non-covalent modifications [162].

9.3.1. Covalent Modification of the Surface of EXs

Click chemistry utilizes covalent interactions between an alkyne and azide residue to form a stable triazole linkage, which can be applied to attach targeting moieties on the surface of EXs [162,163]. One of the most common examples of a chemical conjugation method that uses covalent attachments is the modification of the EX's surface with branched polyethylene glycol (PEG), termed PEGylation [164]. Interestingly, to target sigma receptor overexpressing lung cancer cells, EXs were modified with an aminoethylanisamide-PEG moiety, which served as a targeting ligand for the sigma receptor [165]. In addition, c(RGDyK), a peptide that has a high affinity for integrin $\alpha_V\beta_3$, which is expressed in reactive cerebral vascular endothelial cells after ischemia, was conjugated to the surface of MSC-derived EXs via click chemistry [166]. c(RGDyK)-labeled EXs exhibited an eleven-fold tropism to the lesioned region of the ischemic brain compared to scrambled c(RGDyK) peptide-labeled EXs [166]. We are not aware of the use of a covalent modification of the surface of EXs for the targeted delivery of therapeutic EXs to the brain to treat PD.

9.3.2. Non-Covalent Modification of the Surface of EXs

The exosomal membrane can also be engineered via non-covalent methods, such as receptor–ligand binding, electrostatic interaction, and hydrophobic insertion [167,168]. Transferrin was used to conjugate superparamagnetic magnetite colloidal nanocrystal clusters to the surface of EXs by binding to transferrin receptors expressed on the EXs [169]. The electrostatic interaction approach to conjugate targeting moieties to EXs involves interactions of cationic species with negatively charged functional groups on the EX membrane [168]. This method has been used to attach cationic lipids and a pH-sensitive fusogenic peptide to the negatively charged membrane of EXs [170]. These fusogenic peptide-expressing EXs exhibited increased binding to the endosomal membrane after endocytosis, which facilitated the intracellular delivery of cargo [170]. The substance 1,2-dioleoyl-sn-glycero-3-phosphoethanolamine-N-hydroxysuccinimide (DOPE-NHS) is a hydrophobic chemical that can be used to conjugate targeting peptides into exosomal membranes. For targeting EXs to the heart, stem cell-derived EXs were conjugated with cardiac homing peptide via a DOPE-NHS linker, which resulted in EX accumulation in the heart [171]. We are not aware of the use of receptor-ligand binding, electrostatic interaction, and hydrophobic insertion methods for the targeted delivery of therapeutic EXs to the brain to treat PD.

10. Conclusions

EXs play key roles in intercellular communication by delivering biologically active cargo to nearby or distant recipient cells. The cargo delivered by EXs can have a harmful or beneficial effect on the recipient cell. EXs spread α-syn pathology in the olfactory bulb and the gut, then throughout the PD brain, by transferring pathogenic, misfolded forms of α-syn from diseased cells to healthy cells. Pathogenic, misfolded forms of α-syn are transferred via EXs to and from neurons, astrocytes, and microglia. This sets in motion a cascade of events whereby astrocytes and microglia are activated and then secrete ROS and pro-inflammatory cytokines and chemokines into the extracellular space, which contributes to the degeneration of neurons (Figure 1). Researchers have attempted to minimize or ameliorate the pathogenic effects of α-syn-containing EXs by (a) targeting proteins that play a role in EX biogenesis; (b) developing methods aimed at the removal of α-syn-containing EXs from circulation; (c) inhibiting EX uptake by recipient cells; and (d) loading EXs with therapeutic cargo and delivering them to the brain (Figure 2). Advantages of EXs as carriers of therapeutic agents into the diseased brain include their ability to readily cross the BBB, their potential for targeted delivery of therapeutic cargo over a long distance, and their immune resistance. In addition, a wide variety of cargo, including hydrophilic and lipophilic small therapeutic compounds, siRNA, miRNA, and proteins can be loaded into EXs. The choice of loading method depends on the objective of the study and an assessment of the advantages and disadvantages of each (Table 1). Regardless of the loading method, the loading of therapeutic agents into EXs often results in greater stability, increased bioavailability, protection (e.g., from degradation), and reduced immunogenicity. Genetic modification of EX-producing cells and/or EXs and chemical modification of EXs have emerged as powerful approaches for the targeted delivery of therapeutics to neurons and/or glia. Thus, EXs hold great promise for the development of next-generation therapeutics for the treatment of PD.

Funding: This research received no external funding.

Institutional Review Board Statement: Not applicable.

Informed Consent Statement: Not applicable.

Data Availability Statement: Not applicable.

Conflicts of Interest: The author declares no conflict of interest.

References

1. Zaborowski, M.P.; Balaj, L.; Breakefield, X.O.; Lai, C.P. Extracellular Vesicles: Composition, Biological Relevance, and Methods of Study. *Bioscience* **2015**, *65*, 783–797. [CrossRef] [PubMed]
2. Yáñez-Mó, M.; Siljander, P.R.; Andreu, Z.; Zavec, A.B.; Borràs, F.E.; Buzas, E.I.; Buzas, K.; Casal, E.; Cappello, F.; Carvalho, J.; et al. Biological properties of extracellular vesicles and their physiological functions. *J. Extracell. Vesicles* **2015**, *4*, 27066. [CrossRef] [PubMed]

3. Borges, F.T.; Reis, L.A.; Schor, N. Extracellular vesicles: Structure, function, and potential clinical uses in renal diseases. *Braz. J. Med. Biol. Res.* **2013**, *46*, 824–830. [CrossRef]
4. Bebelman, M.P.; Smit, M.J.; Pegtel, D.M.; Baglio, S.R. Biogenesis and function of extracellular vesicles in cancer. *Pharmacol. Ther.* **2018**, *188*, 1–11. [CrossRef]
5. Raposo, G.; Stoorvogel, W. Extracellular vesicles: Exosomes, microvesicles, and friends. *J. Cell Biol.* **2013**, *200*, 373–383. [CrossRef]
6. Cai, H.; Reinisch, K.; Ferro-Novick, S. Coats, tethers, Rabs, and SNAREs work together to mediate the intracellular destination of a transport vesicle. *Dev. Cell* **2007**, *12*, 671–682. [CrossRef] [PubMed]
7. Wickman, G.; Julian, L.; Olson, M.F. How apoptotic cells aid in the removal of their own cold dead bodies. *Cell Death Differ.* **2012**, *19*, 735–742. [CrossRef]
8. van Niel, G.; D'Angelo, G.; Raposo, G. Shedding light on the cell biology of extracellular vesicles. *Nat. Rev. Mol. Cell Biol.* **2018**, *19*, 213–228. [CrossRef] [PubMed]
9. Keerthikumar, S.; Chisanga, D.; Ariyaratne, D.; Al Saffar, H.; Anand, S.; Zhao, K.; Samuel, M.; Pathan, M.; Jois, M.; Chilamkurti, N.; et al. ExoCarta: A Web-Based Compendium of Exosomal Cargo. *J. Mol. Biol.* **2016**, *428*, 688–692. [CrossRef]
10. Riazifar, M.; Pone, E.J.; Lotvall, J.; Zhao, W. Stem Cell Extracellular Vesicles: Extended Messages of Regeneration. *Annu. Rev. Pharmacol. Toxicol.* **2017**, *57*, 125–154. [CrossRef] [PubMed]
11. Familtseva, A.; Jeremic, N.; Tyagi, S.C. Exosomes: Cell-created drug delivery systems. *Mol. Cell. Biochem.* **2019**, *459*, 1–6. [CrossRef]
12. Cocucci, E.; Meldolesi, J. Ectosomes and exosomes: Shedding the confusion between extracellular vesicles. *Trends Cell Biol.* **2015**, *25*, 364–372. [CrossRef] [PubMed]
13. Meldolesi, J. Exosomes and Ectosomes in Intercellular Communication. *Curr. Biol.* **2018**, *28*, R435–R444. [CrossRef] [PubMed]
14. Lebouvier, T.; Chaumette, T.; Paillusson, S.; Duyckaerts, C.; Bruley des Varannes, S.; Neunlist, M.; Derkinderen, P. The second brain and Parkinson's disease. *Eur. J. Neurosci.* **2009**, *30*, 735–741. [CrossRef] [PubMed]
15. Marras, C.; Beck, J.C.; Bower, J.H.; Roberts, E.; Ritz, B.; Ross, G.W.; Abbott, R.D.; Savica, R.; Van Den Eeden, S.K.; Willis, A.W.; et al. Prevalence of Parkinson's disease across North America. *NPJ Park. Dis.* **2018**, *4*, 21. [CrossRef] [PubMed]
16. Spillantini, M.G.; Schmidt, M.L.; Lee, V.M.; Trojanowski, J.Q.; Jakes, R.; Goedert, M. Alpha-synuclein in Lewy bodies. *Nature* **1997**, *388*, 839–840. [CrossRef] [PubMed]
17. Kalia, L.V.; Lang, A.E. Parkinson's disease. *Lancet* **2015**, *386*, 896–912. [CrossRef] [PubMed]
18. Chaudhuri, K.R.; Healy, D.G.; Schapira, A.H.; National Institute for Clinical, E. Non-motor symptoms of Parkinson's disease: Diagnosis and management. *Lancet Neurol.* **2006**, *5*, 235–245. [CrossRef]
19. Liu, W.; Zhang, Q.; Xing, H.; Gao, G.; Liu, J.; Huang, Y.; Yang, H. Characterization of a Novel Monoclonal Antibody for Serine-129 Phosphorylated alpha-Synuclein: A Potential Application for Clinical and Basic Research. *Front. Neurol.* **2022**, *13*, 821792. [CrossRef] [PubMed]
20. Singleton, A.B.; Farrer, M.; Johnson, J.; Singleton, A.; Hague, S.; Kachergus, J.; Hulihan, M.; Peuralinna, T.; Dutra, A.; Nussbaum, R.; et al. alpha-Synuclein locus triplication causes Parkinson's disease. *Science* **2003**, *302*, 841. [CrossRef]
21. Chartier-Harlin, M.C.; Kachergus, J.; Roumier, C.; Mouroux, V.; Douay, X.; Lincoln, S.; Levecque, C.; Larvor, L.; Andrieux, J.; Hulihan, M.; et al. Alpha-synuclein locus duplication as a cause of familial Parkinson's disease. *Lancet* **2004**, *364*, 1167–1169. [CrossRef]
22. Ibanez, P.; Bonnet, A.M.; Debarges, B.; Lohmann, E.; Tison, F.; Pollak, P.; Agid, Y.; Durr, A.; Brice, A. Causal relation between alpha-synuclein gene duplication and familial Parkinson's disease. *Lancet* **2004**, *364*, 1169–1171. [CrossRef]
23. Polymeropoulos, M.H.; Lavedan, C.; Leroy, E.; Ide, S.E.; Dehejia, A.; Dutra, A.; Pike, B.; Root, H.; Rubenstein, J.; Boyer, R.; et al. Mutation in the alpha-synuclein gene identified in families with Parkinson's disease. *Science* **1997**, *276*, 2045–2047. [CrossRef] [PubMed]
24. Conway, K.A.; Lee, S.J.; Rochet, J.C.; Ding, T.T.; Williamson, R.E.; Lansbury, P.T., Jr. Acceleration of oligomerization, not fibrillization, is a shared property of both alpha-synuclein mutations linked to early-onset Parkinson's disease: Implications for pathogenesis and therapy. *Proc. Natl. Acad. Sci. USA* **2000**, *97*, 571–576. [CrossRef] [PubMed]
25. Choi, W.; Zibaee, S.; Jakes, R.; Serpell, L.C.; Davletov, B.; Crowther, R.A.; Goedert, M. Mutation E46K increases phospholipid binding and assembly into filaments of human alpha-synuclein. *FEBS Lett.* **2004**, *576*, 363–368. [CrossRef] [PubMed]
26. Pan, K.M.; Baldwin, M.; Nguyen, J.; Gasset, M.; Serban, A.; Groth, D.; Mehlhorn, I.; Huang, Z.; Fletterick, R.J.; Cohen, F.E.; et al. Conversion of alpha-helices into beta-sheets features in the formation of the scrapie prion proteins. *Proc. Natl. Acad. Sci. USA* **1993**, *90*, 10962–10966. [CrossRef] [PubMed]
27. Chu, Y.; Kordower, J.H. The prion hypothesis of Parkinson's disease. *Curr. Neurol. Neurosci. Rep.* **2015**, *15*, 28. [CrossRef] [PubMed]
28. Kordower, J.H.; Brundin, P. Propagation of host disease to grafted neurons: Accumulating evidence. *Exp. Neurol.* **2009**, *220*, 224–225. [CrossRef]
29. Olanow, C.W.; Brundin, P. Parkinson's disease and alpha synuclein: Is Parkinson's disease a prion-like disorder? *Mov. Disord.* **2013**, *28*, 31–40. [CrossRef]
30. Lee, H.J.; Patel, S.; Lee, S.J. Intravesicular localization and exocytosis of alpha-synuclein and its aggregates. *J. Neurosci.* **2005**, *25*, 6016–6024. [CrossRef] [PubMed]

31. Alvarez-Erviti, L.; Seow, Y.; Schapira, A.H.; Gardiner, C.; Sargent, I.L.; Wood, M.J.; Cooper, J.M. Lysosomal dysfunction increases exosome-mediated alpha-synuclein release and transmission. *Neurobiol. Dis.* **2011**, *42*, 360–367. [CrossRef] [PubMed]
32. Surguchev, A.A.; Emamzadeh, F.N.; Surguchov, A. Cell Responses to Extracellular alpha-Synuclein. *Molecules* **2019**, *24*, 305. [CrossRef] [PubMed]
33. Borghi, R.; Marchese, R.; Negro, A.; Marinelli, L.; Forloni, G.; Zaccheo, D.; Abbruzzese, G.; Tabaton, M. Full length alpha-synuclein is present in cerebrospinal fluid from Parkinson's disease and normal subjects. *Neurosci. Lett.* **2000**, *287*, 65–67. [CrossRef] [PubMed]
34. El-Agnaf, O.M.; Salem, S.A.; Paleologou, K.E.; Cooper, L.J.; Fullwood, N.J.; Gibson, M.J.; Curran, M.D.; Court, J.A.; Mann, D.M.; Ikeda, S.; et al. Alpha-synuclein implicated in Parkinson's disease is present in extracellular biological fluids, including human plasma. *FASEB J.* **2003**, *17*, 1945–1947. [CrossRef] [PubMed]
35. Grey, M.; Dunning, C.J.; Gaspar, R.; Grey, C.; Brundin, P.; Sparr, E.; Linse, S. Acceleration of alpha-synuclein aggregation by exosomes. *J. Biol. Chem.* **2015**, *290*, 2969–2982. [CrossRef] [PubMed]
36. Desplats, P.; Lee, H.J.; Bae, E.J.; Patrick, C.; Rockenstein, E.; Crews, L.; Spencer, B.; Masliah, E.; Lee, S.J. Inclusion formation and neuronal cell death through neuron-to-neuron transmission of alpha-synuclein. *Proc. Natl. Acad. Sci. USA* **2009**, *106*, 13010–13015. [CrossRef]
37. Hansen, C.; Angot, E.; Bergstrom, A.L.; Steiner, J.A.; Pieri, L.; Paul, G.; Outeiro, T.F.; Melki, R.; Kallunki, P.; Fog, K.; et al. alpha-Synuclein propagates from mouse brain to grafted dopaminergic neurons and seeds aggregation in cultured human cells. *J. Clin. Investig.* **2011**, *121*, 715–725. [CrossRef]
38. Emmanouilidou, E.; Melachroinou, K.; Roumeliotis, T.; Garbis, S.D.; Ntzouni, M.; Margaritis, L.H.; Stefanis, L.; Vekrellis, K. Cell-produced alpha-synuclein is secreted in a calcium-dependent manner by exosomes and impacts neuronal survival. *J. Neurosci.* **2010**, *30*, 6838–6851. [CrossRef] [PubMed]
39. Ngolab, J.; Trinh, I.; Rockenstein, E.; Mante, M.; Florio, J.; Trejo, M.; Masliah, D.; Adame, A.; Masliah, E.; Rissman, R.A. Brain-derived exosomes from dementia with Lewy bodies propagate alpha-synuclein pathology. *Acta Neuropathol. Commun.* **2017**, *5*, 46. [CrossRef] [PubMed]
40. Burbidge, K.; Rademacher, D.J.; Mattick, J.; Zack, S.; Grillini, A.; Bousset, L.; Kwon, O.; Kubicki, K.; Simon, A.; Melki, R.; et al. LGALS3 (galectin 3) mediates an unconventional secretion of SNCA/alpha-synuclein in response to lysosomal membrane damage by the autophagic-lysosomal pathway in human midbrain dopamine neurons. *Autophagy* **2022**, *18*, 1020–1048. [CrossRef] [PubMed]
41. Han, C.; Xiong, N.; Guo, X.; Huang, J.; Ma, K.; Liu, L.; Xia, Y.; Shen, Y.; Li, J.; Jiang, H.; et al. Exosomes from patients with Parkinson's disease are pathological in mice. *J. Mol. Med.* **2019**, *97*, 1329–1344. [CrossRef] [PubMed]
42. di Domenico, A.; Carola, G.; Calatayud, C.; Pons-Espinal, M.; Munoz, J.P.; Richaud-Patin, Y.; Fernandez-Carasa, I.; Gut, M.; Faella, A.; Parameswaran, J.; et al. Patient-Specific iPSC-Derived Astrocytes Contribute to Non-Cell-Autonomous Neurodegeneration in Parkinson's Disease. *Stem Cell Rep.* **2019**, *12*, 213–229. [CrossRef]
43. Lee, H.J.; Suk, J.E.; Bae, E.J.; Lee, S.J. Clearance and deposition of extracellular alpha-synuclein aggregates in microglia. *Biochem. Biophys. Res. Commun.* **2008**, *372*, 423–428. [CrossRef]
44. Liu, J.; Zhou, Y.; Wang, Y.; Fong, H.; Murray, T.M.; Zhang, J. Identification of proteins involved in microglial endocytosis of alpha-synuclein. *J. Proteome Res.* **2007**, *6*, 3614–3627. [CrossRef] [PubMed]
45. Guo, M.; Wang, J.; Zhao, Y.; Feng, Y.; Han, S.; Dong, Q.; Cui, M.; Tieu, K. Microglial exosomes facilitate alpha-synuclein transmission in Parkinson's disease. *Brain* **2020**, *143*, 1476–1497. [CrossRef] [PubMed]
46. Chang, C.; Lang, H.; Geng, N.; Wang, J.; Li, N.; Wang, X. Exosomes of BV-2 cells induced by alpha-synuclein: Important mediator of neurodegeneration in PD. *Neurosci. Lett.* **2013**, *548*, 190–195. [CrossRef]
47. Iannaccone, S.; Cerami, C.; Alessio, M.; Garibotto, V.; Panzacchi, A.; Olivieri, S.; Gelsomino, G.; Moresco, R.M.; Perani, D. In vivo microglia activation in very early dementia with Lewy bodies, comparison with Parkinson's disease. *Park. Relat. Disord.* **2013**, *19*, 47–52. [CrossRef]
48. Ouchi, Y.; Yoshikawa, E.; Sekine, Y.; Futatsubashi, M.; Kanno, T.; Ogusu, T.; Torizuka, T. Microglial activation and dopamine terminal loss in early Parkinson's disease. *Ann. Neurol.* **2005**, *57*, 168–175. [CrossRef] [PubMed]
49. Imamura, K.; Hishikawa, N.; Sawada, M.; Nagatsu, T.; Yoshida, M.; Hashizume, Y. Distribution of major histocompatibility complex class II-positive microglia and cytokine profile of Parkinson's disease brains. *Acta Neuropathol.* **2003**, *106*, 518–526. [CrossRef]
50. Batchelor, P.E.; Porritt, M.J.; Martinello, P.; Parish, C.L.; Liberatore, G.T.; Donnan, G.A.; Howells, D.W. Macrophages and Microglia Produce Local Trophic Gradients That Stimulate Axonal Sprouting Toward but Not beyond the Wound Edge. *Mol. Cell. Neurosci.* **2002**, *21*, 436–453. [CrossRef]
51. Bruck, D.; Wenning, G.K.; Stefanova, N.; Fellner, L. Glia and alpha-synuclein in neurodegeneration: A complex interaction. *Neurobiol. Dis.* **2016**, *85*, 262–274. [CrossRef] [PubMed]
52. Stefanova, N.; Fellner, L.; Reindl, M.; Masliah, E.; Poewe, W.; Wenning, G.K. Toll-like receptor 4 promotes alpha-synuclein clearance and survival of nigral dopaminergic neurons. *Am. J. Pathol.* **2011**, *179*, 954–963. [CrossRef] [PubMed]
53. Fellner, L.; Irschick, R.; Schanda, K.; Reindl, M.; Klimaschewski, L.; Poewe, W.; Wenning, G.K.; Stefanova, N. Toll-like receptor 4 is required for alpha-synuclein dependent activation of microglia and astroglia. *Glia* **2013**, *61*, 349–360. [CrossRef] [PubMed]

54. Su, X.; Federoff, H.J.; Maguire-Zeiss, K.A. Mutant alpha-synuclein overexpression mediates early proinflammatory activity. *Neurotox. Res.* **2009**, *16*, 238–254. [CrossRef]
55. Alvarez-Erviti, L.; Couch, Y.; Richardson, J.; Cooper, J.M.; Wood, M.J. Alpha-synuclein release by neurons activates the inflammatory response in a microglial cell line. *Neurosci. Res.* **2011**, *69*, 337–342. [CrossRef]
56. Roodveldt, C.; Labrador-Garrido, A.; Gonzalez-Rey, E.; Fernandez-Montesinos, R.; Caro, M.; Lachaud, C.C.; Waudby, C.A.; Delgado, M.; Dobson, C.M.; Pozo, D. Glial innate immunity generated by non-aggregated alpha-synuclein in mouse: Differences between wild-type and Parkinson's disease-linked mutants. *PLoS ONE* **2010**, *5*, e13481. [CrossRef] [PubMed]
57. Rojanathammanee, L.; Murphy, E.J.; Combs, C.K. Expression of mutant alpha-synuclein modulates microglial phenotype in vitro. *J. Neuroinflamm.* **2011**, *8*, 44. [CrossRef]
58. Zhang, W.; Wang, T.; Pei, Z.; Miller, D.S.; Wu, X.; Block, M.L.; Wilson, B.; Zhang, W.; Zhou, Y.; Hong, J.S.; et al. Aggregated alpha-synuclein activates microglia: A process leading to disease progression in Parkinson's disease. *FASEB J.* **2005**, *19*, 533–542. [CrossRef]
59. Reynolds, A.D.; Glanzer, J.G.; Kadiu, I.; Ricardo-Dukelow, M.; Chaudhuri, A.; Ciborowski, P.; Cerny, R.; Gelman, B.; Thomas, M.P.; Mosley, R.L.; et al. Nitrated alpha-synuclein-activated microglial profiling for Parkinson's disease. *J. Neurochem.* **2008**, *104*, 1504–1525. [CrossRef]
60. Hirsch, E.C.; Vyas, S.; Hunot, S. Neuroinflammation in Parkinson's disease. *Park. Relat. Disord.* **2012**, *18* (Suppl. S1), S210–S212. [CrossRef]
61. El Andaloussi, S.; Mager, I.; Breakefield, X.O.; Wood, M.J. Extracellular vesicles: Biology and emerging therapeutic opportunities. *Nat. Rev. Drug Discov.* **2013**, *12*, 347–357. [CrossRef] [PubMed]
62. Knott, C.; Stern, G.; Kingsbury, A.; Welcher, A.A.; Wilkin, G.P. Elevated glial brain-derived neurotrophic factor in Parkinson's diseased nigra. *Park. Relat. Disord.* **2002**, *8*, 329–341. [CrossRef]
63. Mythri, R.B.; Venkateshappa, C.; Harish, G.; Mahadevan, A.; Muthane, U.B.; Yasha, T.C.; Srinivas Bharath, M.M.; Shankar, S.K. Evaluation of markers of oxidative stress, antioxidant function and astrocytic proliferation in the striatum and frontal cortex of Parkinson's disease brains. *Neurochem. Res.* **2011**, *36*, 1452–1463. [CrossRef]
64. Sandhu, J.K.; Gardaneh, M.; Iwasiow, R.; Lanthier, P.; Gangaraju, S.; Ribecco-Lutkiewicz, M.; Tremblay, R.; Kiuchi, K.; Sikorska, M. Astrocyte-secreted GDNF and glutathione antioxidant system protect neurons against 6OHDA cytotoxicity. *Neurobiol. Dis.* **2009**, *33*, 405–414. [CrossRef]
65. Hirsch, E.C.; Hunot, S.; Hartmann, A. Neuroinflammatory processes in Parkinson's disease. *Park. Relat. Disord.* **2005**, *11* (Suppl. S1), S9–S15. [CrossRef]
66. Vila, M.; Jackson-Lewis, V.; Guegan, C.; Wu, D.C.; Teismann, P.; Choi, D.K.; Tieu, K.; Przedborski, S. The role of glial cells in Parkinson's disease. *Curr. Opin. Neurol.* **2001**, *14*, 483–489. [CrossRef] [PubMed]
67. Wakabayashi, K.; Hayashi, S.; Yoshimoto, M.; Kudo, H.; Takahashi, H. NACP/alpha-synuclein-positive filamentous inclusions in astrocytes and oligodendrocytes of Parkinson's disease brains. *Acta Neuropathol.* **2000**, *99*, 14–20. [CrossRef]
68. Halliday, G.M.; Stevens, C.H. Glia: Initiators and progressors of pathology in Parkinson's disease. *Mov. Disord.* **2011**, *26*, 6–17. [CrossRef]
69. Klegeris, A.; Giasson, B.I.; Zhang, H.; Maguire, J.; Pelech, S.; McGeer, P.L. Alpha-synuclein and its disease-causing mutants induce ICAM-1 and IL-6 in human astrocytes and astrocytoma cells. *FASEB J.* **2006**, *20*, 2000–2008. [CrossRef] [PubMed]
70. Mulcahy, L.A.; Pink, R.C.; Carter, D.R. Routes and mechanisms of extracellular vesicle uptake. *J. Extracell. Vesicles* **2014**, *3*, 24641. [CrossRef]
71. Hessvik, N.P.; Llorente, A. Current knowledge on exosome biogenesis and release. *Cell. Mol. Life Sci.* **2018**, *75*, 193–208. [CrossRef]
72. Gurung, S.; Perocheau, D.; Touramanidou, L.; Baruteau, J. The exosome journey: From biogenesis to uptake and intracellular signalling. *Cell Commun. Signal.* **2021**, *19*, 47. [CrossRef] [PubMed]
73. Baietti, M.F.; Zhang, Z.; Mortier, E.; Melchior, A.; Degeest, G.; Geeraerts, A.; Ivarsson, Y.; Depoortere, F.; Coomans, C.; Vermeiren, E.; et al. Syndecan-syntenin-ALIX regulates the biogenesis of exosomes. *Nat. Cell Biol.* **2012**, *14*, 677–685. [CrossRef]
74. Song, L.; Tang, S.; Han, X.; Jiang, Z.; Dong, L.; Liu, C.; Liang, X.; Dong, J.; Qiu, C.; Wang, Y.; et al. KIBRA controls exosome secretion via inhibiting the proteasomal degradation of Rab27a. *Nat. Commun.* **2019**, *10*, 1639. [CrossRef] [PubMed]
75. Hsu, C.; Morohashi, Y.; Yoshimura, S.; Manrique-Hoyos, N.; Jung, S.; Lauterbach, M.A.; Bakhti, M.; Gronborg, M.; Mobius, W.; Rhee, J.; et al. Regulation of exosome secretion by Rab35 and its GTPase-activating proteins TBC1D10A-C. *J. Cell Biol.* **2010**, *189*, 223–232. [CrossRef] [PubMed]
76. Ostrowski, M.; Carmo, N.B.; Krumeich, S.; Fanget, I.; Raposo, G.; Savina, A.; Moita, C.F.; Schauer, K.; Hume, A.N.; Freitas, R.P.; et al. Rab27a and Rab27b control different steps of the exosome secretion pathway. *Nat. Cell Biol.* **2010**, *12* (Suppl. S11–S13), 19–30. [CrossRef]
77. Bobrie, A.; Krumeich, S.; Reyal, F.; Recchi, C.; Moita, L.F.; Seabra, M.C.; Ostrowski, M.; Thery, C. Rab27a supports exosome-dependent and -independent mechanisms that modify the tumor microenvironment and can promote tumor progression. *Cancer Res.* **2012**, *72*, 4920–4930. [CrossRef] [PubMed]
78. Catalano, M.; O'Driscoll, L. Inhibiting extracellular vesicles formation and release: A review of EV inhibitors. *J. Extracell. Vesicles* **2020**, *9*, 1703244. [CrossRef]
79. Jiang, T.; Xu, C.; Gao, S.; Zhang, J.; Zheng, J.; Wu, X.; Lu, Q.; Cao, L.; Yang, D.; Xu, J.; et al. Cathepsin L-containing exosomes from alpha-synuclein-activated microglia induce neurotoxicity through the P2X7 receptor. *NPJ Park. Dis.* **2022**, *8*, 127. [CrossRef]

80. Tsutsumi, R.; Hori, Y.; Seki, T.; Kurauchi, Y.; Sato, M.; Oshima, M.; Hisatsune, A.; Katsuki, H. Involvement of exosomes in dopaminergic neurodegeneration by microglial activation in midbrain slice cultures. *Biochem. Biophys. Res. Commun.* **2019**, *511*, 427–433. [CrossRef]
81. Zhu, C.; Bilousova, T.; Focht, S.; Jun, M.; Elias, C.J.; Melnik, M.; Chandra, S.; Campagna, J.; Cohn, W.; Hatami, A.; et al. Pharmacological inhibition of nSMase2 reduces brain exosome release and alpha-synuclein pathology in a Parkinson's disease model. *Mol. Brain* **2021**, *14*, 70. [CrossRef] [PubMed]
82. Nishida-Aoki, N.; Tominaga, N.; Takeshita, F.; Sonoda, H.; Yoshioka, Y.; Ochiya, T. Disruption of Circulating Extracellular Vesicles as a Novel Therapeutic Strategy against Cancer Metastasis. *Mol. Ther.* **2017**, *25*, 181–191. [CrossRef]
83. Zhao, H.; Yang, L.; Baddour, J.; Achreja, A.; Bernard, V.; Moss, T.; Marini, J.C.; Tudawe, T.; Seviour, E.G.; San Lucas, F.A.; et al. Tumor microenvironment derived exosomes pleiotropically modulate cancer cell metabolism. *eLife* **2016**, *5*, e10250. [CrossRef]
84. Kawamoto, T.; Ohga, N.; Akiyama, K.; Hirata, N.; Kitahara, S.; Maishi, N.; Osawa, T.; Yamamoto, K.; Kondoh, M.; Shindoh, M.; et al. Tumor-derived microvesicles induce proangiogenic phenotype in endothelial cells via endocytosis. *PLoS ONE* **2012**, *7*, e34045. [CrossRef] [PubMed]
85. Lima, L.G.; Chammas, R.; Monteiro, R.Q.; Moreira, M.E.; Barcinski, M.A. Tumor-derived microvesicles modulate the establishment of metastatic melanoma in a phosphatidylserine-dependent manner. *Cancer Lett.* **2009**, *283*, 168–175. [CrossRef]
86. Plebanek, M.P.; Mutharasan, R.K.; Volpert, O.; Matov, A.; Gatlin, J.C.; Thaxton, C.S. Nanoparticle Targeting and Cholesterol Flux Through Scavenger Receptor Type B-1 Inhibits Cellular Exosome Uptake. *Sci. Rep.* **2015**, *5*, 15724. [CrossRef] [PubMed]
87. Dass, B.; Kordower, J.H. Gene therapy approaches for the treatment of Parkinson's disease. *Handb. Clin. Neurol.* **2007**, *84*, 291–304. [CrossRef] [PubMed]
88. Cha, Y.; Park, T.Y.; Leblanc, P.; Kim, K.S. Current Status and Future Perspectives on Stem Cell-Based Therapies for Parkinson's Disease. *J. Mov. Disord.* **2023**, *16*, 22–41. [CrossRef]
89. Mushahary, D.; Spittler, A.; Kasper, C.; Weber, V.; Charwat, V. Isolation, cultivation, and characterization of human mesenchymal stem cells. *Cytom. Part A* **2018**, *93*, 19–31. [CrossRef]
90. Yeo, G.E.C.; Ng, M.H.; Nordin, F.B.; Law, J.X. Potential of Mesenchymal Stem Cells in the Rejuvenation of the Aging Immune System. *Int. J. Mol. Sci.* **2021**, *22*, 5749. [CrossRef]
91. Cui, G.H.; Wu, J.; Mou, F.F.; Xie, W.H.; Wang, F.B.; Wang, Q.L.; Fang, J.; Xu, Y.W.; Dong, Y.R.; Liu, J.R.; et al. Exosomes derived from hypoxia-preconditioned mesenchymal stromal cells ameliorate cognitive decline by rescuing synaptic dysfunction and regulating inflammatory responses in APP/PS1 mice. *FASEB J.* **2018**, *32*, 654–668. [CrossRef] [PubMed]
92. Cui, Y.; Ma, S.; Zhang, C.; Cao, W.; Liu, M.; Li, D.; Lv, P.; Xing, Q.; Qu, R.; Yao, N.; et al. Human umbilical cord mesenchymal stem cells transplantation improves cognitive function in Alzheimer's disease mice by decreasing oxidative stress and promoting hippocampal neurogenesis. *Behav. Brain Res.* **2017**, *320*, 291–301. [CrossRef] [PubMed]
93. Li, X.; Tan, J.; Xiao, Z.; Zhao, Y.; Han, S.; Liu, D.; Yin, W.; Li, J.; Li, J.; Wanggou, S.; et al. Transplantation of hUC-MSCs seeded collagen scaffolds reduces scar formation and promotes functional recovery in canines with chronic spinal cord injury. *Sci. Rep.* **2017**, *7*, 43559. [CrossRef] [PubMed]
94. Chelluboina, B.; Dinh, D.H.; Veeravalli, K.K. Transdifferentiation of differentiated stem cells contributes to remyelination. *Stem Cell Res. Ther.* **2015**, *6*, 191. [CrossRef] [PubMed]
95. Shao, Z.H.; Wang, P.J.; Li, M.H.; Zhang, W.; Zheng, S.Q.; Zhao, X.H.; Wang, G.L.; Shang, M.Y.; Mao, X.Q. Effects of mesenchymal stem cell transplantation on growth of liver cancer: Experiment with rats. *Zhonghua Yi Xue Za Zhi* **2009**, *89*, 491–496.
96. Zeltz, C.; Primac, I.; Erusappan, P.; Alam, J.; Noel, A.; Gullberg, D. Cancer-associated fibroblasts in desmoplastic tumors: Emerging role of integrins. *Semin. Cancer Biol.* **2020**, *62*, 166–181. [CrossRef]
97. Yousefi Dehbidi, M.; Goodarzi, N.; Azhdari, M.H.; Doroudian, M. Mesenchymal stem cells and their derived exosomes to combat COVID-19. *Rev. Med. Virol.* **2022**, *32*, e2281. [CrossRef]
98. Kurozumi, K.; Nakamura, K.; Tamiya, T.; Kawano, Y.; Kobune, M.; Hirai, S.; Uchida, H.; Sasaki, K.; Ito, Y.; Kato, K.; et al. BDNF gene-modified mesenchymal stem cells promote functional recovery and reduce infarct size in the rat middle cerebral artery occlusion model. *Mol. Ther.* **2004**, *9*, 189–197. [CrossRef]
99. Matthay, M.A.; Pati, S.; Lee, J.W. Concise Review: Mesenchymal Stem (Stromal) Cells: Biology and Preclinical Evidence for Therapeutic Potential for Organ Dysfunction Following Trauma or Sepsis. *Stem Cells* **2017**, *35*, 316–324. [CrossRef]
100. Yan, Y.C.; Li, Y.H.; Xiao, B.G.; Wang, J.; Xi, J.Y.; Yu, W.B. Cellular and Molecular Mechanisms Underly the Combined Treatment of Fasudil and Bone Marrow Derived-Neuronal Stem Cells in a Parkinson's Disease Mouse Model. *Mol. Neurobiol.* **2022**, *60*, 1826–1835. [CrossRef]
101. Li, Y.; Li, Z.; Gu, J.; Xu, X.; Chen, H.; Gui, Y. Exosomes isolated during dopaminergic neuron differentiation suppressed neuronal inflammation in a rodent model of Parkinson's disease. *Neurosci. Lett.* **2022**, *771*, 136414. [CrossRef] [PubMed]
102. Phinney, D.G.; Pittenger, M.F. Concise Review: MSC-Derived Exosomes for Cell-Free Therapy. *Stem Cells* **2017**, *35*, 851–858. [CrossRef]
103. Teixeira, C.P.; Florencio-Silva, R.; Sasso, G.R.S.; Carbonel, A.A.F.; Simoes, R.S.; Simoes, M.J. Soy isoflavones protect against oxidative stress and diminish apoptosis in ovary of middle-aged female rats. *Gynecol. Endocrinol.* **2019**, *35*, 586–590. [CrossRef] [PubMed]
104. Weiss, J.L.; Ng, L.K.; Chase, T.N. Long-lasting dyskinesia induced by levodopa. *Lancet* **1971**, *1*, 1016–1017. [CrossRef] [PubMed]
105. Kang, U.J.; Fahn, S. Management of tardive dyskinesia. *Ration. Drug Ther.* **1988**, *22*, 1–7.

106. Huot, P.; Johnston, T.H.; Koprich, J.B.; Fox, S.H.; Brotchie, J.M. The pharmacology of L-DOPA-induced dyskinesia in Parkinson's disease. *Pharmacol. Rev.* **2013**, *65*, 171–222. [CrossRef]
107. Kuwabara, H.; Cumming, P.; Yasuhara, Y.; Leger, G.C.; Guttman, M.; Diksic, M.; Evans, A.C.; Gjedde, A. Regional striatal DOPA transport and decarboxylase activity in Parkinson's disease. *J. Nucl. Med.* **1995**, *36*, 1226–1231.
108. Samanta, S.; Rajasingh, S.; Drosos, N.; Zhou, Z.; Dawn, B.; Rajasingh, J. Exosomes: New molecular targets of diseases. *Acta Pharmacol. Sin.* **2018**, *39*, 501–513. [CrossRef]
109. Gomez-Molina, C.; Sandoval, M.; Henzi, R.; Ramirez, J.P.; Varas-Godoy, M.; Luarte, A.; Lafourcade, C.A.; Lopez-Verrilli, A.; Smalla, K.H.; Kaehne, T.; et al. Small Extracellular Vesicles in Rat Serum Contain Astrocyte-Derived Protein Biomarkers of Repetitive Stress. *Int. J. Neuropsychopharmacol.* **2019**, *22*, 232–246. [CrossRef]
110. Bunggulawa, E.J.; Wang, W.; Yin, T.; Wang, N.; Durkan, C.; Wang, Y.; Wang, G. Recent advancements in the use of exosomes as drug delivery systems. *J. Nanobiotechnol.* **2018**, *16*, 81. [CrossRef]
111. Qu, M.; Lin, Q.; Huang, L.; Fu, Y.; Wang, L.; He, S.; Fu, Y.; Yang, S.; Zhang, Z.; Zhang, L.; et al. Dopamine-loaded blood exosomes targeted to brain for better treatment of Parkinson's disease. *J. Control. Release* **2018**, *287*, 156–166. [CrossRef] [PubMed]
112. Haney, M.J.; Klyachko, N.L.; Zhao, Y.; Gupta, R.; Plotnikova, E.G.; He, Z.; Patel, T.; Piroyan, A.; Sokolsky, M.; Kabanov, A.V.; et al. Exosomes as drug delivery vehicles for Parkinson's disease therapy. *J. Control. Release* **2015**, *207*, 18–30. [CrossRef] [PubMed]
113. Vilaca-Faria, H.; Salgado, A.J.; Teixeira, F.G. Mesenchymal Stem Cells-derived Exosomes: A New Possible Therapeutic Strategy for Parkinson's Disease? *Cells* **2019**, *8*, 118. [CrossRef]
114. Xin, H.; Li, Y.; Buller, B.; Katakowski, M.; Zhang, Y.; Wang, X.; Shang, X.; Zhang, Z.G.; Chopp, M. Exosome-mediated transfer of miR-133b from multipotent mesenchymal stromal cells to neural cells contributes to neurite outgrowth. *Stem Cells* **2012**, *30*, 1556–1564. [CrossRef]
115. Lee, E.J.; Choi, Y.; Lee, H.J.; Hwang, D.W.; Lee, D.S. Human neural stem cell-derived extracellular vesicles protect against Parkinson's disease pathologies. *J. Nanobiotechnol.* **2022**, *20*, 198. [CrossRef] [PubMed]
116. Shao, H.; Im, H.; Castro, C.M.; Breakefield, X.; Weissleder, R.; Lee, H. New Technologies for Analysis of Extracellular Vesicles. *Chem. Rev.* **2018**, *118*, 1917–1950. [CrossRef]
117. Ren, J.; He, W.; Zheng, L.; Duan, H. From structures to functions: Insights into exosomes as promising drug delivery vehicles. *Biomater. Sci.* **2016**, *4*, 910–921. [CrossRef]
118. Johnsen, K.B.; Gudbergsson, J.M.; Skov, M.N.; Pilgaard, L.; Moos, T.; Duroux, M. A comprehensive overview of exosomes as drug delivery vehicles—Endogenous nanocarriers for targeted cancer therapy. *Biochim. Biophys. Acta* **2014**, *1846*, 75–87. [CrossRef]
119. Gong, C.; Tian, J.; Wang, Z.; Gao, Y.; Wu, X.; Ding, X.; Qiang, L.; Li, G.; Han, Z.; Yuan, Y.; et al. Functional exosome-mediated co-delivery of doxorubicin and hydrophobically modified microRNA 159 for triple-negative breast cancer therapy. *J. Nanobiotechnol.* **2019**, *17*, 93. [CrossRef]
120. Yuan, D.; Zhao, Y.; Banks, W.A.; Bullock, K.M.; Haney, M.; Batrakova, E.; Kabanov, A.V. Macrophage exosomes as natural nanocarriers for protein delivery to inflamed brain. *Biomaterials* **2017**, *142*, 1–12. [CrossRef]
121. Sheykhhasan, M.; Amini, R.; Soleimani Asl, S.; Saidijam, M.; Hashemi, S.M.; Najafi, R. Neuroprotective effects of coenzyme Q10-loaded exosomes obtained from adipose-derived stem cells in a rat model of Alzheimer's disease. *Biomed. Pharmacother.* **2022**, *152*, 113224. [CrossRef]
122. Fuhrmann, G.; Serio, A.; Mazo, M.; Nair, R.; Stevens, M.M. Active loading into extracellular vesicles significantly improves the cellular uptake and photodynamic effect of porphyrins. *J. Control. Release* **2015**, *205*, 35–44. [CrossRef] [PubMed]
123. Oskouie, M.N.; Aghili Moghaddam, N.S.; Butler, A.E.; Zamani, P.; Sahebkar, A. Therapeutic use of curcumin-encapsulated and curcumin-primed exosomes. *J. Cell. Physiol.* **2019**, *234*, 8182–8191. [CrossRef]
124. Haney, M.J.; Zhao, Y.; Jin, Y.S.; Li, S.M.; Bago, J.R.; Klyachko, N.L.; Kabanov, A.V.; Batrakova, E.V. Macrophage-Derived Extracellular Vesicles as Drug Delivery Systems for Triple Negative Breast Cancer (TNBC) Therapy. *J. Neuroimmune Pharmacol.* **2020**, *15*, 487–500. [CrossRef]
125. Wang, H.; Sui, H.; Zheng, Y.; Jiang, Y.; Shi, Y.; Liang, J.; Zhao, L. Curcumin-primed exosomes potently ameliorate cognitive function in AD mice by inhibiting hyperphosphorylation of the Tau protein through the AKT/GSK-3beta pathway. *Nanoscale* **2019**, *11*, 7481–7496. [CrossRef] [PubMed]
126. Yong, T.; Zhang, X.; Bie, N.; Zhang, H.; Zhang, X.; Li, F.; Hakeem, A.; Hu, J.; Gan, L.; Santos, H.A.; et al. Tumor exosome-based nanoparticles are efficient drug carriers for chemotherapy. *Nat. Commun.* **2019**, *10*, 3838. [CrossRef]
127. Lou, G.; Song, X.; Yang, F.; Wu, S.; Wang, J.; Chen, Z.; Liu, Y. Exosomes derived from miR-122-modified adipose tissue-derived MSCs increase chemosensitivity of hepatocellular carcinoma. *J. Hematol. Oncol.* **2015**, *8*, 122. [CrossRef] [PubMed]
128. Kojima, R.; Bojar, D.; Rizzi, G.; Hamri, G.C.; El-Baba, M.D.; Saxena, P.; Auslander, S.; Tan, K.R.; Fussenegger, M. Designer exosomes produced by implanted cells intracerebrally deliver therapeutic cargo for Parkinson's disease treatment. *Nat. Commun.* **2018**, *9*, 1305. [CrossRef]
129. Sayeed, N.; Sugaya, K. Exosome mediated Tom40 delivery protects against hydrogen peroxide-induced oxidative stress by regulating mitochondrial function. *PLoS ONE* **2022**, *17*, e0272511. [CrossRef]
130. Kim, G.; Kim, M.; Lee, Y.; Byun, J.W.; Hwang, D.W.; Lee, M. Systemic delivery of microRNA-21 antisense oligonucleotides to the brain using T7-peptide decorated exosomes. *J. Control. Release* **2020**, *317*, 273–281. [CrossRef]
131. Ran, N.; Gao, X.; Dong, X.; Li, J.; Lin, C.; Geng, M.; Yin, H. Effects of exosome-mediated delivery of myostatin propeptide on functional recovery of mdx mice. *Biomaterials* **2020**, *236*, 119826. [CrossRef] [PubMed]

132. Pi, F.; Binzel, D.W.; Lee, T.J.; Li, Z.; Sun, M.; Rychahou, P.; Li, H.; Haque, F.; Wang, S.; Croce, C.M.; et al. Nanoparticle orientation to control RNA loading and ligand display on extracellular vesicles for cancer regression. *Nat. Nanotechnol.* **2018**, *13*, 82–89. [CrossRef] [PubMed]
133. Jeong, K.; Yu, Y.J.; You, J.Y.; Rhee, W.J.; Kim, J.A. Exosome-mediated microRNA-497 delivery for anti-cancer therapy in a microfluidic 3D lung cancer model. *Lab Chip* **2020**, *20*, 548–557. [CrossRef]
134. Nie, H.; Xie, X.; Zhang, D.; Zhou, Y.; Li, B.; Li, F.; Li, F.; Cheng, Y.; Mei, H.; Meng, H.; et al. Use of lung-specific exosomes for miRNA-126 delivery in non-small cell lung cancer. *Nanoscale* **2020**, *12*, 877–887. [CrossRef] [PubMed]
135. Li, Z.; Zhou, X.; Wei, M.; Gao, X.; Zhao, L.; Shi, R.; Sun, W.; Duan, Y.; Yang, G.; Yuan, L. In Vitro and in Vivo RNA Inhibition by CD9-HuR Functionalized Exosomes Encapsulated with miRNA or CRISPR/dCas9. *Nano Lett.* **2019**, *19*, 19–28. [CrossRef]
136. Shtam, T.A.; Kovalev, R.A.; Varfolomeeva, E.Y.; Makarov, E.M.; Kil, Y.V.; Filatov, M.V. Exosomes are natural carriers of exogenous siRNA to human cells in vitro. *Cell Commun. Signal.* **2013**, *11*, 88. [CrossRef]
137. Li, Y.J.; Wu, J.Y.; Wang, J.M.; Hu, X.B.; Cai, J.X.; Xiang, D.X. Gemcitabine loaded autologous exosomes for effective and safe chemotherapy of pancreatic cancer. *Acta Biomater.* **2020**, *101*, 519–530. [CrossRef]
138. Sancho-Albero, M.; Rubio-Ruiz, B.; Perez-Lopez, A.M.; Sebastian, V.; Martin-Duque, P.; Arruebo, M.; Santamaria, J.; Unciti-Broceta, A. Cancer-derived exosomes loaded with ultrathin palladium nanosheets for targeted bioorthogonal catalysis. *Nat. Catal.* **2019**, *2*, 864–872. [CrossRef]
139. Kim, M.S.; Haney, M.J.; Zhao, Y.; Mahajan, V.; Deygen, I.; Klyachko, N.L.; Inskoe, E.; Piroyan, A.; Sokolsky, M.; Okolie, O.; et al. Development of exosome-encapsulated paclitaxel to overcome MDR in cancer cells. *Nanomedicine* **2016**, *12*, 655–664. [CrossRef]
140. Tian, Y.; Li, S.; Song, J.; Ji, T.; Zhu, M.; Anderson, G.J.; Wei, J.; Nie, G. A doxorubicin delivery platform using engineered natural membrane vesicle exosomes for targeted tumor therapy. *Biomaterials* **2014**, *35*, 2383–2390. [CrossRef]
141. Alvarez-Erviti, L.; Seow, Y.; Yin, H.; Betts, C.; Lakhal, S.; Wood, M.J. Delivery of siRNA to the mouse brain by systemic injection of targeted exosomes. *Nat. Biotechnol.* **2011**, *29*, 341–345. [CrossRef] [PubMed]
142. Izco, M.; Blesa, J.; Schleef, M.; Schmeer, M.; Porcari, R.; Al-Shawi, R.; Ellmerich, S.; de Toro, M.; Gardiner, C.; Seow, Y.; et al. Systemic Exosomal Delivery of shRNA Minicircles Prevents Parkinsonian Pathology. *Mol. Ther.* **2019**, *27*, 2111–2122. [CrossRef]
143. Kalimuthu, S.; Gangadaran, P.; Rajendran, R.L.; Zhu, L.; Oh, J.M.; Lee, H.W.; Gopal, A.; Baek, S.H.; Jeong, S.Y.; Lee, S.W.; et al. A New Approach for Loading Anticancer Drugs Into Mesenchymal Stem Cell-Derived Exosome Mimetics for Cancer Therapy. *Front. Pharmacol.* **2018**, *9*, 1116. [CrossRef]
144. Luan, X.; Sansanaphongpricha, K.; Myers, I.; Chen, H.; Yuan, H.; Sun, D. Engineering exosomes as refined biological nanoplatforms for drug delivery. *Acta Pharmacol. Sin.* **2017**, *38*, 754–763. [CrossRef]
145. Podolak, I.; Galanty, A.; Sobolewska, D. Saponins as cytotoxic agents: A review. *Phytochem. Rev.* **2010**, *9*, 425–474. [CrossRef]
146. Jeyaram, A.; Lamichhane, T.N.; Wang, S.; Zou, L.; Dahal, E.; Kronstadt, S.M.; Levy, D.; Parajuli, B.; Knudsen, D.R.; Chao, W.; et al. Enhanced Loading of Functional miRNA Cargo via pH Gradient Modification of Extracellular Vesicles. *Mol. Ther.* **2020**, *28*, 975–985. [CrossRef]
147. Wei, H.; Chen, J.; Wang, S.; Fu, F.; Zhu, X.; Wu, C.; Liu, Z.; Zhong, G.; Lin, J. A Nanodrug Consisting Of Doxorubicin And Exosome Derived From Mesenchymal Stem Cells For Osteosarcoma Treatment In Vitro. *Int. J. Nanomed.* **2019**, *14*, 8603–8610. [CrossRef] [PubMed]
148. Sun, D.; Zhuang, X.; Xiang, X.; Liu, Y.; Zhang, S.; Liu, C.; Barnes, S.; Grizzle, W.; Miller, D.; Zhang, H.G. A novel nanoparticle drug delivery system: The anti-inflammatory activity of curcumin is enhanced when encapsulated in exosomes. *Mol. Ther.* **2010**, *18*, 1606–1614. [CrossRef]
149. Zhou, Y.Z.; Alany, R.G.; Chuang, V.; Wen, J. Optimization of PLGA nanoparticles formulation containing L-DOPA by applying the central composite design. *Drug Dev. Ind. Pharm.* **2013**, *39*, 321–330. [CrossRef] [PubMed]
150. Kupiec-Weglinski, J.W.; Austyn, J.M.; Morris, P.J. Migration patterns of dendritic cells in the mouse. Traffic from the blood, and T cell-dependent and -independent entry to lymphoid tissues. *J. Exp. Med.* **1988**, *167*, 632–645. [CrossRef]
151. Wiklander, O.P.; Nordin, J.Z.; O'Loughlin, A.; Gustafsson, Y.; Corso, G.; Mager, I.; Vader, P.; Lee, Y.; Sork, H.; Seow, Y.; et al. Extracellular vesicle in vivo biodistribution is determined by cell source, route of administration and targeting. *J. Extracell. Vesicles* **2015**, *4*, 26316. [CrossRef] [PubMed]
152. Chivet, M.; Javalet, C.; Laulagnier, K.; Blot, B.; Hemming, F.J.; Sadoul, R. Exosomes secreted by cortical neurons upon glutamatergic synapse activation specifically interact with neurons. *J. Extracell. Vesicles* **2014**, *3*, 24722. [CrossRef] [PubMed]
153. Webb, R.L.; Kaiser, E.E.; Scoville, S.L.; Thompson, T.A.; Fatima, S.; Pandya, C.; Sriram, K.; Swetenburg, R.L.; Vaibhav, K.; Arbab, A.S.; et al. Human Neural Stem Cell Extracellular Vesicles Improve Tissue and Functional Recovery in the Murine Thromboembolic Stroke Model. *Transl. Stroke Res.* **2018**, *9*, 530–539. [CrossRef] [PubMed]
154. Yang, T.; Martin, P.; Fogarty, B.; Brown, A.; Schurman, K.; Phipps, R.; Yin, V.P.; Lockman, P.; Bai, S. Exosome delivered anticancer drugs across the blood-brain barrier for brain cancer therapy in Danio rerio. *Pharm. Res.* **2015**, *32*, 2003–2014. [CrossRef]
155. Richardson, J.J.; Ejima, H. Surface Engineering of Extracellular Vesicles through Chemical and Biological Strategies. *Chem. Mater.* **2019**, *31*, 2191–2201. [CrossRef]
156. Liang, Y.; Duan, L.; Lu, J.; Xia, J. Engineering exosomes for targeted drug delivery. *Theranostics* **2021**, *11*, 3183–3195. [CrossRef]
157. Vakhshiteh, F.; Atyabi, F.; Ostad, S.N. Mesenchymal stem cell exosomes: A two-edged sword in cancer therapy. *Int. J. Nanomed.* **2019**, *14*, 2847–2859. [CrossRef]

158. Zhang, M.; Zang, X.; Wang, M.; Li, Z.; Qiao, M.; Hu, H.; Chen, D. Exosome-based nanocarriers as bio-inspired and versatile vehicles for drug delivery: Recent advances and challenges. *J. Mater. Chem. B.* **2019**, *7*, 2421–2433. [CrossRef]
159. Lentz, T.L.; Burrage, T.G.; Smith, A.L.; Crick, J.; Tignor, G.H. Is the acetylcholine receptor a rabies virus receptor? *Science* **1982**, *215*, 182–184. [CrossRef]
160. Kumar, P.; Wu, H.; McBride, J.L.; Jung, K.E.; Kim, M.H.; Davidson, B.L.; Lee, S.K.; Shankar, P.; Manjunath, N. Transvascular delivery of small interfering RNA to the central nervous system. *Nature* **2007**, *448*, 39–43. [CrossRef]
161. Zhang, L.; Wu, T.; Shan, Y.; Li, G.; Ni, X.; Chen, X.; Hu, X.; Lin, L.; Li, Y.; Guan, Y.; et al. Therapeutic reversal of Huntington's disease by in vivo self-assembled siRNAs. *Brain* **2021**, *144*, 3421–3435. [CrossRef] [PubMed]
162. Smyth, T.; Petrova, K.; Payton, N.M.; Persaud, I.; Redzic, J.S.; Graner, M.W.; Smith-Jones, P.; Anchordoquy, T.J. Surface functionalization of exosomes using click chemistry. *Bioconjugate Chem.* **2014**, *25*, 1777–1784. [CrossRef]
163. Nwe, K.; Brechbiel, M.W. Growing applications of "click chemistry" for bioconjugation in contemporary biomedical research. *Cancer Biother. Radiopharm.* **2009**, *24*, 289–302. [CrossRef] [PubMed]
164. Susa, F.; Limongi, T.; Dumontel, B.; Vighetto, V.; Cauda, V. Engineered Extracellular Vesicles as a Reliable Tool in Cancer Nanomedicine. *Cancers* **2019**, *11*, 1979. [CrossRef] [PubMed]
165. Kim, M.S.; Haney, M.J.; Zhao, Y.; Yuan, D.; Deygen, I.; Klyachko, N.L.; Kabanov, A.V.; Batrakova, E.V. Engineering macrophage-derived exosomes for targeted paclitaxel delivery to pulmonary metastases: In vitro and in vivo evaluations. *Nanomedicine* **2018**, *14*, 195–204. [CrossRef]
166. Tian, T.; Zhang, H.X.; He, C.P.; Fan, S.; Zhu, Y.L.; Qi, C.; Huang, N.P.; Xiao, Z.D.; Lu, Z.H.; Tannous, B.A.; et al. Surface functionalized exosomes as targeted drug delivery vehicles for cerebral ischemia therapy. *Biomaterials* **2018**, *150*, 137–149. [CrossRef]
167. Armstrong, J.P.; Holme, M.N.; Stevens, M.M. Re-Engineering Extracellular Vesicles as Smart Nanoscale Therapeutics. *ACS Nano* **2017**, *11*, 69–83. [CrossRef]
168. Nel, A.E.; Madler, L.; Velegol, D.; Xia, T.; Hoek, E.M.; Somasundaran, P.; Klaessig, F.; Castranova, V.; Thompson, M. Understanding biophysicochemical interactions at the nano-bio interface. *Nat. Mater.* **2009**, *8*, 543–557. [CrossRef]
169. Qi, H.; Liu, C.; Long, L.; Ren, Y.; Zhang, S.; Chang, X.; Qian, X.; Jia, H.; Zhao, J.; Sun, J.; et al. Blood Exosomes Endowed with Magnetic and Targeting Properties for Cancer Therapy. *ACS Nano* **2016**, *10*, 3323–3333. [CrossRef]
170. Nakase, I.; Futaki, S. Combined treatment with a pH-sensitive fusogenic peptide and cationic lipids achieves enhanced cytosolic delivery of exosomes. *Sci. Rep.* **2015**, *5*, 10112. [CrossRef]
171. Vandergriff, A.; Huang, K.; Shen, D.; Hu, S.; Hensley, M.T.; Caranasos, T.G.; Qian, L.; Cheng, K. Targeting regenerative exosomes to myocardial infarction using cardiac homing peptide. *Theranostics* **2018**, *8*, 1869–1878. [CrossRef] [PubMed]

biomedicines

MDPI

Review

Regenerative Effects of Exosomes-Derived MSCs: An Overview on Spinal Cord Injury Experimental Studies

Giovanni Schepici, Serena Silvestro and Emanuela Mazzon *

IRCCS Centro Neurolesi "Bonino-Pulejo", Via Provinciale Palermo, Contrada Casazza, 98124 Messina, Italy
* Correspondence: emanuela.mazzon@irccsme.it; Tel.: +39-090-60128172

Abstract: Spinal cord injury (SCI) is a devastating condition usually induced by the initial mechanical insult that can lead to permanent motor and sensory deficits. At present, researchers are investigating potential therapeutic strategies to ameliorate the neuro-inflammatory cascade that occurs post-injury. Although the use of mesenchymal stromal/stem (MSCs) as a potential therapy in application to regenerative medicine promoted anti-inflammatory and neuroprotective effects, several disadvantages limit their use. Therefore, recent studies have reported the effects of exosomes-derived MSCs (MSC-EXOs) as an innovative therapeutic option for SCI patients. It is noteworthy that MSC-EXOs can maintain the integrity of the blood-spinal cord barrier (BSCB), promoting angiogenic, proliferative, and anti-oxidant effects, as well as immunomodulatory, anti-inflammatory, and antiapoptotic properties. Therefore, in this study, we summarized the preclinical studies reported in the literature that have shown the effects of MSC-EXOs as a new molecular target to counteract the devastating effects of SCI.

Keywords: exosomes; spinal cord injury; mesenchymal stromal/stem; blood-spinal cord barrier integrity

1. Introduction

Spinal cord injury (SCI) is a disabling condition that causes partial or complete sensorial and motor deficits. Usually, SCI is the result of an initial mechanical insult, followed by a cascade of structural and neuroinflammatory changes. To ameliorate the damaging events that occur after SCI, researchers have been evaluating the potential of mesenchymal stromal/stem cells (MSCs) as therapeutic agents in application to regenerative medicine. Despite the fact that experimental studies that have used MSCs have proven their beneficial effects on SCI, there are several limitations regarding the application of MSCs as therapeutic agents for humans. Therefore, it is necessary to identify new agents for regenerative medicine application [1].

MSCs exert their therapeutic effects through the release of extracellular vesicles (EVs), a group of membranous vesicles that are cell-derived and 30–1000 nanometer in size, composed of lipid bilayers and secreted into the extracellular space [2]. EVs have been found in biological fluids, including cerebro-spinal fluid (CSF), blood, urine breast milk, saliva, amniotic fluid, and synovial fluid [3]. In addition to MSCs, EVs are also produced by several cell types, such as B cells, NK cells, T cells, erythrocytes, platelets, epithelial cells, endothelial cells, dendritic cells, neurons, oligodendrocytes, Schwann cells, muscle cells, cancer cells and embryonic cells [4]. Based on their size and biogenesis, three comprehensive classes of EVs are known: exosomes, microvesicles (MVs) and apoptotic bodies. Apoptotic bodies are vesicles of 50–2000 nm in size that result from cell death. MVs are vesicles of 150–1000 nm in diameter, obtained by direct budding from cytoplasmic membrane. Exosomes are endosomal vesicles of size 40–150 nm in diameter generated by the fusion of multivesicular bodies (MVBs) with the cell membrane that are released into the extracellular environment [4,5].

It was demonstrate that EVs exert the capacity of transferring biological molecules such as proteins, nucleic acids and lipids without direct cell-to-cell contact [6]. Thanks to their inclusion, morphology and ability to act as carriers to reach injury sites through biological barriers, EVs could be useful for the diagnosis and treatment of diseases [7]. Consequently, advancing technologies in regenerative medicine have led researchers to the isolation and application of exosomes-derived MSCs (MSC-EXOs).

In this regard, it has been demonstrated that MSC-EXOs exerts MSCs physiological functions including anti-inflammatory, restorative, regenerative and immunomodulatory potential. Therefore, due to their specific properties, researchers have investigated MSC-EXOs as a potential therapeutic application for the treatment of permanent disability conditions such as SCI [7,8].

The aim of this review is to summarize the preclinical studies that have reported the effects of MSC-EXOs as a possible therapeutic strategy for SCI.

2. Methodology

Publications between 2017 and 2022 are taken into consideration for this review. PubMed and Scopus were used to retrieve the publications that corresponds to the key-words: "MSCs derived exosomes" and "spinal cord injury".

Studies that have evaluated the role of MSCs-derived exosomes in promoting SCI repair and reducing functional deficits were selected. The Prisma flow diagram illustrates the article selection process (Figure 1).

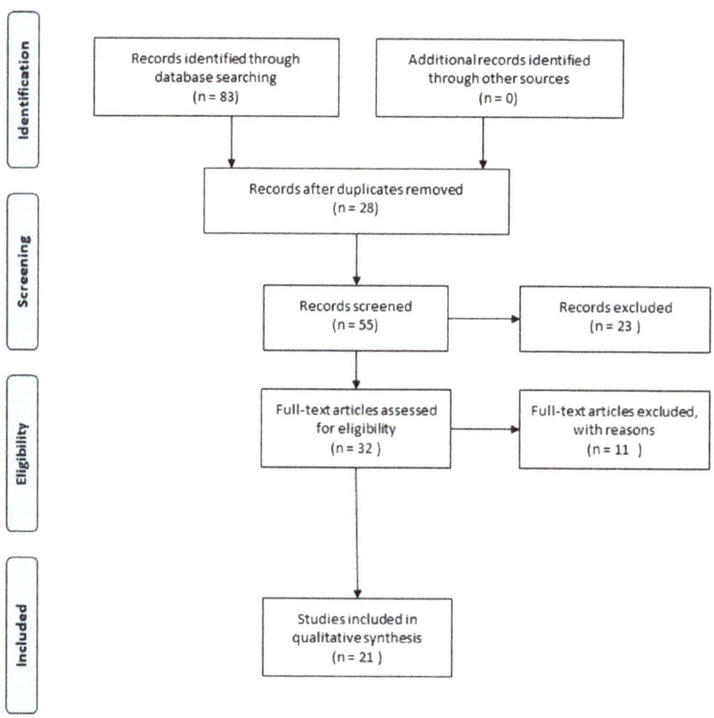

Figure 1. The Prisma flow diagram illustrates the methodology that was used to select the in vivo and in vitro studies used for the writing of the review. Duplicate articles were excluded from the total of the studies that were found. Conversely, articles that highlight the role of MSCs derived exosomes in promoting injury repair and restoring functional deficits are described (The PRISMA Statement is published in [9].

3. Spinal Cord Injury (SCI)

SCI is a devastating injury to the spinal cord that leads to temporary or permanent changes into the spinal cord, as well as the partial or complete loss of motor, autonomic and sensory function [10,11]. SCI is common in males below 30 years of age [12,13]. The hallmarks of SCI are generally paralysis (paraplegia or quadriplegia), with sensory dysfunction below the injury level [14]. It has been demonstrated that SCI can induce the loss of connection between the brain and peripheral nervous system, in turn negatively influencing the majority of basic bodily functions, including breathing, sexual function, hormone release, as well as bowel and bladder functions [15].

Mechanical insult due to physical forces, including compression or contusion, can lead to the transection or stretching of the spinal column with consequent spinal cord disruption, thus promoting the primary injury [16–18].

"Primary injury" is an irreversible process that occurs immediately following injury to the spinal cord, leading the axonal membranes to rupture and the release of materials that inhibit axonal regeneration, including the neurite outgrowth inhibitor protein A, oligodendrocyte myelin glycoprotein, chondroitin sulfate proteoglycan and myelin-associated glycoprotein [19,20].

The subsequent phase of SCI is known as "secondary injury", in which a cascade of events are triggered, leading to progressive neuronal tissue damage and the exacerbation of neurological deficits [21]. The secondary lesion is divided into an acute, a subacute, and a chronic phase [22]. The acute phase is characterized by progressive hemorrhage, edema, ischemia, thrombosis, an increase in oxidative stress, apoptosis, cell necrosis, as well as the release of inflammatory cytokines due to the rupture of the blood-spinal cord barrier (BSCB) [11]. Secondary injury negatively regulates cell survival, leading to an increase in the lesion into the spinal cord in the rostrocaudal directions [23]. Indeed, it has been shown that, among the mechanisms of secondary injury, the major contribution is provided by inflammation due to macrophages, T-cells, microglia and neutrophils infiltration into the site of the lesion, thus promoting the blood-marrow barrier rupture [24]. These cells generate an inflammatory environment mediated by the release of interleukin (IL)-1β, IL-6, and tumor necrosis factor-α (TNFα). It is noteworthy that the inflammatory cytokines reach their peak 6–12 h after injury and stay in circulation for four days [25]. The acute phase is followed by the subacute phase; this is characterized by ionic homeostasis imbalance, which is responsible for an increase in intracellular calcium, which in turn promotes mitochondrial dysfunction and cell death [26,27]. In particular, oligodendrocyte death promotes the axon demineralization process [28]. The mitochondrial changes induce DNA oxidative damage, oxidation of proteins, and lipid peroxidation, leading to reactive oxygen species (ROS) and reactive nitrogen species (RNS) production with further exacerbation of the tissue damage [29]. The expansion of the damage prompts the chronic phase wherein the activation of astrocytes produces excessive levels of the extracellular matrix and increases neuronal apoptosis. This process triggers cystic cavity formation, axonal death and the maturation of the glial scar [30,31]. Consequently, scar formation, tissue necrosis, and cavity can interfere with cell regenerative processes, such as axonal regeneration, which compromises the functional recovery and therapeutic regenerative potential [32]. While in the early phase of secondary injury, the glial scar exerts a positive role in containing inflammation, both removing debris and regenerating BSCB. In the later phase of injury, axonal growth inhibitors and scars can interfere with neuronal regeneration (Figure 2) [33].

Although advances in SCI management have led to an improvement in patients' quality of life, their recovery remains limited [34].

In this regard, the current treatments, including surgical decompression [35], spinal cord pressure monitoring [36], corticosteroids [37,38] and hemodynamic therapy [39], do not completely restore the function of the damaged spinal cord; thus, it is necessary to find new therapeutic treatments for SCI management, such as MSC-EXOs.

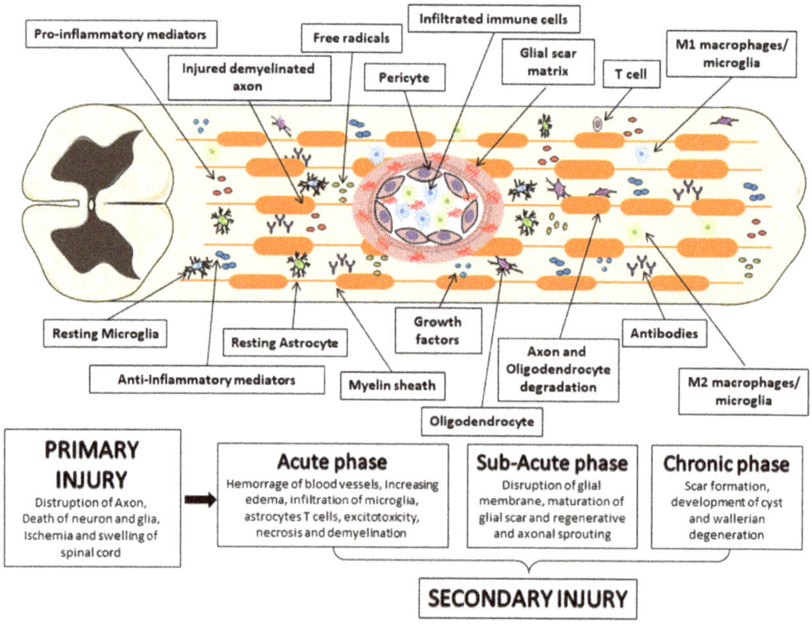

Figure 2. Pathophysiology of spinal cord injury (SCI). This schematic diagram illustrates the phase of SCI and its pathophysiology. Immediately after primary injury, the activation of resident astrocytes and microglia, and the subsequent infiltration of blood immune cells, induce an important neuroinflammatory response. This acute neuroinflammatory response plays a key role in the secondary injury mechanisms in the sub-acute and chronic phases that lead to cell death and tissue degeneration, as well as the formation of the glial scar, axonal degeneration and demyelination. During the acute phase, monocyte-derived macrophages occur in the central area of the injury to scavenge tissue damage. In these phases, the loss of oligodendrocytes leads to axonal demyelination, followed by spontaneous remyelination. Instead, astrocytes and pericytes, normally present in the spinal cord parenchyma, after damage proliferate and migrate to the site of injury and contribute to the formation of the glial scar. The image was created using the image bank of Servier Medical Art (Available online: http://smart.servier.com/, accessed on 1 December 2022), licensed under a Creative Commons Attribution 3.0 Unported License (Available online: https://creativecommons.org/licenses/by/3.0/, accessed on 1 December 2022).

4. MSC-EXOs

Exosomes are natural nanomaterials enclosed by a lipid bilayer membrane that contains phosphatidylserine, cholesterol, sphingomyelin and ceramide. It is noteworthy that exosomes play an important role in cellular communication through the transport of genetic information and bioactive substances, including proteins, nucleic acids and lipids, to create paths for communication between cells. In this regard, it was reported that exosomes could maintain the homeostasis of the CNS crossed with the BBB and communicate through the miRNA proteins in the neurovascular unit [40].

Exosomes are widely distributed in some body fluids, such as blood, cerebrospinal fluid, urine, amniotic fluid, pericardial effusion, milk and saliva [41]. Additionally, exosomes express surface proteins, including membrane transport/fusion proteins and heat shock proteins (HSPs). Despite electron microscopy being the golden standard method for exosome identification, the presence of CD9, CD63, and CD81 favors their identification [42]. Several techniques for the isolation of exosomes from different sources have been developed [43]. Ultracentrifugation is the most used isolation method and is based on the density difference and particle size. Additionally, it is a simple and cost-effective method that allows for isolating a high amount of exosomes [43,44]. The size-exclusion chromatography and ultrafiltration are isolation methods that lead to the biomolecule's separation, according to their size [45]. Additionally, immunocapture techniques are exosome isolation methods based on the interactions between the antibodies and proteins present in the exosome's surface [46]. Polymer precipitation is an isolation method based on the solubility exosome changes [47]. Another method used to isolate and purify exosomes involves the use of microfluidic technologies in order to obtain high purity and sensitivity [43].

As exosomes are membrane-coated nanoparticles, their use as vehicles for drug delivery, as well as in immune modulation and tissue regeneration, are being investigated. Hence, techniques that employ the modification of exosomes to increase their targeting efficiency and cross-biological membranes could be useful for biomedical applications. At present, the gold standard technique for modifying the surface of nanoparticles is poly (ethylene glycol) (PEG) coating, which has led to improved pharmacokinetics through the stability and immunogenicity of the nanoparticles in vivo compared to uncoated nanoparticles. Despite this, it was reported that PEG-coated nanoparticles mediate complement activation and recognition by PEG-specific IgM antibodies with an increase in blood clearance by the liver and hypersensitivity in vivo. Therefore, integrated cell cloaking nanotherapeutics that exploit the biomimetic intrinsic properties of cell membranes could enhance the increment of the nanoparticles in the target tissue. In this regard, it was reported that macrophage membrane-coated nanoparticles improved their accumulation in inflammatory sites. Additionally, prolonged circulation in vivo was also shown in red blood cell membrane-coated nanoparticles. Moreover, to improve the integrated cell cloaking nanotherapeutic techniques for potential clinical applications, the combination of genetic, chemical and physical engineering and nanotherapeutic platforms, including mesoporous silica nanoparticles, magnetic nanoparticles and metal-organic framework, is providing promising results both in regenerative medicine and cancer immunotherapy [48].

Exosome biogenesis is achieved through plasma membrane invagination and the generation of intracellular MVBs with intraluminal vesicles (ILVs). The endocytic pathway, which involves the donor cell, is followed by the transport of intravesicular and transmembrane proteins from the Golgi complex, to lead to the formation of early endosomes [49]. Subsequently, the differentiation and maturation of early endosomes into late endosomes occurs [50]. Morphological and physical changes can identify the transition into late endosomes. In this regard, it has been reported that early endosomes show a tubular shape and are found in the external portion of the cytoplasm. In contrast, late endosomes are spherical and located near the nucleus [51]. Additionally, late endosomes are degraded by binding to lysosomes, plasma membranes or autophagosomes to release the ILVs into the extracellular environment as exosomes [52]. The interaction of exosomes with the recipient cells can occur through their surface receptor molecules and ligands. It has been demonstrated that, after secretion, some exosomes stay on the cell membranes of the donor cells, while the remaining ones interact with the recipient cells [53]. Exosome internalization is a process related to caveolae, raft or clathrin-dependent endocytosis. Additionally, it has been reported that phagocytosis and micropinocytosis can also be considered as methods of internalization. Therefore, exosome internalization that targets recipient cells can be interesting as a potential therapeutic application in regenerative medicine [54,55]. In comparison to MSCs, exosomes have both higher safety and stronger plasticity, deeming them potentially useful in clinical application to Central Nervous System (CNS) injuries [56,57].

As it has been demonstrated that the differentiation of MSCs towards a neural lineage in the damaged brain only includes a limited number of cells, the regenerative potential of MSCs could be more related to their paracrine activity, which is performed by exosomes [44,45].

In addition to the features of MSCs, MSC-EXOs are known for their immunomodulatory, anti-inflammatory, antiapoptotic, angiogenic, proliferative and antioxidant effects [58]. Moreover, MSC-EXOs offer several benefits, including accessible storage, high stability and low immunogenicity [59,60]. MSC-EXOs are cystic vesicle cup-shaped structures with a diameter of 30–100 nm, containing lipids, proteins and RNA [13,14]. The lipid bilayer is important in stabilizing biological activities and maintaining the integrity of the exosomes, while protein modification on the surface leads to an improvement in targeting and recognition of the exosomes. Additionally, the presence of nucleic acids, such as microRNAs (miRNAs), is important in intercellular communication [61,62].

Despite their biogenesis being common to other sources, it has been reported that MSC-EXOs show no differences in terms of their isolation, conservation and morphological characteristics. Moreover, MSC-EXOs have demonstrated the ability to produce more exosomes than other cell lines [15,16]. In addition to the common surface markers CD9 and CD81, MSC-EXOs express some specific adhesion molecules, including CD29, CD44 and CD73, present on the MSCs membrane [17].

Therefore, based on their paracrine effects, MSC-EXOs could be useful to improve functional recovery, as well as being used as a cell-free therapeutic strategy [63].

5. MSC-EXOs as a Potential Therapeutic Tool in SCI

MSC-EXOs are easier to collect and store and possess poor ethical restrictions compared to MSCs. For this reason, researchers have been evaluating the potential therapeutic effects of MSC-EXOs in SCI experimental studies [64]. Several experimental studies have reported that MSC-EXOs can exert anti-inflammatory and anti-apoptotic effects, promote axonal regeneration and macrophage polarization, as well as protect the BSCB from spinal cord damage [65–67]. The functional recovery of SCI patients is related to pro-inflammatory and anti-inflammatory environments, as well as relative levels of pro-inflammatory cytokines and anti-inflammatory factors [68,69]. In this regard, it has been demonstrated that the intravenous injection of human umbilical cord MSC-EXOs inhibited the expression of proinflammatory cytokines IL-1β, IL-6 and the formation of scars, and promoted motor function recovery in a SCI rat model [70].

Neuroinflammation plays an important role in secondary injuries of SCI. It has been demonstrated that neuroinflammation leads to the activation of resident immune cells and is mediated by a protein complex-inflammasome known as the nucleotide-binding domain-like receptor protein 3 (NLRP3) inflammasome. NLRP3 is located in the cytoplasm and regulates the natural immune response [71]. It is noteworthy that an increase in NLRP3 inflammasome activity in a SCI mice model has been reported [72]. Additionally, the inhibition of NLRP3 inflammasome activation led to functional recovery in SCI rats, thus confirming the important role of NLRP3 inflammasome in the control of the inflammatory events that occur in SCI [72,73]. Similarly, it has been shown that the systematic administration of epidural fat MSC-EXOs induced injury reduction and improved neural function recovery in SCI rats, according to a molecular mechanism that led to the suppression of NLRP3 inflammasomes activation and a reduction in inflammatory cytokines. Additionally, an increase in B cell lymphoma-2 (Bcl-2) and a decrease in Bcl-2 associated X protein (Bax) was observed [65].

As SCI leads to the activation of both the classic and alternative complement pathways, thus exacerbating the inflammatory reaction, the inhibition of nuclear factor kappa-light-chain-enhancer of activated B cells (NF-κB) may be a possible strategy for minimizing inflammation in secondary injury and for promoting functional recovery [74]. Consequently, the interaction of complements C1q and C3 to the NF-κB signalling pathway could explain this [75]. Additionally, it has been observed that the C3 complement protein a (key marker of A1 astrocytes) upregulates NF-κB in a dependent manner [76]. In this respect, in a SCI rats model, the administration of bone marrow MSC-EXOs led to a reduction in A1 astrocytes through the downregulation of NFκB P65 [77].

In addition, macrophages are involved in the inflammatory process that occurs in secondary injuries of SCI. Researchers have demonstrated the potential therapeutic effect of MSC-EXOs in macrophage polarization [78]. It is known that macrophages can switch from the pro-inflammatory phenotype M1 to the anti-inflammatory M2 one [79]. Following injury, myelin damage at the initial SCI site leads to the infiltration of the macrophage via chemotaxis [80]. M1 macrophages induce the production of pro-inflammatory cytokines, including TNF-α, IFN-γ, IL-6, ROS and nitric oxide, with harmful effects to the injured spinal cord [78]. In contrast, M2 macrophages exert anti-inflammatory effects through IL-10 release and promote axonal regeneration [80,81]. Hence, the persistence of M1 macrophages induces a severe inflammatory state in SCI and causes further damage to the injured spinal cord. Consequently, it is necessary promote strategies that lead to the polarization of macrophages from the M1 phenotype to the M2 type [82]. The intravenous administration of MSC-EXOs targets M2 macrophages in the injured spinal cord in order to release EVs by MSCs and to improve SCI [83].

It is worth noting that the BSCB plays an important role both in the normal function of the nervous system and in maintaining its integrity. The BSCB is formed by the basement membrane, capillary endothelial cells, astrocyte foot processes and pericytes. Therefore, the BSCB could be a potential therapeutic target for SCI [84]. After SCI, the rupture of the BSCB induces the destruction of the blood vessels at the site of injury and causes a consequent increment both of permeability and toxic materials into the injured spinal cord, leading to edema and neuronal cell death [85]. Additionally, pericytes, as a part of the neurovascular unit, are involved in the formation and maintenance of the blood vessels' properties, as well as BSCB integrity [86]. It is noteworthy that pericytes and several vascular wall cells could induce vessel wall fragility and, thus, the development of spinal vascular shunts and arteriovenous malformations (AVMs), as well as intracerebral hemorrhage [87]. Pericytes play an important role in maintaining vessel stability and angiogenesis through crosstalk with angiopoietin signalling. In this regard, it was reported that Angiopoietin-2, in the presence of the vascular endothelial growth factor (VEGF), can promote vessels formation [88]. The therapeutic potential of MSCs-EXOs in SCI could also occur via the NF-κB p65 pathway, thus inhibiting the migration of pericytes and, promoting BSCB integrity, axonal regeneration and improved motor function, as well as leading to a reduction in neuronal cell apoptosis [66]. Additionally, it has been reported that pericyte from EXOs reduced cell apoptosis, improved microcirculation and protected the BSCB in SCI mice [89].

The importance of miRNAs, such as miRNA-21, miRNA-133 and miRNA-126, as potential therapeutic targets for SCI has recently been proposed [90].

Therefore, thanks to their characteristics, EXOs could cross the BSCB, enhancing the effects of miRNAs, and potentially be used as carriers to miRNAs at the SCI site [91].

Moreover, during tissue damage, an increase in miRNA-21 expression has been highlighted, with a reduction in neuronal apoptosis via the phosphatase and tensin homolog (PTEN)-protein kinase B (Akt) signalling pathway, as well as the modulation of the expression levels of protein-related apoptosis, including Bcl-2, Bax, caspase-3 and caspase-9 [92,93]. Additionally, it has been reported that the downregulation of miRNA-133b led to a reduction in neuronal axonal regeneration and prevented the recovery of motor function [94]. It is worth noting that a decrease in miRNA-126 after SCI has been shown, while an increase in miRNA-126 led to a reduction in inflammation and improved functional recovery and angiogenesis [95].

6. MSC-EXOs as a Potential Therapeutic Tool in SCI Experimental Studies

Several experimental studies have investigated the effects of MSC-EXO as a potential therapeutic strategy for SCI.

Sung et al. evaluated the efficacy of MSCs-EXOs from human epidural adipose tissue (hEpi AD), isolated by tangential flow filtration and characterized by flow cytometry, in addition to nanoparticle tracking analysis. HEpi ADMSCs-EXOs were administrated intravenously, both at low and high concentrations, in SCI-Sprague Dawley (SD) rats and induced by the compression method. The study results demonstrated that the hEpi ADMSCs-EXOs led to a reduction in the inflammatory responses, as well as improved spinal functions. Histopathological and immunohistochemical analyzes of Iba-1 and glial fibrillary acid protein (GFAP) in rat spinal cords demonstrated that the administration of high and low concentrations of hEpi ADMSCs-EXOs reduced neuroinflammation. Overall, an increase in the brain-derived neurotrophic factor (BDNF) level in the spinal cord of rats after the administration of high MSCs-EXOs concentrations was significantly reduced in the SCI vehicle group. In addition, VEGF, an important neurotrophic factor for the survival of spinal neurons, was higher in the spinal cords of the treated mice. Additionally, a reduction in the pro-inflammatory cytokines IL-1β, IL-2 and TNF-α in the MSCs-EXOs groups was highlighted. It is noteworthy that mRNA sequencing analysis of the spinal cord tissue demonstrated that the administration of hEpi ADMSCs-EXOs reduced the SCI-induced inflammatory responses by targeting the immune response and neurogenesis-related genes, thus suggesting that MSCs-EXOs could be useful to improve neurological recovery in SCI [96].

In contrast, Zhou et al. evaluated the effects of bone marrow (BM) MSC-EXOs both in vivo and in vitro. In order to perform the in vivo model, the authors used SD rats induced with the impact method and subsequently treated with BMMSC-EXOs. The in vivo results demonstrated that the transplant of the BMMSC-EXOs led to a reduction in myelin loss and neuronal cell death, and improved both the myelin arrangement and locomotor functional recovery. Moreover, the transplant of the BMMSC-EXOs reduced edema and caspase-1 expression, and inhibited the pericyte pyroptosis and IL-1β release, thus maintaining BSCB integrity. To confirm the in vitro results, microvascular pericytes isolated from a rat's spinal cord were induced with IFN-γ 100 ng/mL plus TNF-α; 10 ng/mL and transfected with lipopolysaccharide (LPS) 1 μg/mL, premixed with Lipofectamine, as well as co-incubated with or without adenosine triphosphate (ATP) 5 mM. Additionally, to test the protective effect of the MSCs-EXOs, pericytes were co-incubated with or without BMMSCs-EXOs (100 μg/mL). The exposure of pericytes to IFN-γ + TNF-α + LPS + Lipofectamine + ATP led to the upregulation of pro-caspase 1 and Nod1 inflammasome, as well as the release of IL-1β. In addition, the treatment with BMMSCs-EXOs effectively inhibited Nod1 inflammasome and pyroptosis in the pericytes, promoting the inhibition of IL-1β release and the upregulation of pro-caspase 1. Therefore, overall, the data suggest that the use of BMMSCs-EXOs improved the integrity of the BSCB after SCI through pericyte pyroptosis inhibition [97].

Zhang et al. also demonstrated the potential therapeutic effects of exosomes derived from human placental MSCs (hPMSCs-EXOs) in SCI. The hPMSCs-EXOs, extracted by sequential centrifugation, displayed proangiogenic effects both in vitro and in vivo. Male mice induced by the contusive SCI model were administered with hPMSCs-EXOs (200 μg/μL) into the SCI epicenter. The in vivo results reported that the transplant of hPMSCs-EXOs led to improved locomotor and sensory function recovery, as well as promoting the new vessel formation and angiogenesis, as shown by a subset of endothelial cells near the injury site that took up the labelled hPMSCs-EXOs. Additionally, to develop the in vitro model and simulate ischemia in SCI, Human Umbilical Vein Endothelial Cells (HUVECs) were cultivated in oxygen-glucose deprivation (OGD) conditions scratching was performed, and they were divided into experimental groups. The in vitro results highlighted that treatment with hPMSCs-EXOs promoted tube formation by endothelial cells, thus confirming the proangiogenic effects of hPMSCs-EXOs. Although is not yet known whether endothelial cells can uptake MSCs-EXOs in the injured area, it is possible that endothelial cells can only uptake MSCs-EXOs at certain stages of their development. Therefore, further studies are required to elucidate the underlying mechanisms [98].

PTEN-AKT-mTOR pathway activation could also promote neurogenesis and axonal regeneration, leading to a reduction in glial scarring and thus be potentially useful for SCI treatment. As miR-26a could activate the PTEN-AKT-mTOR pathway, Chen et al. investigated the effects of BM-MSCs transfected with the mimics of miR-26a, from which the exosomes were harvested. After transfection, the expression level of miR-26a in the exosomes was significantly increased. Then, PC12 cells were incubated with miR-26a overexpressing exosomes (BMMSCs-EXOs-miR-26a) for 48 h. In vitro, BMMSCs-EXOs-miR-26a promoted neurofilament generation in the PC12 cells by downregulating PTEN expression and consequently increasing the phosphorylation of Phosphoinositide 3-kinases

(PI3Ks), AKT and the mammalian target of rapamycin (mTOR) proteins. Targeting the PTEN-AKT-mTOR pathway increased NF generation and nerve regeneration. In addition, in vivo, in the SCI rat model, the injection of BMMSCs-EXOs-miR-26a reduced the injury in the damaged area and ameliorated the functional recovery. Following SCI, miR-26a-overexpressing BMMSC-EXOs improved axonal regeneration, as also shown by the upregulation of neurofilament and β-tubulin-3. Therefore, miR-26a could activate the PTEN-AKT-mTOR pathway and promote axonal regeneration and neurogenesis [99].

Recently, several studies have investigated the potential role of MSCs-EXOs as a miRNAs source in SCI experimental studies. In this regard, Li et al. studied the effects of BMMSCs-derived EXOs transfected with miR-544. Following extradural compression to induce the SCI model, SD rats were treated with BMMSCs-EXOs containing miR-544. The BMMSCs-EXOs transfected with miR-544 improved the neural functional recovery in SCI rats. Additionally, it has been evidenced that overexpressing miR-544 can alleviate the inflammatory response after SCI, evaluated by proinflammatory cytokines reduction including TNF-α, IL-1α, IL-17B and IL-36β [100].

As miRNAs represent the most abundant nucleotides in exosomes, they are receiving increasing attention from researchers. In this regard, Wang et al. identified the expression profiles of exosomal miRNAs derived from human umbilical cord mesenchymal/stromal stem cells (hUCMSCs). MiR-199a-3p and miR-145-5p were the most abundant miRNAs identified in the hUCMSC-EXOs. Furthermore, bioinformatic analysis showed that these miRNAs regulate TrkA turnover, as there seems to be a direct relationship between miR-199a-3p and Cblb, miR-145-5p and Cbl. In this regard, the role of exosomal miR-199a-3p/145-5p on neuronal differentiation through the regulation of the *Cblb* and Cbl genes was explored. To evaluate the synergistic effects of miR-199a-3p/145-5p in EXOs, hUCMSCs were co-transfected with miR-199a-3p/145-5p antisense RNA and the EXO were isolated. To simulate the inflammatory environment and promote the neurite outgrowth that occurs after SCI, an injury model was developed. The PC12 cells were induced with LPS 11 μg/mL, highlighting both the reduction in cell differentiation and miR-199a-3p/145-5p expression. It is noteworthy that when the PC12 cells were pre-treated with hUCMSCs-EXOs co-transfected with miR-199a-3p/145-5p, an increase in PC12 cell differentiation by modulation of the nerve growth factor (NGF)/TrkA pathway differentiation was observed. Moreover, the overexpression of neuronal markers, including β-tubulin-3, heavy-chain neurofilament (NF-H) and Neuronal Nuclei (NeuN) was shown. On the contrary, the knockdown of miR-199a-3p/145-5p in MSCs-EXOs partially abolished the protective effect of the exosomal miRNAs in the PC12 cells. In addition, bioinformatic analysis followed by Western blotting and QRT-PCR analysis demonstrated that miR-199a-3p and miR-145-5p targeted, respectively, the Cblb and Cbl genes, leading to the modulation of TrkA ubiquitination. To confirm the data obtained, the authors performed the study in an in vivo model of SCI. In addition, the in vivo results demonstrated that the injection of EXOs led to an antiapoptotic effect at the lesion site; this effect was partially attributed to the exosomal miR-199a-3p/145-5p that upregulated TrkA expression. Additionally, it has been reported that hUCMSCs-EXOs co-transfected with miR-199a-3p/145-5p infusion improved locomotor function in SCI rats and reduced inflammation [101].

Obesity is considered a metabolic disorder that reshapes the MSCs and their EVs; in this regard, Ji et al. evaluated the protective effects of miR-21 transfected in MSCs-EXOs derived from obese rats. To perform the study, SD rats were induced by laminectomy and were administrated with MSCs-EXOs 24 h after surgery. It has been demonstrated that MSCs-EXOs derived from obese rats did not exert a beneficial effect on the recovery of hindlimb locomotor function and a decrease in miR-21 levels was also observed compared to the group induced with MSCs-EXOs from the control rats. The involvement of miR-21 in SCI's protective effects has been demonstrated by treating MSCs derived from obese rats with miR-21 mimics. MSC-EXOs isolated from obese rats transfected with miR-21 mimic decreased cell apoptosis and injury, and improved locomotor function. Additionally, it has been reported that obesity-related insulin resistance promoted miR-21 deficiency in MSCs-EXOs purified from obese rats. Therefore, it has been suggested that miR-21 could be a potential target for SCI treatment [102]. In addition, Kang et al. investigated the effect of miR-21 on SCI, as well as their underlying molecular mechanisms. It has been demonstrated that miR-21 targets the phosphatase and tensin homolog (PTEN). Indeed, after injury, an increase in miR-21 expression and a consequent reduction in PTEN was observed. To induce an experimental study and investigate the role of miR-21, the authors used MSC-EXOs transfected by miR-21 or PTEN siRNA. The MSC-EXOs transfected by miR-21 or PTEN siRNA led to a reduction in neuronal loss and improved functional recovery after SCI. In this regard, RT-PCR, Western Blot and bioinformatics analysis reported that miR-21m through the inhibition of PTEN/PDCD4, suppressed neuronal death. Additionally, the therapeutic potential of miR-21 has been shown in SH-SY5Y and U251 cells transfected with MSC-EXOs transfected by miR-21 or PTEN small interfering RNA (siRNA). In addition, in vitro, the treatment increased cell viability and suppressed cell death by the miR-21/PTEN/PDCD4 signalling pathway [103]. MiR-21 is known to have the ability to phosphorylate PTEN, which is important in SCI as its silencing in SCI mice was shown to induce cortical neuron growth and increased levels of the mammalian target of rapamycin (mTOR) [104]. In addition, Wang et al. demonstrated the effects of EXOs isolated from PC12 cells or MSCs transfected with phosphatase and tensin homolog pseudogene 1 (PTENP1) short hairpin RNA (shRNA). The EXOs transfected with PTENP1 shRNA led to a reduction in apoptosis both in the SH-SY5Y and U251 cells, according to a mechanism that involved the overexpression of miR-21 and miR-19b, as well as the downregulation of PTENP1 and PTEN. Moreover, the in vitro results were also confirmed in SCI SD rats induced by a contusive model. The in vivo results confirmed the reduction in neuronal apoptosis 28 days after the transplant in the experimental groups treated with transfected EXOs. Therefore, MSC-EXOs transfected with PTENP1 shRNA, through the modulation of miR-19b and miR-21 expression, could be proposed as a new tool for post-SCI recovery [105]. The therapeutic potential of miR-21 and miR-19b derived from hMSCs-EXOs has also been highlighted by Xu et al. The in vitro results demonstrated that, after 48 h, the treatment with EXOs isolated from the supernatant of MSCs and PC12 cells differentiated, led to an increase in miR-21 and miR-19b expression, as well as a decrease in PTEN expression in SH-SY5Y and U251 cells. Therefore, treatment with PC12 cells/MSC-EXOs exerts an inhibitory effect on neuron cell apoptosis. Additionally, the authors evaluated the role of the miR-21/miR-19b pathway in an SCI rat model. The intravenous administration of PC12 cells/MSC-EXOs led to an improvement in functional recovery, as well as reduced neuronal apoptosis in SCI animals. Moreover, it has been confirmed that miR-21 and miR-19b derived from hMSCs-EXOs exerts neuroprotective effects by regulating PTEN expression [106].

Huang et al. investigated the effects of EXOs derived from miR-126-modified MSCs on SCI both in vivo and in vitro. The in vivo results demonstrated that, 28 days after injury, the intravenous administration of labelled miR-126 EXOs led to a reduction in lesion volume and improved functional recovery in SD rats induced by moderate contusion injuries. In addition, in vitro, labelled miR-126 EXOs improved the angiogenesis and migration of HUVECs through the inhibition of Sprouty-related EVH1 domain-containing protein 1 (SPRED1) and phosphoinositide-3-kinase regulatory subunit 2 (PIK3R2), i.e., two targets of miR-126 EXOs. Indeed, it was reported both in vitro and in vivo that treatment with miR-126 EXOs led to a suppression of SPRED1 and PIK3R2 expression and, conversely, an increase in VEGF. These data highlight the potential therapeutic capacity of MSC-EXOs to efficiently transfer miRNAs to the injured spinal cord, thus proving to be a novel potential therapeutic strategy for treating SCI [107].

These data demonstrate the protective role of miRNAs in regeneration and neurogenesis, highlighting their potential use as a treatment for SCI. In this regard, we investigated whether systemic injections of MSC-EXOs transfected with miR-133b, a miRNA already known for its neuroprotective effects in SCI, could reduce spinal cord damage. The study demonstrated that, five days after the transplant, the animals systemically injected with miR-133b EXOs showed an improvement in the recovery of hindlimb function compared to control groups. Moreover, both a reduction in the injury volume and the neuronal cell loss, as well as an increase in the axonal regeneration in the miR-133b EXOs group, were reported. Furthermore, four days following SCI, miR-133b EXOs increased extracellular-signal-regulated kinase (ERK) 1/2 phosphorylation by targeting Ras homolog gene family member A (RhoA) and thus avoiding neuronal cell death. In addition, miR-133b EXOs led to the activation of the signal transducer and activator of transcription 3 (STAT3) and cAMP-response element binding protein (CREB), thus promoting the neuronal cell survival and axonal regeneration; this highlighting once more the potential role of MSC-EXOs transfected with miRNAs [108]. In contrast, Jiang et al. demonstrated the effects of MSC-EXOs transfected with miR-145-5p in an SCI experimental study. The MSC-EXOs transfected with miR-145-5p led to inflammation reduction and improved the animal's functional recovery according to a mechanism that involved the Toll-Like Receptor (TLR)4/NF-κB signalling pathway modulation. In order to confirm the MSC-EXOs effects on cell viability, apoptosis and inflammation, the authors induced an inflammation model in PC12 cells through LPS (5 μg/mL) and then incubated it with 10 μg of MSC-EXOs transfected with miR-145-5p. It is noteworthy that the Western Blot analysis demonstrated that MSC-EXOs containing miR-145-5p reduced the inflammation, as well as the TLR4/NF-κB pathway activation in the PC12 cells [109]. In line with the previous results, Lu et al. demonstrated that the transplant of BMSCs-EXOs reduced neuronal cell death and improved motor recovery through a mechanism that preserved the BSCB integrity. In this regard, it has been shown that the administration of BMSCs-EXOs suppressed the migratory potential of pericytes, thus promoting BSCB integrity via the NF-κB p65 pathway. To confirm the in vivo results and to simulate the pathological environment of SCI in vitro, pericytes isolated from SD rats were exposed to OGD/reperfusion conditions and treated with BMSCs-EVs. In addition, in vitro, treatment with BMMSCs-EVs reduced the migration of pericytes and thus preserved the integrity of the BSCB via NF-κB p65 pathway modulation [66]. It is worth noting that the NF-κB pathway has been related to A1 astrocyte activation and the inflammatory response after SCI. Therefore, with this aim, Wang et al. investigated the inhibitory effects of MSCs-EXOs on the activation of astrocytes following SCI. The intravenous administration of both MSC-EXOs and MSCs led to a decrease in A1 astrocytes activation through the inhibition of the nuclear translocation of NF-κB p65, induced by SCI in the ventral horn of the spinal cord. Moreover, it has been shown that the administration of MSC-EXOs or MSCs reduced pro-inflammatory cytokine levels, including TNFα, IL-1α and IL-1β in the ventral spinal cord after SCI, as well as a decrease in the injury area and improved functional recovery in SCI rats. Additionally, the infusion of MSC-EXOs or MSCs in SCI rats also exerts neuroprotective and anti-apoptotic effects, as shown by the increase in the Myelin Basic Protein (MBP), Synaptophysin (Syn) and Neuronal Nuclei (NeuN). In addition, the in vitro exposure to MSCs-EXOs and MSCs reduced the proportion of SCI-induced A1 astrocytes, most likely through the inhibition of NFκB p65 nuclear translocation [77].

In compliance with this study, Liu et al. demonstrated the efficacy of MSC-EXOs in the suppression of A1 neurotoxic reactive astrocytes activation post-SCI. The BMMSCs-EXOs treatment led to a reduction in A1 neurotoxic reactive astrocytes and suppressed neuronal apoptosis. Through the proangiogenic effects, 28 days after SCI, the treatment with BMMSCs-EXOs promoted axonal regeneration and functional behavioral recovery, as well as reduced glial scar formation, lesion size and inflammation. To confirm the results obtained, the authors performed several in vitro functional assays. In line with the in vivo results, the incubation of HUVEC led to the proliferation, migration and tube formation of HUVEC. The BMMSC-EXOs pre-treatment led to a reduction in the release of LPS-induced nitric oxide in the microglia after 24, 48, 72, and 96 h. Moreover, it has been reported that BMMSCs-EXOs reduced neuronal cell death in the primary neurons induced by treatment with glutamate for 24 h [110]. Taken together, these results suggest that the application of BMMSC-EXOs treatment, which represses A1 neurotoxic reactive astrocytes activation, may be a promising strategy for SCI.

The results of the aforementioned studies demonstrate the potential beneficial effects of MSCs and their MSC-exosome in models of acute SCI. As intravenously administered MSCs are known to not reach the site of injury, it has already been observed that small EVs characterized as exosomes by the trafficking of bone marrow-derived MSCs (MSC-smallEVs) reach the site of injury and target the type M2 macrophages in the injured spinal cord. In this regard, as smallEVs are smaller and more stable and storable than living cells, Nakazaki et al. hypothesized that the infusion of MSC-smallEVs could overcome the many problems associated with cell infusion. Indeed, the transplant of MSC-smallEVs led to BSCB stabilization and improved functional recovery compared to the control animal groups. Additionally, the authors observed that labelled MSCs-EVs have been associated specifically with M2 macrophages and are co-localized with exosome markers, such as CD63, in the lesion site. Moreover, it has been reported that the infusion of EVs increased the expression of M2 macrophage markers, TGF-β and TGF-β receptors, and reduced BSCB permeability. The in vitro results confirm that MSC-sEVs are only taken up by cells when polarized to an M2 phenotype with IL-4 treatment. On the contrary, the cells stimulated to an M1 phenotype did not show a detectable uptake of the EXOs. Overall, these data suggest that MSC-sEVs promote a cascade of cellular responses that improve functional recovery in SCI. Finally, MSC-smallEVs, by targeting M2 macrophages, activate the TGF-β signalling pathway, thus exerting therapeutic effects in SCI. Therefore, contrary to MSCs which could cause risks related to pulmonary embolism, the results of this study demonstrate that multiple administrations of MSC-sEV could be safe. These data highlight how the intravenous administration of MSC-sEV can represent an important non-cellular therapeutic approach for the management of this pathology [111].

In this regard, Lankford et al. evaluated the possible mechanism of action of MSC-EXOs in SCI by studying the tissue distribution and cellular targeting of 1,1-dioctadecyl-3,3,3,3-tetramethylindotricarbocyanine iodide (DiR) fluorescently labelled MSC-EXOs at 3 h and 24 h after intravenous infusion in SCI rats. The DiR labelled MSCs-EXOs were detected in the lesion site in M2 macrophages that express the marker CD206. Therefore, the data suggest that the MSCs-EXOs' regulation of the macrophage's action into the lesion site can contribute to the therapeutic effects of EXOs released by MSCs. MSC-EXOs targeting M2-type macrophages at the site of SCI support the idea that EXOs, released from MSCs, may mediate at least some of the therapeutic effects of the intravenous administration of MSCs [83].

To improve the therapeutic potential of EXOs as a possible clinical application on SCI, researchers are developing different strategies. At present, MSC-secreted nano-sized EXOs have demonstrated an important potential to promote functional behavioral recovery after SCI. As normoxic conditions that occur in vitro differ from the hypoxic micro-environment in vivo, Liu et al. evaluated the effects of MSCs-EXOs under hypoxic (HEXOs) or normoxic (EXOs) conditions, as well as their underlying mechanism. miR-216a-5p is most enriched in HExos and is potentially involved in the microglial polarization of HExos-mediated. The authors isolated EXOs from BMSCs cultivated in normoxic or hypoxic conditions and they transfected them with miR-216a-5p mimics or miR-216a-5p inhibitors, as well as being co-incubated for 24 h with the microglial cell line BV-2 or primary microglia, both induced with LPS to reproduce microglial neuroinflammation in vitro. Although no morphological differences have been shown in experimental groups treated with hypoxic or normoxic conditions, both a greater protein concentration and of the easy up-take of EXOs labelled by microglial cells have been highlighted in HEXOs groups. Moreover, an increase in anti-inflammatory cytokines, as well as a decrease in pro-inflammatory cytokines, both in BV2 cells and primary microglia treated with overexpressed miR-216a-5p-HEXOs (miROE-HEXOs), has been demonstrated. On the contrary, it has been reported that the knockdown of miR-216a-5p in HEXOs (miRKD-HEXOs) could reduce the beneficial effects seen with HExos. Additionally, the authors used C57BL/6 male mice induced by laminectomy and a spinal cord impactor, as well as immediately after SCI infused by tail vein injection with EXOs 200 μg precipitated in 200 μL PBS, or an equal volume of PBS (200 μL). The in vivo results demonstrated that the administration of HEXOs promoted functional behavioral recovery after SCI compared to the EXOs mice group. It has been reported that the transplant of HEXOs led to a shift in the polarization of the microglial/macrophage from the M1 to M2 phenotype. Additionally, it has been confirmed that miR-216a-5p overexpression facilitated the polarization of the microglia/macrophage from the M1 to M2 phenotype. As TLR4 has been identified as a target of exosomal miR-216a-5p, the TLR4/NF-κB/PI3K/AKT signalling pathway can be involved in the microglial polarization modulation. In conclusion, the combination of miRNAs and MSC-EXOs derived from hypoxic conditions could be a minimally invasive approach for SCI treatment [112].

Although there are numerous advantages over MSCs, both EXOs and MSC-derived nanovesicles (N-NVs) do not show the ability to target diseased organs after systemic administration. In this regard, Lee et al. developed and evaluated the effects of macrophage membrane-fused umbilical cord blood-derived MSCs (MF-MSCs). As macrophage membranes contain several binding molecules, including α4β1 integrin, as well as receptors of inflammatory cytokines, MF-NVs by neuroprotective, anti-inflammatory and angiogenic effects, they could improve the efficacy of NVs on SCI. To mimic the ischemic conditions in the spinal cord, HUVECs underwent hypoxia and MF-NVs were added. The in vitro results demonstrated a greater targeting efficiency of MF-NVs for HUVECs cultivated in hypoxic-conditioned. Moreover, the intravenous administration of MF-NVs led to an improvement in the functional recovery in SCI C57BL/6 mice induced by the compression model 1 h after injury and were injected again seven days post-injury. Moreover, the injection of NVs reduced the acute inflammation and cellular damage that occur after SCI. In addition, three days post-injury, the proliferative and remodelling phases that are involved in angiogenesis were observed. As has been reported in the previous studies, the NVs membrane coated from immunocytes, including neutrophils and macrophages, could likely remove inflammatory cytokines, such as IL1β and TNFα, so to explain the targeting mechanism of MF-NVs [113]. Thus, potentiated exosome-mimetic nanovesicles appear as potential therapeutical strategies for SCI management.

In addition, in order to improve the release and integration of EXOs, Li et al. used an innovative implantation strategy related to human MSCs-EXOs immobilized in a peptide-modified adhesive hydrogel (pGel). Otherwise from systemic treatment, MSCs-EXOs immobilized in a pGel contain exosome-encapsulated in an extracellular matrix are able to be inserted in the damaged nervous system, leading to a mitigation of the SCI microenvironment. Before performing the in vivo study, the authors evaluated the delivery capacity of MSCs-EXOs encapsulated in pGel compared to the hyaluronic acid hydrogel group. To induce the in vivo study, SD rats underwent laminectomy, and the spinal cord was transected. Following the lesion, the animals were implanted with human MSCs-EXOs (100 μg) that had been suspended in PBS (20 μL) and injected into the pGel (60 μL). The study results demonstrate the efficacy of the transplant in functional recovery and urinary protection. Finally, 28 days after the Exo-pGel transplants, the exert regenerative effects leading to lesion reduction and an increase in myelin sheaths were observed, thus explaining the improved locomotor functions [100].

The results of all of these studies (Table 1) show the beneficial effects of MSC-EXOs transplantation in neuron tissue regeneration and motor function recovery, as shown in Figure 3. The clinical data and experimental animal reports show that exosomes, in particular exosomal miRNAs, are closely associated with SCI. For this reason, MSC-EXOs could have potential applications in several diseases and may be a promising hope for SCI management. Indeed, MSC-EXOs can cross the BSCB, reducing both neuroinflammation and neuronal apoptosis, thus promoting vascular remodelling, neurogenesis, microglia activation and axonal regeneration in the nervous system and protecting the BSCB.

Table 1. Synthesis of the studies that evaluate the role of MSC-EXOs in several in vivo and in vitro models of SCI.

Cell Therapy	Dose	Rout of Administration	Intervention	Results	Type of Study	Ref.
hEpi ADMSCs-EXOs	1×10^9 and 5×10^9 particles in 0.2 mL PBS	Intravenous administration	Immediately after SCI was induced, the hEpi ADMSCs-EXOs were injected into the animals and the same amount was administered again after 3 days.	The hEpi ADMSC-EXOs injection improved SCI and reduced the inflammatory response of spinal cord injury through the regulation of various cytokines and targeting immune response and neurogenesis-related genes in the spinal cord tissue. Conversely, Increased the expression of neurotrophin factors such as BDNF and VEGF.	In vivo	[96]
BMMSCs-EXOs	200 μg/mL, ~1×10^6	Intravenous administration	BMMSCs-EXOs were administered 30 min and 1 day after SCI	The BMSC-EXOs counteracted neuronal cell death, and reduced myelin loss, improving myelin disposition. Furthermore, the treatment increased pericytic/endothelial cell coverage on the vascular wall, inhibited caspase 1 and IL-1β expression, decreased blood-spinal barrier leakage, and promoted accelerated functional recovery in rats. with SCI. In addition, in vivo exposure to BMSC-EXOs it reduced pericyte pyroptosis and increased its survival rate.	In vivo	[97]
	100 μg/mL	Pericytes co-incubation and exposure to BMSCs-EXOs	Pericytes were co-incubated with or without BMSCs-EXOs for 8 h before exposure to a compound stimulus of IFN-γ + TNF-α + LPS + Lipofectamine + ATP		In vitro	
hPMSCs-EXOs	200 μg/μL	Intrathecal injection	Exosomes were directly injected by stereotactic injection into the epicenter of the SCI after damage	The hPMSCs-Exos have proangiogenic effects on endothelial cells inducing tube formation. In addition, in vivo, the hPMSCs-Exos treatment enhanced angiogenesis in the SCI rats and promoted functional recovery.	In vivo	[98]
	100 μg/mL	HUVECs SCI model exposed to hPMSCs-EXOs	HUVECs have been cultivated in OGD conditions and undergo scratch in order to induce the SCI model and subsequently exposed to hPMSCs-EXOs		In vitro	
BMMSCs-EXOs-miR-26a	20 μg/ml	Intravenous administration	BM-MSCs were transfected with the mimics of miR-26a, and the exosomes were collected. Subsequently, PC12 cells were incubated with BMMSCs-EXOs-miR-26a for 48 h.	BMMSCs-Exos-miR-26a induced neurofilament generation in vitro reducing PTEN expression and increasing the PI3K, AKT, and mTOR proteins phosphorylation. In vivo, treatment enhanced axonal regeneration, and neurogenesis, conversely, it reduced glial scarring and improved functional recovery through PTEN/AKT/mTOR signaling cascades.	In vitro	[99]
	200 μg in 200 μL PBS	PC12 cells incubated with BMMSCs-EXOs-miR-26a	Immediately following SCI, the rats received an injection of BMMSCs-EXOs-miR-26a via tail vein injection.		In vivo	

Table 1. *Cont.*

Cell Therapy	Dose	Rout of Administration	Intervention	Results	Type of Study	Ref.
BMMSCs-EXOs containing miR-544	100 μg diluted in 0.5 mL PBS	Intravenous administration	24 h after SCI, the rat model was induced, the animals received an injection of BMMSCs-EXOs containing miR-544 via tail vein injection.	BMMSCs-EXOs containing miR-544 reduced inflammation and improved both neuronal survival and consequently promoted functional recovery after SCI	In vivo	[100]
hUCMSCs-EXOs co-transfected with miR-199a-3p/145-5p	0, 1, 3, 5, 7, 10, 13, 15, 17, 20, 25 μg/mL	PC12 cells incubated with hUCMSCs-EXOs co-transfected with miR-199a-3p/145-5p	After being pretreated with hUCMSCs-EXOs or with hUCMSCs-EXOs co-transfected with miR-199a-3p/145-5p, the PC12 cells were treated with LPS (11 μg/mL) in order to establish an injury model.	Administration of hUCMSCs-EXOs co-transfected with miR-199a-3p/145-5p to neurons of SCI rats upregulated TrkA expression at the site of injury. Consequently, the downstream pathways of NGF/TrkA and Akt were inactivated. Thus, the treatment promoted locomotor recovery in SCI rats indicating that hUC-MSC-EXOs may be a promising treatment strategy for SCI.	In vitro	[101]
	200 μg	Intravenous administration	SD rats were induced with laminectomy and subsequently underwent artery clamp to trigger acute trauma. After the SCI model was induced, the animals were injected via the tail vein with hUCMSCs-EXOs or hUCMSCs-EXOs co-transfected with miR-199a-3p/145-5p		In vivo	
MSC-EXOs isolated from obese rats transfected with miR-21	100 mg in 0.5 mL of PBS	Intravenous administration	The animals were treated with MSC-EXOs isolated from obese rats transfected with miR-21 mimic or without transfection 24 h after injury	The MSC-EXOs isolated from obese rats, due to a reduction in the levels of miR-21, as a result of insulin resistance, do not exert protective effects against skiing. On the contrary, the MSC-EXOs transfected with miR-21 Mimic showed an increase in the level of miR-21 in MSC-EXOs isolated from obese rats decreased cell apoptosis and area of injury, thus recovering their protective effects against this pathology.	In vivo	[97]
MSC-EXOs transfected with miR-21	-	Intravenous administration	Immediately following SCI, the rats received an injection of MSC-EXOs transfected with miR-21 via tail vein injection.	The MSC-EXOs transfected with miR-21 protected neuronal cells from SCI-induced apoptosis and improved the functional recovery after injury by the miR-21/PTEN/PDCD4 signaling pathway	In vivo	[98]
	-	SH-SY5Y and U251 incubated with MSC-EXOs transfected with miR-21 or PTEN siRNA	SH-SY5Y and U251 cells were firstly transfected with miR-21, or PTEN siRNA using Lipofectamine 2000 and subsequently were treated MSC-EXOs transfected with miR-21 or PTEN siRNA for 48 h		In vitro	
PC12 cells/ /MSC-EXOs co-transfected with miR-21/miR-19b	-	SH-SY5Y and U251 incubated with PC12 cells/MSC-EXOs co-transfected with miR-21/miR-19b	SH-SY5Y and U251 cells were transfected with miR-21, miR-19, or PTEN siRNA using Lipofectamine 2000 and subsequently were treated with PC12 cells/MSC-EXOs transfected with miR-21/miR-19b for 48 h.	PC12 cells/MSC-EXOs transfected with miR-21/miR-19b suppressed the apoptosis of neuron cells by downregulating the PTEN expression.	In vitro	[105]

Table 1. *Cont.*

Cell Therapy	Dose	Rout of Administration	Intervention	Results	Type of Study	Ref.
	-	Intravenous administration	After SCI, the animals were treated with PC12 cells derived EXOs or with MSC-EXOs transfected with miR-21/miR-19 or PTEN siRNA.		In vivo	
PC12 cells/MSC-EXOs		SH-SY5Y and U251 incubated with PC12 cells/MSC-EXOs	SH-SY5Y and U251 cells were co-transfected with miR-21 and wild type/mutant PTEN mRNA or miR-19b and wild type/mutant PTEN mRNA using Lipofectamine 2000 for 48 h	In EXOs derived from MSCs and PC12 cells, the elevated expression of miR-21 and miR19b reduced PTEN expression and attenuated apoptosis in neuronal cells confirming the therapeutic effects of PC12 cells/MSC-EXOs by downregulating the expression of PTEN.	In vitro	[106]
		Intravenous administration	After SCI, the animals were treated with PC12 cells derived EXOs or with MSC-EXOs.		In vivo	
MSC-EXOs transfected with miR-126	100 μg, about 1×10^{10} particles diluted in 0.5 mL of PBS	Intravenous administration	Approximately 30 min after injury, the rats were treated with MSC-EXOs transfected with miR-126 or miR-con EXOs via tail vein injection	MSC-EXOs transfected with miR-126 efficiently transferred miR-126 to the site of injury, induced angiogenesis by suppressing SPRED1 and PIK3R2, stimulated neurogenesis, and protected neuronal cell to apoptosis SCI induced.	In vivo	[107]
	10 μg	HUVECs OGD model exposed to hPMSCs-EXOs	First, HUVECs were incubated with miR-con EXOs or miR-126 EXOs for 6 h and subjected to OGD. Then, the cells were incubated with MSC-EXOs for 2 hours		In vitro	
MSC-EXOs transfected with miR-133b	100 μg in 0.5 mL of PBS	Intravenous administration	The animals were treated with MSC-EXOs transfected with miR-133b, 24 h after injury	Systemic administration of miR-133b-transfected EXOs upregulated miR-133b expression at the site of injury and protected neuronal cells from apoptosis and promoted axon regeneration. Part of these effects was mediated by the activation of the ERK1/2, STAT3, and CREB pathways, targeting RhoA which is instead inhibited.	In vivo	[102]
MSC-EXOs transfected with miR-145-5p	100 μg in 0.5 mL of PBS, equivalent to 1×10^{10} particles	Intravenous administration	The animals were treated with MSC-EXOs transfected with miR-145-5p 30 min after injury	MSC-EXOs transfected with miR-145-5p can be useful to reduce the inflammation in SCI by the involvement of TLR4/NF-κB pathway modulation.	In vivo	[109]
	10 μg	PC12 cells incubated with MSCs-EXOs transfected with miR-145-5p	After 24 h, PC12 cells treated with LPS were incubated with MSCs-EXOs containing miR-145-5p for 48 h		In vitro	

Table 1. *Cont.*

Cell Therapy	Dose	Rout of Administration	Intervention	Results	Type of Study	Ref.
BMMSCs-EVs	200 μg/mL	Intravenous administration	BMMSCs-Evs were injected into the tail vein 30 min post-SCI and 1-day post-injury	BMMSC-Evs reduced apoptosis in neuronal cells, promote regeneration, improved motor function, and attenuated the disruption of BSCB and pericyte coverage via NF-κB p65.	In vivo	[63]
	100 μg/mL	Pericytes co-incubation and exposure to BMSCs-Evs	Pericytes were seeded 100 μg/mL of BMMSC-Evs and after were exposed to OGD/reperfusion exposure		In vitro	
BMMSC-EXOs	200 μg/mL, derived from ~1 × 10^6 MSCs	Intravenous administration	30-min post-injury and 1 day after, the animals were infused by tail vain with BMMSCs or with BMMSC-EXOs	Both MSCs and MSC-EXOs administration exerted anti-inflammatory and neuroprotective properties attenuating SCI-induced A1 astrocytes activation via inhibiting nuclear translocation of NFκB p65	In vivo	[77]
	5 × 10^4	Astrocyte co-culture with BMMSCs or BMMSC-EXOs	Astrocytes collected from SCI rats co-cultured with BMMSCs or MSC-EXOs for 48 h		In vitro	
BMMSC-EXOs	200 μg of BMSCs-EXOs precipitated in 200 μL of PBS	Intravenous administration	After SCI, the rats were treated with BMSCs-EXOs via tail vain	The BMMSC-EXOs treatment induced functional behavioral recovery, enhancing blood vessel formation, reducing glial scars, protecting the neuronal cells against apoptosis, increasing axonal regeneration, and decreasing inflammatory response by suppression of the activation of A1 neurotoxic reactive astrocytes.	In vivo	[110]
	100 μg/mL	HUVECs exposed to BMMSCs-EXOs	2 × 10^4 HUVEC cells were seeded and after co-incubated with BMMSC-EXOs for 24 h. It has been tested the effects of BMMSCs-EXOs on nitric oxide production, HUVEC cells, 1 hour before stimulation with 5 ng/mL LPS, microglia 2 × 10^5 cells/mL, have been pretreated with or without BMSCs-EXOs 100 μg/mL		In vitro	
BMMSC-small EVs	2.5 × 10^9 or 8.3 × 10^8	Intravenous administration	On day 7 post-SCI, MSCs or MSC-sEVs suspended in 1 mL DMEM were infused via the femoral vein. On 8- and 9-day post-SCI, 0.2 mL DMEM alone or 1/3 dose MSC-sEVs in 0.2 mL DMEM was infused via the saphenous vein.	Both MSC infusion and fractionated MSC-smallEVs target M2 macrophages and augment TGF-β receptors, activating the TGF-β signaling pathway, thus promoting functional recovery in SCI animals.	In vivo	[111]
BMMSC-EXOs	2.5 × 10^9 in 0.2 mL of PBS	Intravenous administration	One week post-injury, DiR labeled MSC-EXOs were infused into the saphenous veins	Intravenous administration of MSC-EXOs rapidly traffic to the injured and associate specifically with M2 macrophages.	In vivo	[83]

Table 1. *Cont.*

Cell Therapy	Dose	Rout of Administration	Intervention	Results	Type of Study	Ref.
BMMSC-EXOs	200 μg/mL	BV2 exposed to BMMSCs-EXOs under hypoxic or normoxic condition	LPS (1 μg/mL) was co-cultured with BV2 microglia for 24 h followed by the addition of EXOs	Hypoxia preconditioning represents a promising and effective approach to enhancing the therapeutic properties of MSC-EXOs, promoting functional behavioral recovery in the SCI model by shifting microglial polarization from M1 to M2 phenotype in vivo and in vitro.	In vitro	[112]
	200 μg of total protein of EXOs precipitated in 200 μL PBS	Intravenous administration	Mice were subjected to SCI, followed by tail vein injection of EXOs, HEXOs, miR-NCOE-HExos, miROE-HExos, miR-NCKD-HExos, and miRKD-HExos.		In vivo	
N-NVs and MF-NVs	20 μg/mL		PC12 cells and HUVECs were cultured in the media containing 500 μM of H_2O_2 and lipopolysaccharide in a hypoxic incubator for 24 h. To polarize macrophages into the M1 phenotype, RAW 264.7 cells were cultured in the presence of LPS for 24 h in normoxia. After, the cells were treated with N-NVs and MF-NVs (20 μg/mL) for 24 h under hypoxic and polarization culture conditions.	Compared to normal N-NVs, MF-NVs contained a larger quantity of ischemic area-targeting molecules. The MF-NVs enhanced their accumulation in the injured spinal cord. This increased reduced apoptosis and inflammation prevented the axonal loss, increased blood vessel formation, decreased fibrosis, and consequently, improved spinal cord function.	In vitro	[113]
	25 μg of N-NV in 100 μL PBS, and 25 μg of MF-NV in 100 μL PBS	Intravenous administration	N-NVs and MF-NVs intravenously injected to tail vein 1 h and 7 days post-SCI		In vivo	
Human MSC-EXOs immobilized in pGel	100 μg suspended in 20 μL PBS	Topical transplantation	After the lesion, the animals were implanted with human MSCs-EXOs and injected into the pGel (60 μL)	The human MSC-EXOs immobilized in pGel induced nerve tissue repair and functional recovery protecting bladder and kidney tissues from SCI induced-neuronal damage.	In vivo	[100]

Mesenchymal stromal/stem cells: MSCs; human epidural adipose tissue-derived MSCs: hEpi AD–MSCs; exosomes-derived MSCs: MSC-EXOs; phosphate-buffered saline: PBS; Spinal cord injury: SCI; brain-derived neurotrophic factor: BDNF; vascular endothelial growth factor: VEGF; Bone marrow MSCs: BMMSCs; interferon-γ: IFN-γ; tumor necrosis factor α: TNF-α; lipopolysaccharide: LPS; adenosine triphosphate: ATP; interleukin-1β: IL-1β; human placenta-derived MSCs: hPMSCs; Human Umbilical Vein Endothelial Cells: HUVECs; oxygen-glucose deprivation: OGD; Phosphoinositide 3-kinases: PI3Ks; phosphatase and tensin homolog: PTEN; protein kinase B: Akt; mammalian target of rapamycin: mTOR; human umbilical cord: hUC-MSCs; human umbilical cord MSCs: hUCMSCs; nerve growth factor: NGF; extracellular-signal regulated kinase: ERK; signal transducer and activator of transcription 3: STAT3; cAMP-response element binding protein: CREB; Ras homolog gene family member A: RhoA; nuclear factor kappa-light-chain-enhancer of activated B cells: NF-κB; Toll-Like Receptor: TLR; small interfering RNA: siRNA; phosphatase and tensin homolog: PTEN; Sprouty-related EVH1 domain-containing protein 1: SPRED1; and phosphoinositide-3-kinase regulatory subunit 2: PIK3R2; extracellular vesicles: EVs; EVs derived from BMMSCs: BMM-SCs-EVs; blood-spinal cord barrier: BSCB; macrophage membrane-fused exosome-mimetic nanovesicles: MF-NVs; MSC-derived nanovesicles: N-NVs; peptide-modified adhesive hydrogel: pGel; MSCs-EXOs under hypoxic: HEXOs; overexpressed miR-216a-5p-HEXOs: miROE-HEXOs; knockdown of miR-216a-5p in HEXOs: miRKD-HEXOs.

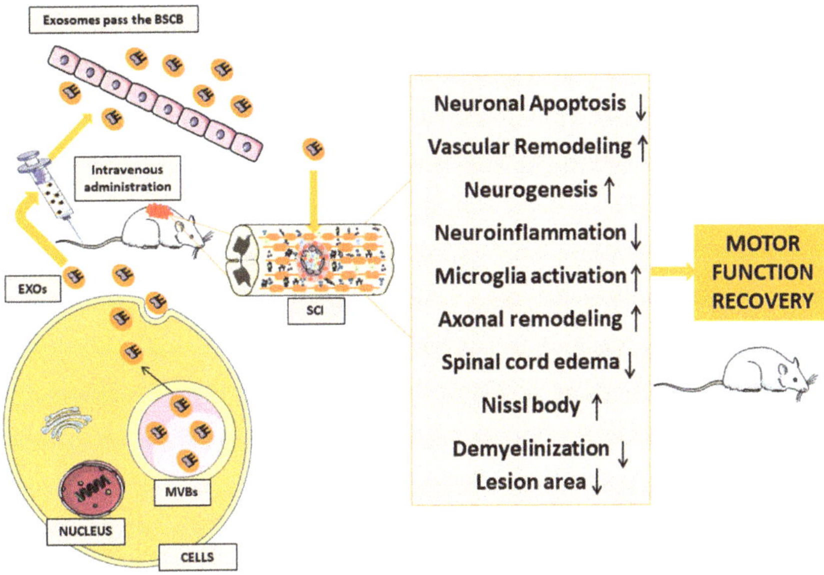

Figure 3. Repair of the nervous system following SCI post exosomes transplantation. Exosomes secreted by donor cells can cross to the blood-brain barrier, reducing both neuroinflammation and neuronal apoptosis, thus promoting vascular remodeling, neurogenesis, microglia activation and axonal remodeling in the nervous system. The image was created using the image bank of Servier Medical Art (Available online: http://smart.servier.com/, accessed on 1 December 2022), licensed under a Creative Commons Attribution 3.0 Unported License (Available online: https://creativecommons.org/licenses/by/3.0/, accessed on 1 December 2022).

7. Challenges and Future Perspectives

For decades, research has focused on regenerative strategies capable of improving the recovery of the injured spinal cord after SCI. Although the transplant of MSCs seems to be a potential treatment for SCI, factors such as tumorigenesis, low survival rate and immune rejection, as well as the lack of direct differentiation of MSCs in neuronal cells, can limit their application to promote spinal cord repair. The study of MSC-EXOs could represent new challenges and opportunities for developing regenerative strategies. However, before MSC-EXOs can be applied to clinical practice, it is necessary to address several challenges related to the source and optimal culture conditions, including isolation, purification, amplification, as well as the optimal dose, frequency and route of EXOs administration. As MSC-EXOs isolated from different tissue sources contain different inclusions, they show different abilities to repair damage. Consequently, the choice of MSC-EXOs should be performed according to the different tissues of origin. Furthermore, in order to not affect the biological activity of EXOs, it is necessary to implement standardized, inexpensive, rapid isolation and purification procedures. Indeed, the different separation methods show significant differences in RNA and protein contents. Hence, the storage, transportation, and preservation of EXOs are fundamental. In order to improve the recovery of the injured spinal cord after SCI, a further challenge is represented by the sufficient MSC-EXOs number to be administered. Consequently, physiological stimuli, as well as chemical and physical pretreatment, including hypoxic preconditioning or cytokine preconditioning, could improve the paracrine effects of MSC-EXOs and regulate the production and release of different factors, as well as of EXOs. Additionally, innovative implantation strategies, such as EXOs-encapsulated in an extracellular matrix, have led to an improvement in the capacity of EXOs inserted into damaged nervous systems. Despite the PEG being the gold-standard technique for modifying the surface of nanoparticles, new techniques, such as integrated cell cloaking nanotherapeutics, are being investigated in order to improve the increment of nanoparticles in the target tissue and, thus, being used as vehicles for drug delivery, immune modulation and tissue regeneration. Although encouraging results are being obtained by methods that combine MSC-EXOs with biological materials, or those that used MSC-EXOs for targeted drug or gene delivery, future studies are needed to investigate them in depth.

8. Conclusions

As the therapeutic effects of MSCs are related to their paracrine activity by the release of proteins, lipids and high levels of miRNAs in their contained MSC-EXOs, modulating the signaling pathways involved in their neuro-regenerative and neuroprotective effects could be a potential tool to treat SCI. Several experimental studies have demonstrated that different miRNAs, including miR-21; miR-19; miR-126; miR-133b; miR-199a-3p/145-5p; miR-26a and miR-544, through modulation of the signaling pathways PTEN/AKT/mTOR, NF-κB p65 or ERK1/2, reduced astrocytes activation and pericytes migration suppressed both neuronal apoptosis and inflammation in SCI. Additionally, an improvement in the functional recovery induced by axonal regeneration, the release of proangiogenic factors and the polarization of macrophages toward the M2 state have been shown, thus promoting BSCB integrity and a reduction in the damage post-SCI. As, at present, there are no standardized methods to isolate and administered MSC-EXOs, it could be useful to investigate new methods to deliver the EXOs directly to the lesion site. Moreover, it is necessary to understand the additional mechanisms involved in the regenerative properties, as well as to establish the efficacy and safety of transplanting EXOs in SCI patients; hence, further studies are required.

Author Contributions: Conceptualization, G.S. and E.M.; writing—original draft preparation, G.S., S.S.; writing—review and editing, G.S., S.S. and E.M.; supervision, E.M. All authors have read and agreed to the published version of the manuscript.

Funding: This study was supported by Current Research Funds 2023, Ministry of Health, Italy.

Institutional Review Board Statement: Not applicable.

Informed Consent Statement: Not applicable.

Data Availability Statement: Not applicable.

Acknowledgments: The authors would like to thank the Ministry of Health, Italy.

Conflicts of Interest: The authors declare no conflict of interest.

References

1. Kim, G.U.; Sung, S.E.; Kang, K.K.; Choi, J.H.; Lee, S.; Sung, M.; Yang, S.Y.; Kim, S.K.; Kim, Y.I.; Lim, J.H.; et al. Therapeutic Potential of Mesenchymal Stem Cells (MSCs) and MSC-Derived Extracellular Vesicles for the Treatment of Spinal Cord Injury. *Int. J. Mol. Sci.* **2021**, *22*, 3672. [CrossRef] [PubMed]
2. Mathieu, M.; Martin-Jaular, L.; Lavieu, G.; Thery, C. Specificities of secretion and uptake of exosomes and other extracellular vesicles for cell-to-cell communication. *Nat. Cell Biol.* **2019**, *21*, 9–17. [CrossRef]
3. Vader, P.; Mol, E.A.; Pasterkamp, G.; Schiffelers, R.M. Extracellular vesicles for drug delivery. *Adv. Drug Deliv. Rev.* **2016**, *106*, 148–156. [CrossRef] [PubMed]
4. Aimaletdinov, A.M.; Gomzikova, M.O. Tracking of Extracellular Vesicles' Biodistribution: New Methods and Approaches. *Int. J. Mol. Sci.* **2022**, *23*, 1312. [CrossRef] [PubMed]
5. Yanez-Mo, M.; Siljander, P.R.; Andreu, Z.; Zavec, A.B.; Borras, F.E.; Buzas, E.I.; Buzas, K.; Casal, E.; Cappello, F.; Carvalho, J.; et al. Biological properties of extracellular vesicles and their physiological functions. *J. Extracell. Vesicles* **2015**, *4*, 27066. [CrossRef]
6. Izadpanah, M.; Seddigh, A.; Ebrahimi Barough, S.; Fazeli, S.A.S.; Ai, J. Potential of Extracellular Vesicles in Neurodegenerative Diseases: Diagnostic and Therapeutic Indications. *J. Mol. Neurosci.* **2018**, *66*, 172–179. [CrossRef]
7. Yang, Z.; Li, Y.; Wang, Z. Recent Advances in the Application of Mesenchymal Stem Cell-Derived Exosomes for Cardiovascular and Neurodegenerative Disease Therapies. *Pharmaceutics* **2022**, *14*, 618. [CrossRef]
8. Sun, Y.; Liu, G.; Zhang, K.; Cao, Q.; Liu, T.; Li, J. Mesenchymal stem cells-derived exosomes for drug delivery. *Stem Cell Res. Ther.* **2021**, *12*, 561. [CrossRef]

9. Moher, D.; Liberati, A.; Tetzlaff, J.; Altman, D.G.; Group, P. Preferred reporting items for systematic reviews and meta-analyses: The PRISMA statement. *PLoS Med.* **2009**, *6*, e1000097. [CrossRef]
10. Aziz, I.; Che Ramli, M.D.; Mohd Zain, N.S.; Sanusi, J. Behavioral and Histopathological Study of Changes in Spinal Cord Injured Rats Supplemented with Spirulina platensis. *Evid.-Based Complement. Altern. Med.* **2014**, *2014*, 871657. [CrossRef]
11. Sykova, E.; Cizkova, D.; Kubinova, S. Mesenchymal Stem Cells in Treatment of Spinal Cord Injury and Amyotrophic Lateral Sclerosis. *Front. Cell Dev. Biol.* **2021**, *9*, 695900. [CrossRef] [PubMed]
12. Singh, A.; Tetreault, L.; Kalsi-Ryan, S.; Nouri, A.; Fehlings, M.G. Global prevalence and incidence of traumatic spinal cord injury. *Clin. Epidemiol.* **2014**, *6*, 309–331. [CrossRef]
13. Kumar, R.; Lim, J.; Mekary, R.A.; Rattani, A.; Dewan, M.C.; Sharif, S.Y.; Osorio-Fonseca, E.; Park, K.B. Traumatic Spinal Injury: Global Epidemiology and Worldwide Volume. *World Neurosurg.* **2018**, *113*, e345–e363. [CrossRef]
14. Chen, W.C.; Liu, W.F.; Bai, Y.Y.; Zhou, Y.Y.; Zhang, Y.; Wang, C.M.; Lin, S.; He, H.F. Transplantation of mesenchymal stem cells for spinal cord injury: A systematic review and network meta-analysis. *J. Transl. Med.* **2021**, *19*, 178. [CrossRef]
15. Liau, L.L.; Looi, Q.H.; Chia, W.C.; Subramaniam, T.; Ng, M.H.; Law, J.X. Treatment of spinal cord injury with mesenchymal stem cells. *Cell Biosci.* **2020**, *10*, 112. [CrossRef] [PubMed]
16. Morales, I.I.; Toscano-Tejeida, D.; Ibarra, A. Non Pharmacological Strategies to Promote Spinal Cord Regeneration: A View on Some Individual or Combined Approaches. *Curr. Pharm. Des.* **2016**, *22*, 720–727. [CrossRef] [PubMed]
17. Tyler, J.Y.; Xu, X.M.; Cheng, J.X. Nanomedicine for treating spinal cord injury. *Nanoscale* **2013**, *5*, 8821–8836. [CrossRef]
18. Rosenzweig, E.S.; McDonald, J.W. Rodent models for treatment of spinal cord injury: Research trends and progress toward useful repair. *Curr. Opin. Neurol.* **2004**, *17*, 121–131. [CrossRef]
19. Kumar, H.; Ropper, A.E.; Lee, S.H.; Han, I. Propitious Therapeutic Modulators to Prevent Blood-Spinal Cord Barrier Disruption in Spinal Cord Injury. *Mol. Neurobiol.* **2017**, *54*, 3578–3590. [CrossRef]
20. Ahuja, C.S.; Nori, S.; Tetreault, L.; Wilson, J.; Kwon, B.; Harrop, J.; Choi, D.; Fehlings, M.G. Traumatic Spinal Cord Injury-Repair and Regeneration. *Neurosurgery* **2017**, *80*, S9–S22. [CrossRef]
21. Alizadeh, A.; Dyck, S.M.; Karimi-Abdolrezaee, S. Traumatic Spinal Cord Injury: An Overview of Pathophysiology, Models and Acute Injury Mechanisms. *Front. Neurol.* **2019**, *10*, 282. [CrossRef]
22. Silva, N.A.; Sousa, N.; Reis, R.L.; Salgado, A.J. From basics to clinical: A comprehensive review on spinal cord injury. *Prog. Neurobiol.* **2014**, *114*, 25–57. [CrossRef]
23. Ramer, L.M.; Ramer, M.S.; Steeves, J.D. Setting the stage for functional repair of spinal cord injuries: A cast of thousands. *Spinal Cord* **2005**, *43*, 134–161. [CrossRef] [PubMed]
24. Zhou, X.; He, X.; Ren, Y. Function of microglia and macrophages in secondary damage after spinal cord injury. *Neural Regen. Res.* **2014**, *9*, 1787–1795. [CrossRef] [PubMed]
25. Nakamura, M.; Houghtling, R.A.; MacArthur, L.; Bayer, B.M.; Bregman, B.S. Differences in cytokine gene expression profile between acute and secondary injury in adult rat spinal cord. *Exp. Neurol.* **2003**, *184*, 313–325. [CrossRef] [PubMed]
26. Zhivotovsky, B.; Orrenius, S. Calcium and cell death mechanisms: A perspective from the cell death community. *Cell Calcium* **2011**, *50*, 211–221. [CrossRef]
27. Park, E.; Velumian, A.A.; Fehlings, M.G. The role of excitotoxicity in secondary mechanisms of spinal cord injury: A review with an emphasis on the implications for white matter degeneration. *J. Neurotrauma* **2004**, *21*, 754–774. [CrossRef]
28. Dong, H.; Fazzaro, A.; Xiang, C.; Korsmeyer, S.J.; Jacquin, M.F.; McDonald, J.W. Enhanced oligodendrocyte survival after spinal cord injury in Bax-deficient mice and mice with delayed Wallerian degeneration. *J. Neurosci.* **2003**, *23*, 8682–8691. [CrossRef]
29. Sugawara, T.; Chan, P.H. Reactive oxygen radicals and pathogenesis of neuronal death after cerebral ischemia. *Antioxid. Redox Signal.* **2003**, *5*, 597–607. [CrossRef]
30. Donnelly, D.J.; Popovich, P.G. Inflammation and its role in neuroprotection, axonal regeneration and functional recovery after spinal cord injury. *Exp. Neurol.* **2008**, *209*, 378–388. [CrossRef]
31. Tran, A.P.; Warren, P.M.; Silver, J. The Biology of Regeneration Failure and Success After Spinal Cord Injury. *Physiol. Rev.* **2018**, *98*, 881–917. [CrossRef]
32. Kwiecien, J.M.; Dabrowski, W.; Dabrowska-Bouta, B.; Sulkowski, G.; Oakden, W.; Kwiecien-Delaney, C.J.; Yaron, J.R.; Zhang, L.; Schutz, L.; Marzec-Kotarska, B.; et al. Prolonged inflammation leads to ongoing damage after spinal cord injury. *PLoS ONE* **2020**, *15*, e0226584. [CrossRef] [PubMed]
33. Yuan, Y.M.; He, C. The glial scar in spinal cord injury and repair. *Neurosci. Bull.* **2013**, *29*, 421–435. [CrossRef]
34. Wilson, J.R.; Forgione, N.; Fehlings, M.G. Emerging therapies for acute traumatic spinal cord injury. *CMAJ* **2013**, *185*, 485–492. [CrossRef] [PubMed]
35. Yang, M.; Yin, X.; Liu, S.; Hui, H.; Yan, L.; He, B.; Hao, D. Letter: Ultra-Early (<12 Hours) Surgery Correlates With Higher Rate of American Spinal Injury Association Impairment Scale Conversion After Cervical Spinal Cord Injury. *Neurosurgery* **2019**, *85*, E399–E400. [CrossRef] [PubMed]
36. Kwon, B.K.; Curt, A.; Belanger, L.M.; Bernardo, A.; Chan, D.; Markez, J.A.; Gorelik, S.; Slobogean, G.P.; Umedaly, H.; Giffin, M.; et al. Intrathecal pressure monitoring and cerebrospinal fluid drainage in acute spinal cord injury: A prospective randomized trial. *J. Neurosurg.* **2009**, *10*, 181–193. [CrossRef] [PubMed]
37. Bracken, M.B. Steroids for acute spinal cord injury. *Cochrane Database Syst. Rev.* **2012**, *1*, CD001046. [CrossRef] [PubMed]

38. Gupta, R.; Bathen, M.E.; Smith, J.S.; Levi, A.D.; Bhatia, N.N.; Steward, O. Advances in the management of spinal cord injury. *J. Am. Acad. Orthop. Surg.* **2010**, *18*, 210–222. [CrossRef]
39. Hawryluk, G.; Whetstone, W.; Saigal, R.; Ferguson, A.; Talbott, J.; Bresnahan, J.; Dhall, S.; Pan, J.; Beattie, M.; Manley, G. Mean Arterial Blood Pressure Correlates with Neurological Recovery after Human Spinal Cord Injury: Analysis of High Frequency Physiologic Data. *J. Neurotrauma* **2015**, *32*, 1958–1967. [CrossRef]
40. Jin, M.; Zhang, S.; Wang, M.; Li, Q.; Ren, J.; Luo, Y.; Sun, X. Exosomes in pathogenesis, diagnosis, and therapy of ischemic stroke. *Front. Bioeng. Biotechnol.* **2022**, *10*, 980548. [CrossRef]
41. Kucuk, N.; Primozic, M.; Knez, Z.; Leitgeb, M. Exosomes Engineering and Their Roles as Therapy Delivery Tools, Therapeutic Targets, and Biomarkers. *Int. J. Mol. Sci.* **2021**, *22*, 9543. [CrossRef] [PubMed]
42. Li, M.; Li, S.; Du, C.; Zhang, Y.; Li, Y.; Chu, L.; Han, X.; Galons, H.; Zhang, Y.; Sun, H.; et al. Exosomes from different cells: Characteristics, modifications, and therapeutic applications. *Eur. J. Med. Chem.* **2020**, *207*, 112784. [CrossRef]
43. Yang, X.X.; Sun, C.; Wang, L.; Guo, X.L. New insight into isolation, identification techniques and medical applications of exosomes. *J. Control. Release* **2019**, *308*, 119–129. [CrossRef] [PubMed]
44. Zhang, Y.; Bi, J.; Huang, J.; Tang, Y.; Du, S.; Li, P. Exosome: A Review of Its Classification, Isolation Techniques, Storage, Diagnostic and Targeted Therapy Applications. *Int. J. Nanomed.* **2020**, *15*, 6917–6934. [CrossRef] [PubMed]
45. Yang, D.; Zhang, W.; Zhang, H.; Zhang, F.; Chen, L.; Ma, L.; Larcher, L.M.; Chen, S.; Liu, N.; Zhao, Q.; et al. Progress, opportunity, and perspective on exosome isolation—Efforts for efficient exosome-based theranostics. *Theranostics* **2020**, *10*, 3684–3707. [CrossRef] [PubMed]
46. Doyle, L.M.; Wang, M.Z. Overview of Extracellular Vesicles, Their Origin, Composition, Purpose, and Methods for Exosome Isolation and Analysis. *Cells* **2019**, *8*, 727. [CrossRef]
47. Antimisiaris, S.G.; Mourtas, S.; Marazioti, A. Exosomes and Exosome-Inspired Vesicles for Targeted Drug Delivery. *Pharmaceutics* **2018**, *10*, 218. [CrossRef]
48. Lee, N.H.; You, S.; Taghizadeh, A.; Taghizadeh, M.; Kim, H.S. Cell Membrane-Cloaked Nanotherapeutics for Targeted Drug Delivery. *Int. J. Mol. Sci.* **2022**, *23*, 2223. [CrossRef]
49. Ding, Y.; Luo, Q.; Que, H.; Wang, N.; Gong, P.; Gu, J. Mesenchymal Stem Cell-Derived Exosomes: A Promising Therapeutic Agent for the Treatment of Liver Diseases. *Int. J. Mol. Sci.* **2022**, *23*, 972. [CrossRef]
50. Juan, T.; Furthauer, M. Biogenesis and function of ESCRT-dependent extracellular vesicles. *Semin. Cell Dev. Biol.* **2018**, *74*, 66–77. [CrossRef]
51. Keller, S.; Sanderson, M.P.; Stoeck, A.; Altevogt, P. Exosomes: From biogenesis and secretion to biological function. *Immunol. Lett.* **2006**, *107*, 102–108. [CrossRef] [PubMed]
52. van Niel, G.; Porto-Carreiro, I.; Simoes, S.; Raposo, G. Exosomes: A common pathway for a specialized function. *J. Biochem.* **2006**, *140*, 13–21. [CrossRef] [PubMed]
53. Muthu, S.; Bapat, A.; Jain, R.; Jeyaraman, N.; Jeyaraman, M. Exosomal therapy-a new frontier in regenerative medicine. *Stem Cell* **2021**, *8*, 7. [CrossRef]
54. Fitzner, D.; Schnaars, M.; van Rossum, D.; Krishnamoorthy, G.; Dibaj, P.; Bakhti, M.; Regen, T.; Hanisch, U.K.; Simons, M. Selective transfer of exosomes from oligodendrocytes to microglia by macropinocytosis. *J. Cell Sci.* **2011**, *124*, 447–458. [CrossRef] [PubMed]
55. Feng, D.; Zhao, W.L.; Ye, Y.Y.; Bai, X.C.; Liu, R.Q.; Chang, L.F.; Zhou, Q.; Sui, S.F. Cellular internalization of exosomes occurs through phagocytosis. *Traffic* **2010**, *11*, 675–687. [CrossRef]
56. Riazifar, M.; Mohammadi, M.R.; Pone, E.J.; Yeri, A.; Lasser, C.; Segaliny, A.I.; McIntyre, L.L.; Shelke, G.V.; Hutchins, E.; Hamamoto, A.; et al. Stem Cell-Derived Exosomes as Nanotherapeutics for Autoimmune and Neurodegenerative Disorders. *ACS Nano* **2019**, *13*, 6670–6688. [CrossRef]
57. Cui, G.H.; Wu, J.; Mou, F.F.; Xie, W.H.; Wang, F.B.; Wang, Q.L.; Fang, J.; Xu, Y.W.; Dong, Y.R.; Liu, J.R.; et al. Exosomes derived from hypoxia-preconditioned mesenchymal stromal cells ameliorate cognitive decline by rescuing synaptic dysfunction and regulating inflammatory responses in APP/PS1 mice. *FASEB J.* **2018**, *32*, 654–668. [CrossRef]
58. Pashoutan Sarvar, D.; Shamsasenjan, K.; Akbarzadehlaleh, P. Mesenchymal Stem Cell-Derived Exosomes: New Opportunity in Cell-Free Therapy. *Adv. Pharm. Bull.* **2016**, *6*, 293–299. [CrossRef]
59. Kalluri, R.; LeBleu, V.S. The biology, function, and biomedical applications of exosomes. *Science* **2020**, *367*, eaau6977. [CrossRef]
60. Fayazi, N.; Sheykhhasan, M.; Soleimani Asl, S.; Najafi, R. Stem Cell-Derived Exosomes: A New Strategy of Neurodegenerative Disease Treatment. *Mol. Neurobiol.* **2021**, *58*, 3494–3514. [CrossRef]
61. Mathivanan, S.; Simpson, R.J. ExoCarta: A compendium of exosomal proteins and RNA. *Proteomics* **2009**, *9*, 4997–5000. [CrossRef]
62. Keerthikumar, S.; Chisanga, D.; Ariyaratne, D.; Al Saffar, H.; Anand, S.; Zhao, K.; Samuel, M.; Pathan, M.; Jois, M.; Chilamkurti, N.; et al. ExoCarta: A Web-Based Compendium of Exosomal Cargo. *J. Mol. Biol.* **2016**, *428*, 688–692. [CrossRef] [PubMed]
63. Chen, B.; Li, Q.; Zhao, B.; Wang, Y. Stem Cell-Derived Extracellular Vesicles as a Novel Potential Therapeutic Tool for Tissue Repair. *Stem Cells Transl. Med.* **2017**, *6*, 1753–1758. [CrossRef]
64. Guy, R.; Offen, D. Promising Opportunities for Treating Neurodegenerative Diseases with Mesenchymal Stem Cell-Derived Exosomes. *Biomolecules* **2020**, *10*, 1320. [CrossRef] [PubMed]
65. Huang, J.H.; Fu, C.H.; Xu, Y.; Yin, X.M.; Cao, Y.; Lin, F.Y. Extracellular Vesicles Derived from Epidural Fat-Mesenchymal Stem Cells Attenuate NLRP3 Inflammasome Activation and Improve Functional Recovery After Spinal Cord Injury. *Neurochem. Res.* **2020**, *45*, 760–771. [CrossRef] [PubMed]

66. Lu, Y.; Zhou, Y.; Zhang, R.; Wen, L.; Wu, K.; Li, Y.; Yao, Y.; Duan, R.; Jia, Y. Bone Mesenchymal Stem Cell-Derived Extracellular Vesicles Promote Recovery Following Spinal Cord Injury via Improvement of the Integrity of the Blood-Spinal Cord Barrier. *Front. Neurosci.* **2019**, *13*, 209. [CrossRef]
67. Yu, T.; Zhao, C.; Hou, S.; Zhou, W.; Wang, B.; Chen, Y. Exosomes secreted from miRNA-29b-modified mesenchymal stem cells repaired spinal cord injury in rats. *Braz. J. Med. Biol. Res.* **2019**, *52*, e8735. [CrossRef] [PubMed]
68. Biglari, B.; Swing, T.; Child, C.; Buchler, A.; Westhauser, F.; Bruckner, T.; Ferbert, T.; Jurgen Gerner, H.; Moghaddam, A. A pilot study on temporal changes in IL-1beta and TNF-alpha serum levels after spinal cord injury: The serum level of TNF-alpha in acute SCI patients as a possible marker for neurological remission. *Spinal Cord* **2015**, *53*, 510–514. [CrossRef]
69. Kwon, B.K.; Streijger, F.; Fallah, N.; Noonan, V.K.; Belanger, L.M.; Ritchie, L.; Paquette, S.J.; Ailon, T.; Boyd, M.C.; Street, J.; et al. Cerebrospinal Fluid Biomarkers To Stratify Injury Severity and Predict Outcome in Human Traumatic Spinal Cord Injury. *J. Neurotrauma* **2017**, *34*, 567–580. [CrossRef]
70. Romanelli, P.; Bieler, L.; Scharler, C.; Pachler, K.; Kreutzer, C.; Zaunmair, P.; Jakubecova, D.; Mrowetz, H.; Benedetti, B.; Rivera, F.J.; et al. Extracellular Vesicles Can Deliver Anti-inflammatory and Anti-scarring Activities of Mesenchymal Stromal Cells After Spinal Cord Injury. *Front. Neurol.* **2019**, *10*, 1225. [CrossRef]
71. Davis, B.K.; Wen, H.; Ting, J.P. The inflammasome NLRs in immunity, inflammation, and associated diseases. *Annu. Rev. Immunol.* **2011**, *29*, 707–735. [CrossRef]
72. Jiang, W.; Li, M.; He, F.; Zhou, S.; Zhu, L. Targeting the NLRP3 inflammasome to attenuate spinal cord injury in mice. *J. Neuroinflamm.* **2017**, *14*, 207. [CrossRef] [PubMed]
73. Jiang, W.; Huang, Y.; He, F.; Liu, J.; Li, M.; Sun, T.; Ren, W.; Hou, J.; Zhu, L. Dopamine D1 Receptor Agonist A-68930 Inhibits NLRP3 Inflammasome Activation, Controls Inflammation, and Alleviates Histopathology in a Rat Model of Spinal Cord Injury. *Spine* **2016**, *41*, E330–E334. [CrossRef]
74. Anderson, A.J.; Robert, S.; Huang, W.; Young, W.; Cotman, C.W. Activation of complement pathways after contusion-induced spinal cord injury. *J. Neurotrauma* **2004**, *21*, 1831–1846. [CrossRef] [PubMed]
75. Fraser, D.A.; Arora, M.; Bohlson, S.S.; Lozano, E.; Tenner, A.J. Generation of inhibitory NFkappaB complexes and phosphorylated cAMP response element-binding protein correlates with the anti-inflammatory activity of complement protein C1q in human monocytes. *J. Biol. Chem.* **2007**, *282*, 7360–7367. [CrossRef] [PubMed]
76. Brambilla, R.; Bracchi-Ricard, V.; Hu, W.H.; Frydel, B.; Bramwell, A.; Karmally, S.; Green, E.J.; Bethea, J.R. Inhibition of astroglial nuclear factor kappaB reduces inflammation and improves functional recovery after spinal cord injury. *J. Exp. Med.* **2005**, *202*, 145–156. [CrossRef]
77. Wang, L.; Pei, S.; Han, L.; Guo, B.; Li, Y.; Duan, R.; Yao, Y.; Xue, B.; Chen, X.; Jia, Y. Mesenchymal Stem Cell-Derived Exosomes Reduce A1 Astrocytes via Downregulation of Phosphorylated NFkappaB P65 Subunit in Spinal Cord Injury. *Cell. Physiol. Biochem.* **2018**, *50*, 1535–1559. [CrossRef]
78. Guerrero, A.R.; Uchida, K.; Nakajima, H.; Watanabe, S.; Nakamura, M.; Johnson, W.E.; Baba, H. Blockade of interleukin-6 signaling inhibits the classic pathway and promotes an alternative pathway of macrophage activation after spinal cord injury in mice. *J. Neuroinflamm.* **2012**, *9*, 40. [CrossRef]
79. Mosser, D.M.; Edwards, J.P. Exploring the full spectrum of macrophage activation. *Nat. Rev. Immunol.* **2008**, *8*, 958–969. [CrossRef]
80. Kigerl, K.A.; Gensel, J.C.; Ankeny, D.P.; Alexander, J.K.; Donnelly, D.J.; Popovich, P.G. Identification of two distinct macrophage subsets with divergent effects causing either neurotoxicity or regeneration in the injured mouse spinal cord. *J. Neurosci.* **2009**, *29*, 13435–13444. [CrossRef]
81. David, S.; Kroner, A. Repertoire of microglial and macrophage responses after spinal cord injury. *Nat. Rev. Neurosci.* **2011**, *12*, 388–399. [CrossRef] [PubMed]
82. Sun, G.; Li, G.; Li, D.; Huang, W.; Zhang, R.; Zhang, H.; Duan, Y.; Wang, B. hucMSC derived exosomes promote functional recovery in spinal cord injury mice via attenuating inflammation. *Mater. Sci. Eng. C* **2018**, *89*, 194–204. [CrossRef]
83. Lankford, K.L.; Arroyo, E.J.; Nazimek, K.; Bryniarski, K.; Askenase, P.W.; Kocsis, J.D. Intravenously delivered mesenchymal stem cell-derived exosomes target M2-type macrophages in the injured spinal cord. *PLoS ONE* **2018**, *13*, e0190358. [CrossRef]
84. Reinhold, A.K.; Rittner, H.L. Barrier function in the peripheral and central nervous system-a review. *Pflug. Arch.* **2017**, *469*, 123–134. [CrossRef]
85. Hu, J.; Yu, Q.; Xie, L.; Zhu, H. Targeting the blood-spinal cord barrier: A therapeutic approach to spinal cord protection against ischemia-reperfusion injury. *Life Sci.* **2016**, *158*, 1–6. [CrossRef]
86. Jo, D.H.; Kim, J.H.; Heo, J.I.; Kim, J.H.; Cho, C.H. Interaction between pericytes and endothelial cells leads to formation of tight junction in hyaloid vessels. *Mol. Cells* **2013**, *36*, 465–471. [CrossRef]
87. Lizana, J.; Aliaga, N.; Marani, W.; Escribano, A.; Montemurro, N. Spinal Vascular Shunts: Single-Center Series and Review of the Literature of Their Classification. *Neurol. Int.* **2022**, *14*, 581–599. [CrossRef]
88. Ota, T.; Komiyama, M. Pathogenesis of non-hereditary brain arteriovenous malformation and therapeutic implications. *Interv. Neuroradiol.* **2020**, *26*, 244–253. [CrossRef]
89. Yuan, X.; Wu, Q.; Wang, P.; Jing, Y.; Yao, H.; Tang, Y.; Li, Z.; Zhang, H.; Xiu, R. Exosomes Derived From Pericytes Improve Microcirculation and Protect Blood-Spinal Cord Barrier After Spinal Cord Injury in Mice. *Front. Neurosci.* **2019**, *13*, 319. [CrossRef] [PubMed]
90. Bartel, D.P. MicroRNAs: Genomics, biogenesis, mechanism, and function. *Cell* **2004**, *116*, 281–297. [CrossRef] [PubMed]

91. Ding, S.Q.; Chen, J.; Wang, S.N.; Duan, F.X.; Chen, Y.Q.; Shi, Y.J.; Hu, J.G.; Lu, H.Z. Identification of serum exosomal microRNAs in acute spinal cord injured rats. *Exp. Biol. Med.* **2019**, *244*, 1149–1161. [CrossRef]
92. Buller, B.; Liu, X.; Wang, X.; Zhang, R.L.; Zhang, L.; Hozeska-Solgot, A.; Chopp, M.; Zhang, Z.G. MicroRNA-21 protects neurons from ischemic death. *FEBS J.* **2010**, *277*, 4299–4307. [CrossRef] [PubMed]
93. Han, Z.; Chen, F.; Ge, X.; Tan, J.; Lei, P.; Zhang, J. miR-21 alleviated apoptosis of cortical neurons through promoting PTEN-Akt signaling pathway in vitro after experimental traumatic brain injury. *Brain Res.* **2014**, *1582*, 12–20. [CrossRef] [PubMed]
94. Yu, Y.M.; Gibbs, K.M.; Davila, J.; Campbell, N.; Sung, S.; Todorova, T.I.; Otsuka, S.; Sabaawy, H.E.; Hart, R.P.; Schachner, M. MicroRNA miR-133b is essential for functional recovery after spinal cord injury in adult zebrafish. *Eur. J. Neurosci.* **2011**, *33*, 1587–1597. [CrossRef]
95. Hu, J.; Zeng, L.; Huang, J.; Wang, G.; Lu, H. miR-126 promotes angiogenesis and attenuates inflammation after contusion spinal cord injury in rats. *Brain Res.* **2015**, *1608*, 191–202. [CrossRef]
96. Sung, S.E.; Seo, M.S.; Kim, Y.I.; Kang, K.K.; Choi, J.H.; Lee, S.; Sung, M.; Yim, S.G.; Lim, J.H.; Seok, H.G.; et al. Human Epidural AD-MSC Exosomes Improve Function Recovery after Spinal Cord Injury in Rats. *Biomedicines* **2022**, *10*, 678. [CrossRef]
97. Zhou, Y.; Wen, L.L.; Li, Y.F.; Wu, K.M.; Duan, R.R.; Yao, Y.B.; Jing, L.J.; Gong, Z.; Teng, J.F.; Jia, Y.J. Exosomes derived from bone marrow mesenchymal stem cells protect the injured spinal cord by inhibiting pericyte pyroptosis. *Neural Regen. Res.* **2022**, *17*, 194–202. [CrossRef] [PubMed]
98. Zhang, C.; Zhang, C.; Xu, Y.; Li, C.; Cao, Y.; Li, P. Exosomes derived from human placenta-derived mesenchymal stem cells improve neurologic function by promoting angiogenesis after spinal cord injury. *Neurosci. Lett.* **2020**, *739*, 135399. [CrossRef] [PubMed]
99. Chen, Y.; Tian, Z.; He, L.; Liu, C.; Wang, N.; Rong, L.; Liu, B. Exosomes derived from miR-26a-modified MSCs promote axonal regeneration via the PTEN/AKT/mTOR pathway following spinal cord injury. *Stem Cell Res. Ther.* **2021**, *12*, 224. [CrossRef]
100. Li, L.; Zhang, Y.; Mu, J.; Chen, J.; Zhang, C.; Cao, H.; Gao, J. Transplantation of Human Mesenchymal Stem-Cell-Derived Exosomes Immobilized in an Adhesive Hydrogel for Effective Treatment of Spinal Cord Injury. *Nano Lett.* **2020**, *20*, 4298–4305. [CrossRef]
101. Wang, Y.; Lai, X.; Wu, D.; Liu, B.; Wang, N.; Rong, L. Umbilical mesenchymal stem cell-derived exosomes facilitate spinal cord functional recovery through the miR-199a-3p/145-5p-mediated NGF/TrkA signaling pathway in rats. *Stem Cell Res. Ther.* **2021**, *12*, 117. [CrossRef]
102. Ji, W.; Jiang, W.; Li, M.; Li, J.; Li, Z. miR-21 deficiency contributes to the impaired protective effects of obese rat mesenchymal stem cell-derived exosomes against spinal cord injury. *Biochimie* **2019**, *167*, 171–178. [CrossRef] [PubMed]
103. Kang, J.; Li, Z.; Zhi, Z.; Wang, S.; Xu, G. MiR-21 derived from the exosomes of MSCs regulates the death and differentiation of neurons in patients with spinal cord injury. *Gene Ther.* **2019**, *26*, 491–503. [CrossRef]
104. Meng, F.; Henson, R.; Wehbe-Janek, H.; Ghoshal, K.; Jacob, S.T.; Patel, T. MicroRNA-21 regulates expression of the PTEN tumor suppressor gene in human hepatocellular cancer. *Gastroenterology* **2007**, *133*, 647–658. [CrossRef] [PubMed]
105. Wang, Z.; Song, Y.; Han, X.; Qu, P.; Wang, W. Long noncoding RNA PTENP1 affects the recovery of spinal cord injury by regulating the expression of miR-19b and miR-21. *J. Cell. Physiol.* **2020**, *235*, 3634–3645. [CrossRef] [PubMed]
106. Xu, G.; Ao, R.; Zhi, Z.; Jia, J.; Yu, B. miR-21 and miR-19b delivered by hMSC-derived EVs regulate the apoptosis and differentiation of neurons in patients with spinal cord injury. *J. Cell. Physiol.* **2019**, *234*, 10205–10217. [CrossRef]
107. Huang, J.H.; Xu, Y.; Yin, X.M.; Lin, F.Y. Exosomes Derived from miR-126-modified MSCs Promote Angiogenesis and Neurogenesis and Attenuate Apoptosis after Spinal Cord Injury in Rats. *Neuroscience* **2020**, *424*, 133–145. [CrossRef]
108. Li, D.; Zhang, P.; Yao, X.; Li, H.; Shen, H.; Li, X.; Wu, J.; Lu, X. Exosomes Derived From miR-133b-Modified Mesenchymal Stem Cells Promote Recovery After Spinal Cord Injury. *Front. Neurosci.* **2018**, *12*, 845. [CrossRef]
109. Jiang, Z.; Zhang, J. Mesenchymal stem cell-derived exosomes containing miR-145-5p reduce inflammation in spinal cord injury by regulating the TLR4/NF-kappaB signaling pathway. *Cell Cycle* **2021**, *20*, 993–1009. [CrossRef]
110. Liu, W.; Wang, Y.; Gong, F.; Rong, Y.; Luo, Y.; Tang, P.; Zhou, Z.; Zhou, Z.; Xu, T.; Jiang, T.; et al. Exosomes Derived from Bone Mesenchymal Stem Cells Repair Traumatic Spinal Cord Injury by Suppressing the Activation of A1 Neurotoxic Reactive Astrocytes. *J. Neurotrauma* **2019**, *36*, 469–484. [CrossRef]
111. Nakazaki, M.; Morita, T.; Lankford, K.L.; Askenase, P.W.; Kocsis, J.D. Small extracellular vesicles released by infused mesenchymal stromal cells target M2 macrophages and promote TGF-beta upregulation, microvascular stabilization and functional recovery in a rodent model of severe spinal cord injury. *J. Extracell. Vesicles* **2021**, *10*, e12137. [CrossRef] [PubMed]
112. Liu, W.; Rong, Y.; Wang, J.; Zhou, Z.; Ge, X.; Ji, C.; Jiang, D.; Gong, F.; Li, L.; Chen, J.; et al. Exosome-shuttled miR-216a-5p from hypoxic preconditioned mesenchymal stem cells repair traumatic spinal cord injury by shifting microglial M1/M2 polarization. *J. Neuroinflamm.* **2020**, *17*, 47. [CrossRef] [PubMed]
113. Lee, J.R.; Kyung, J.W.; Kumar, H.; Kwon, S.P.; Song, S.Y.; Han, I.B.; Kim, B.S. Targeted Delivery of Mesenchymal Stem Cell-Derived Nanovesicles for Spinal Cord Injury Treatment. *Int. J. Mol. Sci.* **2020**, *21*, 4185. [CrossRef] [PubMed]

MDPI AG
Grosspeteranlage 5
4052 Basel
Switzerland
Tel.: +41 61 683 77 34

Biomedicines Editorial Office
E-mail: biomedicines@mdpi.com
www.mdpi.com/journal/biomedicines

www.ingramcontent.com/pod-product-compliance
Lightning Source LLC
Chambersburg PA
CBHW061444210926
51850CB00008B/1608

* 9 7 8 3 7 2 5 8 5 5 6 1 2 *